Neuropsychiatric Care for Genetic Syndromes and Other Neurodevelopmental Disorders

Robyn P. Thom • Christopher J. McDougle
Editors

Neuropsychiatric Care for Genetic Syndromes and Other Neurodevelopmental Disorders

What Every Clinician Needs to Know

Springer

Editors
Robyn P. Thom
Lurie Center for Autism
Lexington, MA, USA

Christopher J. McDougle
Lurie Center for Autism
Lexington, MA, USA

ISBN 978-3-031-76271-0 ISBN 978-3-031-76269-7 (eBook)
https://doi.org/10.1007/978-3-031-76269-7

This Springer imprint is published by the registered company Springer Nature Switzerland AG
The registered company address is: Gewerbestrasse 11, 6330 Cham, Switzerland

Preface

Medical advances have led not only to the increased detection of genetic syndromes, but also increased survival of those with neurodevelopmental disorders. With these medical advances, neuropsychiatric symptoms such as anxiety, hyperactivity, depression, insomnia, and irritability are increasingly becoming a predominant predictor of quality of life in this population. Unfortunately, clinicians receive very little formal education or hands on training in the care of individuals with neurodevelopmental disorders. Furthermore, because of language and cognitive differences, the clinical presentation of neuropsychiatric conditions can differ from what is typically observed in the general population. The current gold standard of care for the vast majority of neuropsychiatric symptoms in individuals with neurodevelopmental disorders is based on clinical experience and expert opinion, as few evidence-based treatments or practice guidelines exist.

Despite these challenges, recent research advances in genetic syndromes have begun to outpace that of idiopathic neurodevelopmental disorders. For example, preclinical models of Rett syndrome followed by translational and clinical research led to the Food and Drug Administration (FDA) approval of trofinetide for this syndrome in March of 2023. Since each of these genetic syndromes is rare, practicing clinicians generally do not encounter enough cases to develop comfort and expertise in each of them, or familiarity with novel treatments. Therefore, patients with neurodevelopmental disorders and genetic syndromes often travel to seek highly specialized care, including in order to access research opportunities. However, this creates an inequity for families who are unable to access specialized care for a variety of reasons.

This book is designed as an easy-to-use, clinically oriented, guide for clinicians treating patients with neurodevelopmental disorders and genetic syndromes. It includes chapters on idiopathic autism spectrum disorder and intellectual disability, followed by chapters on 16 genetic syndromes. Each chapter provides an overview of the disorder or syndrome, the signs and symptoms of common psychiatric comorbidities, an approach to the clinical assessment, psychosocial and biological treatment strategies, as well as common medical comorbidities relevant to selecting safe and appropriate pharmacotherapy.

It is our hope that this text provides the reader with the knowledge needed to deliver high-quality clinical care to those with neurodevelopmental disorders and genetic syndromes. And if the book helps lead some readers towards a clinical or research career in this area, then so much the better.

Lexington, MA, USA — Robyn P. Thom
Lexington, MA, USA — Christopher J. McDougle

Contents

1 Idiopathic Autism Spectrum Disorder 1
Hannah M. Carroll, Robyn P. Thom, and Christopher J. McDougle

2 Intellectual Disability 27
Renée M. Green and Ainsley Losh

3 Williams Syndrome 41
Ana Fish, Barbara R. Pober, and Robyn P. Thom

4 Down Syndrome 59
Michelle L. Palumbo, Stephanie Santoro, and Yamini Howe

5 Angelman Syndrome 73
Christopher J. Keary, Nicole Simon, and Amanda Tourjee

6 Prader-Willi Syndrome 91
Julia Katz

7 Fragile X Syndrome 109
Elizabeth Berry-Kravis and Craig Erickson

8 Duplication 15q Syndrome 129
Dana Q. Tran

9 DiGeorge Syndrome 141
Dena Oaklander, Khalid I. Afzal, and Karam Radwan

10 Tuberous Sclerosis Complex 157
David W. Dunn and Lydia J. Fisher

11 Turner Syndrome 171
W. Philip Bartel, Robert Accordino, Bushra Awidi, and Laura M. Prager

12 Rett Syndrome 191
Susanna B. Mierau

13 Phelan–McDermid Syndrome 203
Paige Hickey Townsend, Heli Patel, and Ann M. Neumeyer

14 Smith–Lemli–Opitz Syndrome 229
Kelly K. Noah and Elaine Tierney

15 Smith–Magenis Syndrome 245
Diane Treadwell-Deering, Kevin Kaplan, and Lorraine Potocki

16 Klinefelter Syndrome 261
David S. Hong

17 Lesch–Nyhan Syndrome 269
Lydia J. Fischer and David W. Dunn

18 Cornelia de Lange Syndrome 283
Marco A. Grados, Sid Srivastava, Pratik Agarwal,
and Antonie D. Kline

Index 297

Contributors

Robert Accordino Department of Psychiatry, Weill Cornell Medicine, New York, USA

Khalid I. Afzal Department of Psychiatry and Behavioral Neuroscience, The University of Chicago, Chicago, IL, USA

Pratik Agarwal Lokmanya Tilak Municipal Medical College, Mumbai, India

Bushra Awidi Department of Psychiatry, Massachusetts General Hospital, Boston, MA, USA

W. Philip Bartel University of Pittsburgh School of Medicine, Pittsburgh, PA, USA

Elizabeth Berry-Kravis Departments of Pediatrics, Neurological Sciences, Anatomy and Cell Biology, Rush University Medical Center, Chicago, IL, USA

Hannah M. Carroll UMass Chan Medical School, Worchester, MA, USA

David W. Dunn Department of Psychiatry, Indiana University School of Medicine, Indianapolis, IN, USA
Department of Neurology, Indiana University School of Medicine, Indianapolis, IN, USA

Craig Erickson Division of Child and Adolescent Psychiatry, Cincinnati Children's Hospital Medical Center, Cincinnati, OH, USA

Ana Fish Cambridge Health Alliance, Cambridge, MA, USA

Lydia J. Fisher Department of Psychiatry, Indiana University School of Medicine, Indianapolis, IN, USA

Marco A. Grados Johns Hopkins University School of Medicine, Baltimore, MD, USA

Renée M. Green Lurie Center for Autism, Massachusetts General Hospital, Lexington, MA, USA
Department of Psychiatry, Harvard Medical School, Boston, MA, USA

David S. Hong Department of Psychiatry and Behavioral Sciences, Stanford University, Stanford, CA, USA

Yamini Howe Cortica, Burlington, MA, USA

Kevin Kaplan Department of Developmental Pediatrics, Baylor College of Medicine and Texas Children's Hospital, Houston, TX, USA
Department of Sleep Medicine, Baylor College of Medicine and Texas Children's Hospital, Houston, TX, USA
Department of Molecular and Human Genetics, Baylor College of Medicine and Texas Children's Hospital, Houston, TX, USA

Julia Katz Department of Child and Adolescent Psychiatry and Behavioral Sciences, Children's Hospital of Philadelphia, Philadelphia, PA, USA

Christopher J. Keary Angelman Syndrome Program, Lurie Center for Autism, Massachusetts General Hospital for Children, Boston, MA, USA

Antonie D. Kline Greater Baltimore Medical Center, Baltimore, MD, USA

Ainsley Losh Lurie Center for Autism, Massachusetts General Hospital, Lexington, MA, USA

Christopher J. McDougle Lurie Center for Autism, Lexington, MA, USA

Susanna B. Mierau Lurie Center for Autism, Massachusetts General Hospital, Lexington, MA, USA
Division of Cognitive and Behavioral Neurology, Brigham and Women's Hospital, Boston, MA, USA
Harvard Medical School, Boston, MA, USA

Ann M. Neumeyer Lurie Center for Autism, Massachusetts General Hospital, Lexington, MA, USA

Kelly K. Noah Smith-Lemli-Opitz Foundation, Fargo, ND, USA

Dena Oaklander Department of Psychiatry and Behavioral Neuroscience, The University of Chicago, Chicago, IL, USA

Michelle L. Palumbo Massachusetts General Hospital for Children, Lexington, MA, USA

Heli Patel Lurie Center for Autism, Massachusetts General Hospital, Lexington, MA, USA

Barbara R. Pober Massachusetts General Hospital, Boston, MA, USA

Lorraine Potocki Department of Developmental Pediatrics, Baylor College of Medicine and Texas Children's Hospital, Houston, TX, USA
Department of Sleep Medicine, Baylor College of Medicine and Texas Children's Hospital, Houston, TX, USA
Department of Molecular and Human Genetics, Baylor College of Medicine and Texas Children's Hospital, Houston, TX, USA

Laura M. Prager Department of Psychiatry and Behavioral Science, Boston Children's Hospital, Boston, MA, USA

Karam Radwan Department of Psychiatry and Behavioral Neuroscience, The University of Chicago, Chicago, IL, USA

Stephanie Santoro Massachusetts General Hospital, Boston, MA, USA

Nicole Simon Angelman Syndrome Program, Lurie Center for Autism, Massachusetts General Hospital for Children, Boston, MA, USA

Sid Srivastava Harvard Medical School, Boston, MA, USA

Robyn P. Thom Lurie Center for Autism, Lexington, MA, USA

Elaine Tierney Kennedy Krieger Institute, Baltimore, MD, USA
Department of Psychiatry and Behavioral Sciences, Johns Hopkins University School of Medicine, Baltimore, MD, USA

Amanda Tourjee Angelman Syndrome Program, Lurie Center for Autism, Massachusetts General Hospital for Children, Boston, MA, USA

Paige Hickey Townsend Lurie Center for Autism, Massachusetts General Hospital, Lexington, MA, USA

Dana Q. Tran Massachusetts General Hospital Lurie Center for Autism, Lexington, MA, USA
Harvard Medical School, Boston, MA, USA

Diane Treadwell-Deering Department of Developmental Pediatrics, Baylor College of Medicine and Texas Children's Hospital, Houston, TX, USA
Department of Sleep Medicine, Baylor College of Medicine and Texas Children's Hospital, Houston, TX, USA
Department of Molecular and Human Genetics, Baylor College of Medicine and Texas Children's Hospital, Houston, TX, USA

Idiopathic Autism Spectrum Disorder

1

Hannah M. Carroll, Robyn P. Thom,
and Christopher J. McDougle

1.1 Overview

Autism spectrum disorder (ASD) is a neurodevelopmental disorder characterized by deficits in social communication as well as restricted and repetitive patterns of behavior, interests, or activities [1]. Approximately 1 in 100 children are diagnosed with ASD globally [2]. The prevalence of ASD in the United States is much higher, with a prevalence of 1 in 36 children based on data from the Autism and Developmental Disabilities Monitoring (ADDM) Network [3]. When broken down by sex, global and US prevalence rates estimate that ASD is approximately four times more common in boys than in girls. This male preponderance has been established since the first cases of ASD were reported back in 1943 [4, 5]. Notably, the ADDM reported for the first time that the prevalence of ASD was lower among White children aged 8 years than among other racial and ethnic groups [3]. Data from other national and statewide studies have also shown disparities in diagnosis related to race and minority status [6–9]. The average age of initial diagnosis in the United States is 49 months, or just over 4 years, but initial signs can be detected between 6 and 18 months [3, 10]. There is no single, definitive diagnostic test for ASD. It is typically diagnosed through a comprehensive evaluation process that involves gathering a robust developmental history, clinical observation, and use of autism screening tools [11, 12]. The behaviors and symptoms gathered during the evaluation are then assessed using the diagnostic criteria outlined in the *Diagnostic and Statistical Manual of Mental Disorders, Fifth Edition* (DSM-5) [1].

H. M. Carroll
UMass Chan Medical School, Worchester, MA, USA
e-mail: Hannah.Carroll@umassmed.edu

R. P. Thom · C. J. McDougle (✉)
Lurie Center for Autism, Lexington, MA, USA
e-mail: RTHOM@MGH.HARVARD.EDU; CMCDOUGLE@mgh.harvard.edu

R. P. Thom, C. J. McDougle (eds.), *Neuropsychiatric Care for Genetic Syndromes and Other Neurodevelopmental Disorders*,
https://doi.org/10.1007/978-3-031-76269-7_1

The diagnostic criteria for autism have undergone significant revision since it was first identified in the 1940s by Dr. Leo Kanner and Dr. Hans Asperger [1, 13, 14]. Kanner is credited as the first person to describe autism in 1943 [5]. Around the same time, Hans Asperger identified similar traits in his patients although he put more focus on the presence of extreme intelligence [15]. Both physicians separately recognized the same core symptoms of ASD including social deficits, language impairment in the form of muteness or abnormality of speech, and restrictive and repetitive behaviors. These early findings remain foundational characteristics of ASD today [13, 14].

The first two editions of the DSM, published in 1952 and 1968, respectively, did not recognize autism as a formal diagnostic entity. Rather, autistic symptoms were included under the diagnosis of childhood schizophrenia [13]. In 1980, infantile autism and residual autism were included under a new class of disorders in the DSM-3 labeled as Pervasive Developmental Disorders (PDDs) [16]. Diagnostic criteria for infantile autism included onset before 30 months of age, lack of sociability, deficits in language development, peculiar speech patterns (echolalia, metaphorical language, and pronoun reversal), abnormal responses to various aspects of the environment, and the absence of certain symptoms characteristic of schizophrenia (delusions, hallucinations, and loose associations). There were also diagnoses in the DSM-3 listed as "late-onset" autism (childhood-onset PDD) and "subthreshold" PDD (atypical PDD). Several years later, the DSM-3 was revised and introduced autistic disorder and PDD not-otherwise-specified (PDD-NOS) as replacement diagnoses for infantile autism and "subthreshold" PDD, respectively, with altered diagnostic criteria. Major changes were made when the DSM-4 was published in 1994, including the recognition of Asperger's disorder, Rett's disorder, and childhood disintegrative disorder as discrete diagnoses, in addition to the two previously defined diagnoses: autistic disorder and PDD-NOS [13, 15]. The DSM-4 allowed for an explosion of research papers to be published due to the convergence on a more definitive description of subtypes of autism than the previous versions of the DSM.

The current edition of the DSM, the DSM-5, introduced autism spectrum disorder (ASD) as a replacement for autistic disorder, PDD-NOS, and Asperger's disorder in 2013 [15, 17]. The DSM-5 has two core domains by which ASD is defined: (1) deficits in social communication and (2) restricted and repetitive behaviors and interests [17, 18]. The DSM-5 diagnostic criteria for ASD also include symptom severity specifiers.

The heterogeneity of ASD leads to unique clinical presentations and challenges in each affected individual. Despite the significant differences in each case, every person must share the foundational features of difficulty in social communication and interaction, as well as demonstrate restricted and repetitive behaviors [19, 20]. Diminished social ability in individuals with ASD presents as difficulties with social pragmatics, such as appropriate eye contact, reciprocal conversation, turn-taking, greetings, figurative language, and understanding nonverbal cues [21–23]. Restrictive and repetitive behaviors can range from "lower order" behaviors, such as repetitive motor actions and movements, to "higher order" behaviors, which are characterized by routines, insistence on sameness, and narrowed interests [24]. Sensory stimulation abnormalities have also been considered a core feature of ASD by many researchers, dating back to the original descriptions of the disorder by Dr. Kanner and Dr. Asperger [5, 15, 25, 26]. Individuals with ASD might be hyporesponsive (unaware of sensory input), hyperresponsive (exaggerated response to sensory input), or sensory-seeking (searching for sensory stimulation) [27–29]. Motor abnormalities are not considered core symptoms of ASD but are commonly observed. For example, head lag in infants (the head lagging behind the trunk in a pull-to-sit position) or asymmetry when lying down is commonly observed in children who later go on to receive a diagnosis of ASD [30–32]. Motor delays are commonly reported as one of the first areas of parental concern beginning around 15 months of age [33]. Sensorimotor deficits can lead to difficulties with accuracy, speed, and initiation of eye movements; coordination of eye and body movements; and the ability to integrate visual information into motor learning [32].

Identifying the pathogenesis of ASD has been complicated by its phenotypic variability and genetic complexity. Family studies of ASD have shown that it is highly heritable [34]. One study found that the probability of an ASD diagnosis in individuals with a full sibling with ASD was 12.9% compared to 1.2% for individuals without an autistic sibling [35]. Other studies of idiopathic ASD show that the risk of diagnosis is increased when there is an older sibling with ASD and is even higher when there are two or more children with ASD in the family [36, 37]. In a meta-analysis of twin studies, heritability estimates range from 64 to 91% [38]. Although genes clearly play a role in ASD susceptibility, a genetic cause cannot always be found. Several ASD risk gene loci have been previously identified, but there is insufficient evidence to establish definitive genes that confer ASD specificity [39, 40]. The cause of ASD is likely multifactorial and cannot be attributed to a singular anomaly [34, 41]. Researchers have evaluated the immune system, genetic components, environmental factors, epigenetics, dendritic morphology, and pre−/neo−/postnatal impacts that could contribute to the development of ASD [42–48].

1.2 Signs and Symptoms of Common Psychiatric Comorbidities

1.2.1 Intellectual Disability

Approximately 33% of individuals with ASD have co-occurring intellectual disability (ID) [2, 49, 50]. Intellectual disability (see Chap. 2) is a developmental disorder characterized by intellectual and adaptive functioning deficits [1]. The high level of co-occurrence between ASD and ID suggests possible genetic similarities [51], but research about a shared etiological pathway remains unknown. When assessing for ID in an individual with ASD, there are a number of factors to consider. One is that ASD is often associated with a specific profile of cognitive ability characterized by a higher nonverbal IQ (thinking skills and problem-solving abilities) than verbal IQ (ability to analyze information and solve problems using language-based reasoning) [52]. Other factors include performing poorly on standardized tests due to engaging in interfering behaviors during testing. Similarly, nonverbal or minimally verbal individuals may be deemed "untestable." To ensure that individuals with ASD with potential co-occurring ID are able to perform at their best, it is recommended that a "flexible testing" approach be utilized to best capture the true abilities of the individual [53]. "Flexible testing" may include using short-form versions, taking breaks, allowing parents/caregivers to attend, testing in a more comfortable location, or allowing for alternative response formats for items requiring spoken words [53–55]. Few measures exist that clearly differentiate between ASD and ID. At this time, the best measures for attempting to parcel out symptoms of ASD versus pure ID include the Autism Diagnostic Observation Schedule, second edition (ADOS-2) [56], and the Autism Diagnostic Interview-Revised (ADI-R) [57]. The ADOS-2 and the ADI-R are highly sensitive to the presence of autism symptoms without being influenced by the individual's age, language/speech proficiency, or cognitive ability [58, 59].

1.2.2 Irritability

Irritability in ASD consists of verbal and physical aggression, self-injurious behavior (SIB), and property destruction [60, 61]. It is also the only symptom domain for which there are Food and Drug Administration (FDA) approved drugs: the atypical antipsychotics, risperidone and aripiprazole [62–64]. Irritability is common across the full spectrum of ASD severity [65, 66]. Increased aggressive behaviors have been concurrently associated with greater sleep difficulties [67–69], anxiety [70], and inattention/hyperactivity [71] in children with ASD.

Verbal and physical aggression include behaviors that are threatening or likely to cause harm. Verbal aggression can present as threatening or cursing at another person, whereas physical aggression includes hitting, biting, or throwing objects. Approximately 35–50% of children with ASD demonstrate at least one of the two—verbal or physical aggression—with variable frequency, intensity, and duration [69, 72]. Risk factors for aggression in children with ASD are unique from those found in typically developing children [73]. For example, male sex and certain social factors (i.e., level of parent education and marital status) have been shown to predict aggressive behaviors in typically developing children but not in children with ASD [74, 75]. Language ability, intellectual impairment, and adaptive functioning have been suggested as predictors of aggressive behaviors in ASD [74, 76]. Certain features of ASD, such as the desire to engage in repetitive behaviors, have also been shown to drive aggression in children [77]. Untreated aggression increases the risk of placement in restrictive schools or residences and the use of physical intervention [78] and impairs social relationships [79]. Aggression also results in increased levels of caregiver stress and diminished well-being [80, 81]. It is therefore vital to address aggression in individuals with ASD.

There is limited research that specifically addresses property destruction in individuals with ASD, although it is frequently observed. Breaking toys, destroying decorations, and punching walls are a few common examples. A study conducted on two young children with ASD found that engaging in property destruction was a way for them to gain access to items that could be used to engage in stereotypies (breaking mini blinds, plastic toys, and hangers) [82]. Several other examples of property destruction in both adults and children with ASD have been published with different explanations for what drives these behaviors [83–86]. The destruction of objects could be a way to satisfy sensory-seeking behaviors, or it could also be a way for individuals to cope with feelings of boredom or frustration. For example, the immediate gratification that comes from the novel sensation of breaking a toy or punching through drywall serves as a reinforcer for individuals with ASD who exhibit destructive behaviors when bored [82, 85].

There is a high rate of SIB in ASD with an estimated prevalence of 42% [87, 88]. Self-injurious behaviors refer to a series of aggressive behaviors that an individual inflicts upon themselves and have the potential to result in physical injury. Common forms of SIB include head banging, self-biting, skin scratching, hair pulling, hand mouthing, and hitting oneself against hard objects [88, 89]. In a meta-analysis by Steendfeldt-Kristensen et al. [88], hitting oneself with their own hands was the most common form of self-injury in ASD, followed by skin picking and hitting self on or with objects. In contrast, self-cutting is a rare form of SIB in ASD. Self-injurious behaviors tend to be a long-term and pervasive problem that first appear in childhood and progress into adolescence. Self-injurious behaviors often increase in prevalence and persist well into adulthood [90–92]. It has been postulated that SIB may serve a communicative function that helps individuals obtain social attention, gain access to desired items (i.e., food and toys), escape required tasks (i.e., schoolwork and daily chores), or obtain automatic sensory stimulation [93]. Self-injurious behaviors could also be a manifestation of underlying pain or a mechanism patients use to engage inhibitory pain pathways that alleviate visceral pain [93, 94]. Behavioral risk factors such as impulsivity and overactivity can predict self-injury in ASD [91], but the complexity of communication deficits and medical comorbidities in individuals with ASD make it challenging to identify the etiology of SIB [95, 96].

1.2.3 Attention-Deficit/Hyperactivity Disorder (ADHD)

Attention-deficit/hyperactivity disorder (ADHD) is one of the most common comorbidities in ASD. Estimates of the prevalence of ADHD in individuals with ASD range from 40% to 70% [97, 98]. Children and adolescents with ASD have a higher prevalence of ADHD (47.8%) than adults with ASD (22.4%) [98]. Previous versions of the DSM considered ADHD and ASD mutually exclusive, but the current DSM-5 now allows for co-diagnosis. ADHD alone can contribute to social impairment [99], making it difficult to differentiate between ASD alone, ADHD alone, and co-occurring ASD and ADHD [100, 101]. A prospective longitudinal sample from the United Kingdom (UK) investigating ADHD in adults with ASD also found that parent reports can be clinically useful even at 25 years of age [102]. Diagnostic tests and evaluations are crucial to not only understand an individual's impairment but also inform the selection of targeted treatments [103].

1.2.4 Anxiety

Anxiety disorders are frequently diagnosed at a higher rate in individuals with ASD when compared to the general population. Approximately 40% of children with ASD (aged 6–18 years) suffer from an anxiety disorder, which is nearly double the prevalence of anxiety in children without ASD [104, 105]. The current and lifetime prevalence of anxiety disorders in adults with ASD are 27% and 42%, respectively [106]. A birth cohort study of 31,220 individuals (median age 22.8 years) demonstrated that those with ASD were 3.5 times more likely to have a lifetime history of an anxiety disorder compared to age- and sex-matched controls [107]. Common examples of anxiety symptoms in individuals with ASD include debilitating worry about changes in routine, schedules, and the environment; distress or nervousness in the context of social interactions; and specific fears relating to loud sounds or unusual phobias of mundane objects (e.g., toilets, microwaves, and hairbrushes) [108, 109]. Anxiety in ASD can manifest as social avoidance, compulsions, and verbal rituals. Higher-order repetitive behaviors can become more frequent in anxious individuals with ASD. This could present as pushing in chairs or needing to accomplish tasks in a specific order [109, 110]. Additionally, higher levels of anxiety are associated with more severe symptoms of ASD, as measured by the Children's Social Behavior Questionnaire [111, 112]. It has been postulated that the intolerance of uncertainty may mediate anxiety in youth with ASD [110].

1.2.5 Obsessive-Compulsive Disorder

Obsessive-compulsive disorder (OCD) and ASD are both characterized by repetitive thoughts and repetitive behaviors. However, the restricted and repetitive behaviors of ASD present differently from the behaviors seen in OCD alone. It is important to distinguish repetitive behaviors typically seen in individuals with ASD from repetitive phenomena involved in co-occurring psychiatric disorders. Repetitive thoughts can be broken down into preoccupations, ruminations, obsessions, overvalued ideas, and delusions [113]. The highly restricted and fixated interests of individuals with ASD are classified as preoccupations. These thoughts are generally enjoyable but can become problematic when an individual fixates on their circumscribed interest for extended periods of time [114]. As for repetitive behaviors, subtypes include tics, stereotypies, compulsions, extrapyramidal symptoms (EPS), and automatisms [113]. Stereotypies are commonly seen in individuals with ASD and appear within the first few years of life [115]. Stereotypies in ASD present as hand flapping, body rocking, toe walking, spinning objects, and running objects across one's peripheral vision [116]. Notably, stereotypies are more common and persistent if comorbid ID is present [117].

Obsessive-compulsive disorder is far more prevalent in individuals with ASD compared to the general population. Prevalence estimates of comorbid OCD in individuals with ASD range from 2.6% to 37.2%, likely reflecting the difficulty parsing out obsessions and compulsions from the core repetitive patterns of behavior of

ASD [118–120]. Despite this variability, the literature consistently reports elevated rates of OCD in individuals with ASD compared to the general population [119]. If an individual with ASD has intrusive, unwanted, and distressing thoughts accompanied by ego-dystonic behaviors, then they meet the criteria for obsessions related to OCD [113, 121–123]. Examples of compulsions, separate from the aforementioned stereotypies seen in ASD, might include cleaning, checking, ordering, or hoarding [124, 125].

1.2.6 Depression

A recent meta-analysis found that individuals with ASD are approximately four times more likely to experience depression compared to the general population [126]. Risk factors for depression include older age and average to above-average IQ [127]. It should be noted, however, that it is more difficult to accurately diagnose depression in an individual with limited language and/or cognitive ability. Patients with co-occurring depression might experience significantly lower social motivation, diminished quality of life, heightened gastrointestinal problems, greater anxiety, and increased aggression. Another symptom of depression often seen in individuals with ASD is decreased enjoyment of their specific interests. The diagnosis of depression in ASD can be challenging due to the inherent social communication deficits including difficulty recognizing and expressing emotions. Symptoms of ASD such as apparent social disinterest, decreased pleasure in activities, sleep disturbance, and flat affect may also overlap with symptoms of depression, making it difficult to know which symptoms are attributable to which disorder [106, 127]. Depressive symptoms could, therefore, easily be overlooked as symptoms of ASD by clinicians and parents [128]. There have been some proposed neurobiological mechanisms including serotonin and dopamine gene variants that have been linked to more severe depressive symptoms in children with ASD [127].

1.2.7 Social Skill Deficits

Social deficits tend to appear within the first 2 years of life in children with ASD. Children affected by ASD may not seek out others or share complementary feeling states and are often content being alone. This can present in later years with difficulty sharing the emotional state of others in cooperative games or group settings. Deficits in joint attention development have also been noted as a distinguishing feature in young children with ASD [129–131]. Joint attention is a typical and spontaneous behavior whereby an infant shows enjoyment in sharing an object or event with another person by looking back and forth between the two. The skill is also associated with language acquisition, which is another atypical aspect of development in children with ASD [130]. At around 10–12 months of age, infants with ASD typically will not follow a parent pointing to an object, even with repeatedly calling the child's name or tapping on their shoulder. Between 12 and 16 months, typically developing children are able to point, comment, and share a social experience. Children with ASD fail to point and comment at appropriate times, or they do not show a positive affect or connectedness when they engage in these behaviors [131, 132]. Responding to one's name (orienting to name) is one of the most common deficits in social attention in children with ASD [132, 133]. It is also one of the first symptoms identified by parents as a concern as early as 18 months [134, 135].

1.2.8 Sleep Disorders

Difficulty with sleep onset and/or maintenance occurs in approximately 50–80% of children with ASD, which is significantly higher than the prevalence rate of 11–37% in typically developing children. The underlying cause of sleep disturbances in ASD can be attributed to neurobiological, medical, or behavioral origins. An example of each would be abnormalities in the melatonin pathway, epilepsy and gastrointestinal disturbance during sleep, or resistance to transitioning from daytime to nighttime activities. Several different sleep disorders have been implicated in ASD, including insomnia, sleep disordered breathing, parasomnias, and sleep-related movement disorders (rhythmical movement disorder and restless leg syndrome) [136]. The most common sleep problem reported by parents is insomnia, and studies have shown that insomnia remains the most common sleep disorder among adults with ASD. Sleep disorders may exacerbate behavioral issues of inattention, hyperactivity, and increased repetitive behaviors [137].

1.3 Assessment

The American Academy of Pediatrics recommends screening all children for symptoms of ASD through a combination of developmental surveillance at all well-child visits and standardized autism-specific screening tests at 18 and 24 months of age through primary care. Early symptoms of ASD include not responding to one's name by 12 months, not pointing to objects/showing interest by 14 months, no pretend play by 18 months, and more general symptoms of self-isolation, lack of empathy, delayed speech and language skills, echolalia, obsessive interests, repetitive movements (flapping hands, rocking, and spinning in circles), or unusual reactions to sensory stimuli. Early diagnosis can promote better outcomes through early intervention [138]. The diagnosis typically occurs around 3 years of age since it may be more difficult to recognize mild symptoms of ASD in younger children, especially if they have average or above-average cognitive abilities. Most children will be referred to a specialist, such as a developmental-behavioral or neurodevelopmental pediatrician, psychologist, neurologist, or psychiatrist, for a diagnostic evaluation. General pediatricians and child psychologists who are familiar with the application of the DSM-5 criteria can also make an initial clinical diagnosis to allow for access to early intervention.

The DSM-5 provides three levels of severity and two core domains to consider when making an ASD diagnosis. Level 1 severity indicates "requiring support," level 2 indicates "requiring substantial support," and level 3 indicates "requiring very substantial support." The two core symptom domains of ASD include (1) persistent social deficits and (2) restricted and repetitive patterns of behavior, interests, or activities. Within each domain, certain criteria must be met for a diagnosis. Individuals must have all three symptoms of social deficits, which consist of abnormal social-emotional reciprocity, deficits in nonverbal communicative behaviors used for social interaction, and difficulty developing, maintaining, and understanding relationships. There are four criteria within the domain of restricted and repetitive behaviors, but only two of the four need to be met for a diagnosis. Those criteria are (1) stereotyped or repetitive motor movements, use of objects, or speech; (2) insistence on sameness, inflexible adherence to routines, or ritualized patterns of verbal or nonverbal behavior; (3) highly restricted and fixated interests that are abnormal in intensity or focus; and (4) hyper- or hyporeactivity to sensory input or unusual interests in sensory aspects of the environment. Another facet specified by the DSM-5 is that symptoms must be present in the early developmental period, although symptoms may not fully manifest until later in life.

There is no laboratory test that can be used to make an ASD diagnosis. Rather, careful observation of behaviors, symptoms, and developmental history is necessary to confirm a diagnosis. Genetic testing might inform treatment plans for certain genetic etiologies of ASD [34, 51]. In order to elicit symptoms of ASD, there are a number of surveys and questionnaires that can help to support an initial diagnosis. Common parent-completed questionnaires include the Modified Checklist for Autism in Toddlers (M-CHAT), the Social Responsiveness Scale (SRS), and the Social Communication Questionnaire (SCQ), to name a few [12, 20]. There is also the ADI-R, which is a lengthy parental interview conducted by a trained clinician, which provides a structured report of behaviors associated with ASD. Elevated scores on any of these evaluations may indicate greater severity of symptoms as well as ID, language difficulties, and behavioral dysregulation. Validated structured observation tools used to gather data to corroborate a diagnosis include the ADOS-2 and the Childhood Autism Rating Scale, second edition (CARS-2). No singular tool is appropriate for all clinical scenarios, as they are only meant to support the evaluation of DSM-5 criteria informed by the combination of parent history, clinical observation, and other data.

It should be noted that approximately 9% of children who are diagnosed with ASD in early childhood may no longer meet the full diagnostic criteria for ASD by young adulthood. These children tend to have participated in early intervention, have a history of higher cognitive skills at the age of two years, or show a reduction in their repetitive behaviors over time [139, 140]. This could either be due to an increased likelihood of overdiagnosis at a younger age or earlier identification, allowing for more responsive outcomes to intervention [141]. It is therefore vital to build longitudinal relationships and reassess symptoms throughout development.

1.4 Treatment

1.4.1 Behavioral Interventions

Behavioral interventions are the mainstay treatment for the core symptoms of ASD and work most effectively when started at an early age [11, 133, 138]. Researchers have classified these interventions into two groups: comprehensive treatment models (CTMs) and focused interventions [142, 143]. Comprehensive treatment models focus on core ASD symptoms and have been found to improve language, cognitive, and functional language skills in young children. They use intensive long-term multidisciplinary strategies in naturalistic environments, and there is a lot of flexibility in terms of modes of instruction. For example, different models can be conducted at home or in a classroom, individually or in a group, and provided by instructors or parents. Examples of well-established CTMs include Early Intensive Behavioral Intervention (EIBI) [144]; Early Start Denver Model (ESDM) [145]; Developmental, Individual difference, Relationship-based model (DIR/Floortime, or Greenspan model) [146]; Pivotal Response Training (PRT) [147]; and Treatment and Education of Autistic and related Communication Handicapped Children (TEACCH) [148]. Focused interventions, on the other hand, address a single skill or area of development until the skill is mastered. This is in contrast to the longitudinal aspect of CTMs, but their flexible mode of instruction is generally similar. Examples of focused interventions include social skills training, toilet training, and behavioral strategies such as prompting, ignoring, time delay, reinforcement, discrete trial teaching, and extinction.

1.4.2 Pharmacological Treatment

Although behavioral interventions have been shown to be the most effective modality of treatment when started at an early age, psychopharmacological treatments can also provide significant benefits to patients with ASD. Psychotropic medications are used in approximately two-thirds of adolescents with ASD, particularly in those with co-occurring psychiatric conditions like the ones listed above [149]. A significant proportion of individuals taking psychotropic medications are often prescribed more than one. Most medications are used off-label since there are only two medications approved by the FDA for any condition related to ASD, in this case irritability [62, 63]. There are no FDA-approved medications for common psychiatric comorbidities, such as ADHD or anxiety, for example. A wide range of other drugs are used to treat co-occurring psychiatric conditions with ASD; however, children with ASD tend to be more sensitive to medication effects and more likely to have adverse reactions than those without ASD [64]. Because assessing for treatment effectiveness and tolerability can be challenging in minimally verbal patients, obtaining objective symptom measures from different sources before and after intervention can be helpful.

Selective serotonin reuptake inhibitors (SSRIs) have been studied for the treatment of ASD due to the theory that serotonin dysregulation is associated with symptoms frequently seen in autistic individuals [64, 150, 151]. Positron emission tomography (PET) scans have shown decreased levels of serotonin in the central nervous system of children under 5 years old with ASD, while a separate line of research has identified a deficit of the enzyme that converts tryptophan to serotonin in patients with ASD [152, 153]. Despite these findings, clinical trials have shown inconsistent benefits of SSRIs for improving aggression and the core symptoms of ASD [64, 150]. When improvement of symptoms has been demonstrated in studies of SSRIs, it is typically in adolescents or adults rather than in children [151, 154–159].

Antipsychotics are the most efficacious medications for the treatment of irritability in individuals with ASD [160]. In fact, risperidone and aripiprazole are the only FDA-approved treatments for irritability in ASD in children and adolescents [62, 63]. Clinical trials have found them to be effective in reducing irritability and, to a lesser extent, repetitive behaviors [62, 63, 161]. These medications may have a decreased risk of extrapyramidal symptoms compared to conventional antipsychotics. The most common side effects include fatigue, increased appetite, gastrointestinal symptoms, hyperprolactinemia, weight gain, and sedation. However, more severe side effects—including dyslipidemia, hyperglycemia, metabolic syndrome, and extrapyramidal symptoms or drug-induced movement disorders—are not uncommon and should be considered before deciding to prescribe either of these medications [64].

Alpha-2 agonists, most notably guanfacine, are among the first-line medications considered for treating children with ASD and prominent symptoms of ADHD [162–164]. As previously stated, ADHD is one of the most common co-occurring disorders in individuals with ASD, making it an important psychopharmacological target symptom [100]. In a multisite, randomized clinical trial, extended-release guanfacine for the treatment of ADHD symptoms was compared to placebo in children with ASD. The guanfacine group showed a 43.6% decline in scores on the Aberrant Behavior Checklist (ABC) hyperactivity subscale, whereas the placebo group only showed a 13.2% decrease. Individuals taking guanfacine also showed a positive response rate of 50% ("much improved" or "very much improved" on the Clinical Global Impression-Improvement [CGI-I] scale) compared to 9.4% for placebo [165]. In a follow-up analysis of secondary measures in this same trial of extended-release guanfacine, guanfacine decreased oppositional behavior and, to a more modest degree, repetitive behavior [166]. The most common adverse effects identified in this trial included drowsiness, fatigue, and decreased appetite, making guanfacine a better tolerated drug than many other ADHD medications in ASD [165, 166]. There are limited studies on the use of alpha-2 agonists in ASD, but those that have been published show that this drug class could have positive benefits, including decreased irritability, stereotypy, hyperactivity, inappropriate speech, and hyperarousal behaviors [162, 163, 167–169].

Atomoxetine is a selective norepinephrine reuptake inhibitor approved for the treatment of ADHD in children, adolescents, and adults. Studies of atomoxetine in co-occurring ASD and ADHD demonstrate that it is generally effective in improving symptoms of hyperactivity and inattention in ASD [170–174]. In 2012, Harfterkamp et al. published the results of an 8-week placebo-controlled study of atomoxetine involving a sample of 97 children (aged 6 to 17 years) with ASD and ADHD symptoms. Subjects were randomly assigned to double-blind treatment with 1.2 mg/kg/day of atomoxetine or placebo. The atomoxetine group showed a significantly greater decline in ADHD rating scale scores after treatment. Non-severe adverse events were reported in 81.3% of the atomoxetine group and 65.3% of the placebo group. Nausea, decrease in appetite, fatigue, and early morning awakening were among the most common adverse effects [174].

Stimulants can also be used to treat co-occurring ADHD in ASD but may not be as well tolerated as guanfacine and atomoxetine. Years of efficacy and safety data support the use of stimulant medications (methylphenidate and amphetamines) as preferred first-line medications for ADHD in the general population [175]. Although there are relatively few trials assessing the efficacy and tolerability of stimulant medications for ADHD in ASD, existing data suggest that they may not be as efficacious or well tolerated. In the largest randomized controlled crossover trial examining methylphenidate in children with ASD, approximately 50% of children were considered treatment responders [176], which is considerably lower than the response rate observed in neurotypical children. Eighteen percent of methylphenidate-treated subjects discontinued the study due to adverse effects.

There is a high prevalence of anxiety in ASD, but the antidepressants and anti-anxiety medications used in neurotypical individuals with anxiety have yielded contradictory or nonsignificant results [177]. Two drugs that have shown potentially promising effects on reducing anxiety symptoms in patients with ASD include buspirone, a serotonin $(5\text{-HT})_{1A}$ receptor partial agonist and dopamine (D_2) receptor antagonist, and mirtazapine, a central presynaptic alpha$_2$-adrenergic antagonist that also blocks serotonin $(5\text{-HT})_2$ receptors and norepinephrine reuptake [178–180]. A number of retrospective and open-label studies have been published on these drugs, but there has only been one randomized double-blind placebo-controlled trial of a drug for anxiety in ASD [178]. In this pilot trial of mirtazapine, 30 children aged 5–17 years with ASD and clinically significant anxiety based on the Pediatric Anxiety Rating Scale (PARS) were randomized to either mirtazapine or placebo. Forty-seven percent of participants assigned to mirtazapine were considered treatment responders on the CGI-I. Participants assigned to mirtazapine also showed a statistically significant within-group decrease in anxiety based on the PARS. The study was insufficiently powered to detect a drug-placebo difference. There were no severe adverse events or emergence of suicidality that occurred during the study and no statistically significant difference in adverse effect frequency between mirtazapine and placebo. The most commonly reported adverse effects among the mirtazapine group were sedation/drowsiness, appetite increase, and irritability [178]. This study calls for larger randomized controlled trials powered to provide more definitive evidence of the safety, tolerability, and efficacy of pharmacologic treatments for anxiety in children and adolescents with ASD.

Melatonin is the only drug that has evidence to support its use in treating sleep disorders in ASD. A randomized placebo-controlled trial conducted by Gringras and colleagues investigated the efficacy and safety of pediatric-appropriate, prolonged-release melatonin for insomnia in children and adolescents with ASD [181]. A total of 125 children and adolescents (2–17.5 years of age) whose sleep problems failed to improve with behavioral intervention alone were randomly assigned to receive melatonin or placebo for 13 weeks. Sleep measures included the validated caregivers' sleep and nap diary (SND) and Composite Sleep Disturbance Index (CSDI). The results showed that participants taking melatonin slept for an average of 57.5 min longer and their sleep latency decreased by 39.6 min on average. Those in the placebo group slept 9.14 min longer, and their sleep latency only decreased by 12.5 min. Treatment with melatonin was generally safe; somnolence was the most commonly reported adverse effect. Promising results from other randomized trials of melatonin are summarized in a recent systematic review and meta-analysis from 2022 that included results from 15 trials [182]. The authors concluded that melatonin use in people with ASD is well tolerated and improves total sleep time, sleep latency, and sleep efficiency. They also noted that prolonged-release melatonin is better for maintaining sleep but does not significantly improve wake after sleep onset and night awakening parameters.

1.5 Common Medical Comorbidities

1.5.1 Seizures/Epilepsy

Individuals with ASD are at an elevated risk for seizures of all types [183]. The reported prevalence of epilepsy in ASD has varied from 12.6% to 39.2% [184–188]. The natural history of seizures in ASD differs from that of the general population and other neurodevelopmental disorders, in that they tend to be more treatment-refractory [189, 190]. Aside from genetic abnormalities, recent studies have identified metabolic and mitochondrial disorders, immune dysfunction, mineral and vitamin deficiencies, and exposure to environmental toxins as possible common risk factors for ASD and epilepsy [191]. Clinicians need to exercise caution when prescribing psychotropic medications that could decrease the seizure threshold in individuals with ASD [192].

1.5.2 Gastrointestinal Disorders

The most common gastrointestinal (GI) issues reported in individuals with ASD are chronic constipation, abdominal pain, diarrhea, and encopresis (typically due to constipation) [193]. There is a wide range of prevalence estimates of GI issues reported in individuals with ASD across studies, with some reaching as high as 91%. In fact, seven out of the 11 original patients diagnosed with autism by Dr. Kanner were described as having eating/feeding or dietary problems, indicating a historical association of ASD with GI issues [5]. Other signs of GI inflammation, such as gastroesophageal reflux, bloody stools, vomiting, and gaseousness are elevated in individuals with ASD [194, 195]. Furthermore, increased intestinal permeability is linked to ASD and is hypothesized to affect immune activation [196]. Food allergies, altered dietary nutrient intake, and metabolic disruptions have also been associated with ASD, providing additional support for GI dysfunction as a potential contributor to the manifestation of autistic symptoms in some patients [194, 195].

1.5.3 Immune System Dysregulation

There has been long-standing interest in the role of autoimmune mechanisms and immune dysregulation that may be involved in the relationship between autoimmune disorders and ASD [48, 197–199]. Researchers have uncovered numerous pathways that could explain the immune and autoimmune etiologies of ASD [197, 200, 201]. The mechanisms of these pathways include dysfunction of cytokines, human leukocyte antigens, immunoglobulins, mitochondria, oxidative stress, the immune-gut axis, and epigenetics [197]. These insults to the immune system can occur prenatally and/or postnatally. Maternal infection activates an immunological response that could increase the risk for ASD in offspring as seen in connection with numerous viruses contracted congenitally [48]. Maternal autoimmune dysfunction could also impact the developing offspring through the release of anti-brain autoantibodies. Several studies have looked at blood and plasma samples from mothers and found higher rates of anti-fetal brain antibodies in mothers of children with ASD compared to controls [202–207]. The postnatal environment including inflammation and endogenous autoantibodies may also contribute to atypical neurodevelopment. There is evidence from many studies on the role of inflammation and the immune system in neuropsychiatric illnesses beyond ASD, including bipolar disorder, post-traumatic stress disorder (PTSD), and, most notably, schizophrenia [208–213].

Key Points to Remember

- Autism spectrum disorder (ASD) is a neurodevelopmental disorder characterized by deficits in social communication as well as restricted and repetitive patterns of behavior, interests, or activities.
- ASD has undergone major changes in both nosology and criteria for diagnosis since it was first described by Dr. Leo Kanner in 1943.
- The DSM-5 has two core domains by which ASD is defined: deficits in social communication and restricted and repetitive behaviors and interests.
- A three-tiered scale of severity is included in the DSM-5 for clinicians to delineate the level of support required for each individual diagnosed with ASD due to the vast heterogeneity of phenotypes.
- Early symptoms of ASD include not responding to name by 12 months, not pointing to objects/showing interest by 14 months, no pretend play by 18 months,

and general symptoms of self-isolation, lack of empathy, delayed speech and language skills, echolalia, obsessive interests, repetitive movements (flapping hands, rocking, and spinning in circles), or unusual reactions to sensory perceptions.

- Common psychiatric comorbidities include intellectual disability, ADHD, anxiety, irritability, and depression.
- Medical comorbidities are highly prevalent and include gastrointestinal disorders, seizures, and immune system dysregulation.
- When an ASD diagnosis is suspected based on screenings conducted routinely at 18 months and 24 months, children are referred to a specialist to receive a full diagnosis or can be diagnosed by a pediatrician or general psychologist familiar with DSM-5 diagnostic criteria.
- Careful observation of behaviors, symptoms, and developmental history is used to diagnose ASD based on DSM-5 criteria. Structured surveys, observations, and questionnaires including the M-CHAT, SRS, and SCQ, can help evaluate these criteria.
- Behavioral interventions include comprehensive treatment models that focus on core ASD symptoms to improve language, cognitive, and functional language skills in young children as well as focused interventions that address a single skill or area of development.
- There are two medications approved by the FDA to treat irritability in ASD: the atypical antipsychotics, risperidone and aripiprazole. All other psychotropic drugs are prescribed off-label and are used in approximately two-thirds of adolescents with autism, typically to treat commonly co-occurring psychiatric conditions such as ADHD or anxiety.

References

1. American Psychiatric Association. Diagnostic and statistical manual of mental disorders. American Psychiatric Association; 2013
2. Zeidan J, Fombonne E, Scorah J, Ibrahim A, Durkin MS, Saxena S, et al. Global prevalence of autism: a systematic review update. Autism Res. 2022;15
3. Maenner MJ, Shaw KA, Baio J, Washington A, Patrick M, DiRienzo M, et al. Prevalence of autism spectrum disorder among children aged 8 Years-Autism and developmental disabilities monitoring network, 11 Sites, United States, 2016. MMWR Surveill Summ. 2020;69(4)
4. Napolitano A, Schiavi S, La Rosa P, Rossi-Espagnet MC, Petrillo S, Bottino F, et al. Sex differences in autism spectrum disorder: diagnostic, neurobiological, and behavioral features. Front Psych. 2022;13
5. Kanner L. Autistic disturbances of affective contact. Nerv Child. 1943;2:217–50
6. Wiggins LD, Durkin M, Esler A, Lee LC, Zahorodny W, Rice C, et al. Disparities in documented diagnoses of autism spectrum disorder based on demographic, individual, and service factors. Autism Res. 2020;13(3)
7. Aylward BS, Gal-Szabo DE, Taraman S. Racial, ethnic, and sociodemographic disparities in diagnosis of children with autism spectrum disorder. J Dev Behav Pediatr. 2021;42(8)

8. Goldblum JE, McFayden TC, Bristol S, Putnam OC, Wylie A, Harrop C. Autism prevalence and the intersectionality of assigned sex at birth, race, and ethnicity on age of diagnosis. J Autism Dev Disord. 2023
9. Bishop-Fitzpatrick L, Kind AJH. A scoping review of health disparities in autism spectrum disorder. J Autism Dev Disord. 2017;47(11)
10. Tanner A, Dounavi K. The emergence of autism symptoms prior to 18 months of age: a systematic literature review. J Autism Dev Disord. 2021;51(3)
11. McCarty P, Frye RE. Early detection and diagnosis of autism spectrum disorder: why is it so difficult? Semin Pediatr Neurol. 2020;35
12. Randall M, Egberts KJ, Samtani A, Scholten RJPM, Hooft L, Livingstone N, et al. Diagnostic tests for autism spectrum disorder (ASD) in preschool children. Cochrane Database Syst Rev. 2018
13. Wolff S. The history of autism. Eur Child Adolesc Psychiatry. 2004;13
14. Verhoeff B. Autism in flux: a history of the concept from Leo Kanner to DSM-5. Hist Psychiatry. 2013;24(4)
15. Asperger H. Die Autistisehen Psychopathen im Kindesalter. Arch Psychiatr Nervenkr. 1944;117(1):76–136
16. McEvedy C, Infantile autism. The syndrome and its implications for a neural theory of behaviour. J Psychosom Res. 1965;9(3)
17. Mazefsky CA, McPartland JC, Gastgeb HZ, Minshew NJ. Brief report: comparability of DSM-IV and DSM-5 ASD research samples. J Autism Dev Disord. 2013;43(5)
18. Volkmar FR, McPartland JC. From Kanner to DSM-5: autism as an evolving diagnostic concept. Annu Rev Clin Psychol. 2014;10
19. Mottron L, Bzdok D. Autism spectrum heterogeneity: fact or artifact? Mol Psychiatry. 2020;25
20. Sharma SR, Gonda X, Tarazi FI. Autism spectrum disorder: classification, diagnosis and therapy. Pharmacol Ther. 2018;190
21. Moody CT, Laugeson EA. Social skills training in autism spectrum disorder across the lifespan. Child Adolesc Psychiatr Clin N Am. 2020;29
22. Sasson NJ, Nowlin RB, Pinkham AE. Social cognition, social skill, and the broad autism phenotype. Autism. 2013;17(6)
23. Silveira-Zaldivar T, Özerk G, Özerk K. Developing social skills and social competence in children with autism. Int Electron J Element Educ. 2020;13(3)
24. Harrop C, McConachie H, Emsley R, Leadbitter K, Green J. Restricted and repetitive behaviors in autism spectrum disorders and typical development: cross-sectional and longitudinal comparisons. J Autism Dev Disord. 2014;44(5)
25. Schaaf RC, Mailloux Z, Ridgway E, Berruti AS, Dumont RL, Jones EA, et al. Sensory phenotypes in autism: making a case for the inclusion of sensory integration functions. J Autism Dev Disord. 2022
26. Grapel JN, Cicchetti DV, Volkmar FR. Sensory features as diagnostic criteria for autism: sensory features in autism. Yale J Biol Med. 2015;88(1)
27. Baum SH, Stevenson RA, Wallace MT. Behavioral, perceptual, and neural alterations in sensory and multisensory function in autism spectrum disorder. Prog Neurobiol. 2015;134
28. Neufeld J, Taylor MJ, Lundin Remnélius K, Isaksson J, Lichtenstein P, Bölte S. A co-twin-control study of altered sensory processing in autism. Autism. 2021;25(5)
29. Marco EJ, Hinkley LBN, Hill SS, Nagarajan SS. Sensory processing in autism: a review of neurophysiologic findings. Pediatr Res. 2011;69(5 Part 2)
30. Flanagan JE, Landa R, Bhat A, Bauman M. Head lag in infants at risk for autism: a preliminary study. Am J Occup Ther. 2012;66(5)
31. Matson JL, Mahan S, Fodstad JC, Hess JA, Neal D. Motor skill abilities in toddlers with autistic disorder, pervasive developmental disorder-not otherwise specified, and atypical development. Res Autism Spectr Disord. 2010;4(3)
32. Hannant P, Tavassoli T, Cassidy S. The role of sensorimotor difficulties in autism spectrum conditions. Front Neurol. 2016;7

33. Chawarska K, Paul R, Klin A, Hannigen S, Dichtel LE, Volkmar F. Parental recognition of developmental problems in toddlers with autism spectrum disorders. J Autism Dev Disord. 2007;37(1)
34. Bailey A, Phillips W, Rutter M. Autism: towards an integration of clinical, genetic, neuropsychological, and neurobiological perspectives. J Child Psychol Psychiatry Allied Discip. 1996;37
35. Ozonoff S, Young GS, Carter A, Messinger D, Yirmiya N, Zwaigenbaum L, et al. Recurrence risk for autism spectrum disorders: a baby siblings research consortium study. Pediatrics. 2011;128(3)
36. Folstein S, Rutter M. Infantile autism: A genetic study of 21 twin pairs. J Child Psychol Psychiatry. 1977;18(4)
37. Steffenburg S, Gillberg C, Hellgren L, Andersson L, Gillberg IC, Jakobsson G, et al. A twin study of autism in Denmark, Finland, Iceland, Norway and Sweden. J Child Psychol Psychiatry. 1989;30(3)
38. Tick B, Bolton P, Happé F, Rutter M, Rijsdijk F. Heritability of autism spectrum disorders: a meta-analysis of twin studies. J Child Psychol Psychiatry. 2016;57(5)
39. Myers SM, Challman TD, Bernier R, Bourgeron T, Chung WK, Constantino JN, et al. Insufficient evidence for "autism-specific" genes. Am J Hum Genet. 2020;106
40. Mpoulimari I, Zintzaras E. Identification of chromosomal regions linked to autism-spectrum disorders: a meta-analysis of genome-wide linkage scans. Genet Test Mol Biomarkers. 2022;26(2)
41. Gyawali S, Patra BN. Autism spectrum disorder: Trends in research exploring etiopathogenesis. Psychiatry Clin Neurosci. 2019;73
42. Doi M, Usui N, Shimada S. Prenatal environment and neurodevelopmental disorders. Front Endocrinol. 2022;13
43. Yu L, Wu YM, Wu BL. Genetic architecture, epigenetic influence and environment exposure in the pathogenesis of Autism. Sci China Life Sci. 2015;58
44. Rodriguez-Gomez DA, Garcia-Guaqueta DP, Charry-Sánchez JD, Sarquis-Buitrago E, Blanco M, Velez-van-Meerbeke A, et al. A systematic review of common genetic variation and biological pathways in autism spectrum disorder. BMC Neurosci. 2021;22(1)
45. Watts TJ. The pathogenesis of autism. Clin Med Pathol. 2008;1
46. Zawadzka A, Cieślik M, Adamczyk A. The role of maternal immune activation in the pathogenesis of autism: a review of the evidence, proposed mechanisms and implications for treatment. Int J Mol Sci. 2021;22
47. Abdallah MW, Mortensen EL, Greaves-Lord K, Larsen N, Bonefeld-Jørgensen EC, Nørgaard-Pedersen B, et al. Neonatal levels of neurotrophic factors and risk of autism spectrum disorders. Acta Psychiatr Scand. 2013;128(1)
48. McDougle CJ, Landino SM, Vahabzadeh A, O'Rourke J, Zurcher NR, Finger BC, et al. Toward an immune-mediated subtype of autism spectrum disorder. Brain Res. 2015;1617
49. Shenouda J, Barrett E, Davidow AL, Sidwell K, Lescott C, Halperin W, et al. Prevalence and disparities in the detection of autism without intellectual disability. Pediatrics. 2023;151(2)
50. Matson JL, Shoemaker M. Intellectual disability and its relationship to autism spectrum disorders. Res Dev Disabil. 2009;30
51. Abrahams BS, Geschwind DH. Advances in autism genetics: on the threshold of a new neurobiology. Nat Rev Genet. 2008;9
52. Grondhuis SN, Lecavalier L, Arnold LE, Handen BL, Scahill L, McDougle CJ, et al. Differences in verbal and nonverbal IQ test scores in children with autism spectrum disorder. Res Autism Spectr Disord. 2018;49:47–55
53. Courchesne V, Girard D, Jacques C, Soulières I. Assessing intelligence at autism diagnosis: mission impossible? Testability and cognitive profile of autistic preschoolers. J Autism Dev Disord. 2019;49(3)
54. Minshew NJ, Turner CA, Goldstein G. The application of short forms of the wechsler intelligence scales in adults and children with high functioning autism. J Autism Dev Disord. 2005;35(1)

55. Paynter JM. Assessment of school-aged children with autism spectrum disorder. J Psychol Couns Sch. 2015;25(1)
56. Gotham K, Pickles A, Lord C. Standardizing ADOS scores for a measure of severity in autism spectrum disorders. J Autism Dev Disord. 2009;39(5)
57. Lord C, Rutter M, Le Couteur A. Autism diagnostic interview-revised: a revised version of a diagnostic interview for caregivers of individuals with possible pervasive developmental disorders. J Autism Dev Disord. 1994;24(5)
58. Kanne SM, Gerber AJ, Quirmbach LM, Sparrow SS, Cicchetti DV, Saulnier CA. The role of adaptive behavior in autism spectrum disorders: Implications for functional outcome. J Autism Dev Disord. 2011;41(8)
59. Shumway S, Farmer C, Thurm A, Joseph L, Black D, Golden C. The ADOS calibrated severity score: relationship to phenotypic variables and stability over time. Autism Res. 2012;5(4)
60. Hill AP, Zuckerman KE, Hagen AD, Kriz DJ, Duvall SW, Van Santen J, et al. Aggressive behavior problems in children with autism spectrum disorders: prevalence and correlates in a large clinical sample. Res Autism Spectr Disord. 2014;8(9)
61. Kanne SM, Mazurek MO. Aggression in children and adolescents with ASD: prevalence and risk factors. J Autism Dev Disord. 2011;41(7)
62. McCracken JT, McGough J, Shah B, Cronin P, Hong D, Aman MG, et al. Risperidone in children with autism and serious behavioral problems. N Engl J Med. 2002;347(5)
63. Owen R, Sikich L, Marcus RN, Corey-Lisle P, Manos G, McQuade RD, et al. Aripiprazole in the treatment of irritability in children and adolescents with autistic disorder. Pediatrics. 2009;124(6)
64. Aishworiya R, Valica T, Hagerman R, Restrepo B. An update on psychopharmacological treatment of autism spectrum disorder. Neurotherapeutics. 2022;19(1)
65. Mayes SD, Calhoun SL. Symptoms of autism in young children and correspondence with the DSM. Infants Young Child. 1999;12(2)
66. Mayes SD, Calhoun SL, Murray MJ, Ahuja M, Smith LA. Anxiety, depression, and irritability in children with autism relative to other neuropsychiatric disorders and typical development. Res Autism Spectr Disord. 2011;5(1)
67. Goldman SE, Richdale AL, Clemons T, Malow BA. Parental sleep concerns in autism spectrum disorders: variations from childhood to adolescence. J Autism Dev Disord. 2012;42(4)
68. Mayes SD, Calhoun SL. Variables related to sleep problems in children with autism. Res Autism Spectr Disord. 2009;3(4)
69. Mazurek MO, Kanne SM, Wodka EL. Physical aggression in children and adolescents with autism spectrum disorders. Res Autism Spectr Disord. 2013;7(3)
70. Kim JA, Szatmari P, Bryson SE, Streiner DL, Wilson FJ. The prevalence of anxiety and mood problems among children with autism and Asperger syndrome. Autism. 2000;4(2)
71. Yerys BE, Wallace GL, Sokoloff JL, Shook DA, James JD, Kenworthy L. Attention deficit/hyperactivity disorder symptoms moderate cognition and behavior in children with autism spectrum disorders. Autism Res. 2009;2(6)
72. Farmer CA, Aman MG. Aggressive behavior in a sample of children with autism spectrum disorders. Res Autism Spectr Disord. 2011;5(1)
73. NICHD Early Child Care Research Network. Trajectories of physical aggression from toddlerhood to middle childhood: predictors, correlates, and outcomes. Monogr Soc Res Child Dev. 2004;69(4)
74. Hartley SL, Sikora DM, McCoy R. Prevalence and risk factors of maladaptive behaviour in young children with autistic disorder. J Intellect Disabil Res. 2008
75. Farmer C, Butter E, Mazurek MO, Cowan C, Lainhart J, Cook EH, et al. Aggression in children with autism spectrum disorders and a clinic-referred comparison group. Autism. 2015;19(3)
76. Dominick KC, Davis NO, Lainhart J, Tager-Flusberg H, Folstein S. Atypical behaviors in children with autism and children with a history of language impairment. Res Dev Disabil. 2007;28(2)

77. Reese RM, Richman DM, Belmont JM, Morse P. Functional characteristics of disruptive behavior in developmentally disabled children with and without autism. J Autism Dev Disord. 2005;35(4)
78. Dagnan D, Weston C. Physical intervention with people with intellectual disabilities: the influence of cognitive and emotional variables. J Appl Res Intellect Disabil. 2006;19(2)
79. Gitimoghaddam M, Chichkine N, McArthur L, Sangha SS, Symington V. Applied behavior analysis in children and youth with autism spectrum disorders: a scoping review. Perspect. Behav Sci. 2022
80. Hodgetts S, Nicholas D, Zwaigenbaum L. Home sweet home? families' experiences with aggression in children with autism spectrum disorders. Focus Autism Other Dev Disabl. 2013;28(3)
81. Neece CL, Green SA, Baker BL. Parenting stress and child behavior problems: a transactional relationship across time. Am J Intellect Dev Disabil. 2012;117(1)
82. Fisher WW, Lindauer SE, Alterson CJ, Thompson RH. Assessment and treatment of destructive behavior maintained by stereotypic object manipulation. J Appl Behav Anal. 1998;31(4):513–27
83. Brahm NC, Fast GA, Brown RC. Buspirone for autistic disorder in a woman with an intellectual disability. Ann Pharmacother. 2008;42(1)
84. Mitteer DR, Romani PW, Greer BD, Fisher WW. Assessment and treatment of pica and destruction of holiday decorations. J Appl Behav Anal. 2015;48(4)
85. Reese RM, Richman DM, Zarcone J, Zarcone T. Individualizing functional assessments for children with autism: The contribution of perseverative behavior and sensory disturbances to disruptive behavior. Focus Autism Other Dev Disabl. 2003;18(2)
86. Reese RM, Hellings J, Stephen S. Treatment methods for destructive and aggressive behaviour in people with severe developmental and intellectual disabilities. In: Psychiatric and behavioural disorders in intellectual and developmental disabilities. Cambridge University Press; 2001. p. 269–82
87. Matson JL, Wilkins J, Mac KJ. The relationship of challenging behaviors to severity and symptoms of autism spectrum disorders. J Ment Health Res Intellect Disabil. 2008;2(1)
88. Steenfeldt-Kristensen C, Jones CA, Richards C. The prevalence of self-injurious behaviour in autism: a meta-analytic study. J Autism Dev Disord. 2020;50(11)
89. Minshawi NF, Hurwitz S, Fodstad JC, Biebl S, Morriss DH, McDougle CJ. The association between self-injurious behaviors and autism spectrum disorders. Psychol Res Behav Manag. 2014;7
90. Oliver C, Murphy GH, Corbett JA. Self-injurious behaviour in people with mental handicap: a total population study. J Intellect Disabil Res. 1987;31(2)
91. Laverty C, Oliver C, Moss J, Nelson L, Richards C. Persistence and predictors of self-injurious behaviour in autism: a ten-year prospective cohort study. Mol Autism. 2020;11(1)
92. Oliphant RYK, Smith EM, Grahame V. What is the prevalence of self-harming and suicidal behaviour in under 18s with ASD, with or without an intellectual disability? J Autism Dev Disord. 2020, 50(10):3510–24
93. Minshawi NF, Hurwitz S, Morriss D, McDougle CJ. Multidisciplinary assessment and treatment of self-Injurious behavior in autism spectrum disorder and intellectual disability: Integration of psychological and biological theory and approach. J Autism Dev Disord. 2015;45(6)
94. Peebles KA, Price TJ. Self-injurious behaviour in intellectual disability syndromes: Evidence for aberrant pain signalling as a contributing factor. J Intellect Disabil Res. 2012;56(5)
95. Dempsey J, Dempsey AG, Guffey D, Minard CG, Goin-Kochel RP. Brief report: further examination of self-Injurious behaviors in children and adolescents with autism spectrum disorders. J Autism Dev Disord. 2016;46(5)
96. Gulsrud A, Lin CE, Park MN, Hellemann G, McCracken J. Self-injurious behaviours in children and adults with autism spectrum disorder (ASD). J Intellect Disabil Res. 2018
97. Hours C, Recasens C, Baleyte JM. ASD and ADHD comorbidity: what are we talking about? Front Psych. 2022;13

98. Rong Y, Yang CJ, Jin Y, Wang Y. Prevalence of attention-deficit/hyperactivity disorder in individuals with autism spectrum disorder: A meta-analysis. Res Autism Spectr Disord. 2021;83
99. Thom RP, Keary CJ, Kramer G, Nowinski LA, McDougle CJ. Psychiatric assessment of social impairment across the lifespan. Harv Rev Psychiatry. 2020;28
100. Reiersen AM, Todd RD. Co-occurrence of ADHD and autism spectrum disorders: Phenomenology and treatment. Expert Rev Neurother. 2008;8
101. Antshel KM, Russo N. Autism spectrum disorders and ADHD: Overlapping phenomenology, diagnostic issues, and treatment considerations. Curr Psychiatry Rep. 2019;21
102. Riglin L, Leppert B, Langley K, Thapar AK, O'Donovan MC, Davey Smith G, et al. Investigating attention-deficit hyperactivity disorder and autism spectrum disorder traits in the general population: What happens in adult life? J Child Psychol Psychiatry. 2021;62(4)
103. Hatch B, Kadlaskar G, Miller M. Diagnosis and treatment children and adolescents with autism and ADHD. Psychol Sch. 2023;60(2)
104. Beesdo K, Knappe S, Pine DS. Anxiety and anxiety disorders in children and adolescents: developmental issues and implications for DSM-V. Psychiatr Clin N Am. 2009;32
105. Simonoff E, Pickles A, Charman T, Chandler S, Loucas T, Baird G. Psychiatric disorders in children with autism spectrum disorders: prevalence, comorbidity, and associated factors in a population-derived sample. J Am Acad Child Adolesc Psychiatry. 2008;47(8)
106. Hollocks MJ, Lerh JW, Magiati I, Meiser-Stedman R, Brugha TS. Anxiety and depression in adults with autism spectrum disorder: a systematic review and meta-analysis. Psychol Med. 2019;49
107. Kirsch AC, Huebner ARS, Mehta SQ, Howie FR, Weaver AL, Myers SM, et al. Association of comorbid mood and anxiety disorders with autism spectrum disorder. JAMA Pediatr. 2020;174(1)
108. Grondhuis SN, Aman MG. Assessment of anxiety in children and adolescents with autism spectrum disorders. Res Autism Spectr Disord. 2012;6
109. Kerns CM, Kendall PC, Berry L, Souders MC, Franklin ME, Schultz RT, et al. Traditional and atypical presentations of anxiety in youth with autism spectrum disorder. J Autism Dev Disord. 2014;44(11)
110. Williams S, Leader G, Mannion A, Chen J. An investigation of anxiety in children and adolescents with autism spectrum disorder. Res Autism Spectr Disord. 2015;10
111. White SW, Oswald D, Ollendick T, Scahill L. Anxiety in children and adolescents with autism spectrum disorders. Clin Psychol Rev. 2009;29
112. MacNeil BM, Lopes VA, Minnes PM. Anxiety in children and adolescents with autism spectrum disorders. Res Autism Spectr Disord. 2009;3
113. Thom RP, McDougle CJ. Repetitive thoughts and behaviors in autism spectrum disorder: a symptom-based framework for novel therapeutics. ACS Chem Neurosci. 2023;14
114. Anthony LG, Kenworthy L, Yerys BE, Jankowski KF, James JD, Harms MB, et al. Interests in high-functioning autism are more intense, interfering, and idiosyncratic than those in neurotypical development. Dev Psychopathol. 2013;25(3)
115. Péter Z, Oliphant ME, Fernandez TV. Motor stereotypies: a pathophysiological review. Front Neurosci. 2017;11
116. Cunningham AB, Schreibman L. Stereotypy in autism: the importance of function. Res Autism Spectr Disord. 2008;2(3)
117. Esbensen AJ, Seltzer MM, Lam KSL, Bodfish JW. Age-related differences in restricted repetitive behaviors in autism spectrum disorders. J Autism Dev Disord. 2009;39(1)
118. Martin AF, Jassi A, Cullen AE, Broadbent M, Downs J, Krebs G. Co-occurring obsessive–compulsive disorder and autism spectrum disorder in young people: prevalence, clinical characteristics and outcomes. Eur Child Adolesc Psychiatry. 2020;29(11)
119. Ruscio AM, Stein DJ, Chiu WT, Kessler RC. The epidemiology of obsessive-compulsive disorder in the National Comorbidity Survey Replication. Mol Psychiatry. 2010;15(1)
120. van Steensel FJA, Bögels SM, Perrin S. Anxiety disorders in children and adolescents with autistic spectrum disorders: a meta-analysis. Clin Child Fam Psychol Rev. 2011;14

121. Meier SM, Petersen L, Schendel DE, Mattheisen M, Mortensen PB, Mors O. Obsessive-compulsive disorder and autism spectrum disorders: longitudinal and offspring risk. PLoS One. 2015;10(11)
122. Postorino V, Kerns CM, Vivanti G, Bradshaw J, Siracusano M, Mazzone L. Anxiety disorders and obsessive-compulsive disorder in individuals with autism spectrum disorder. Curr Psychiatry Rep. 2017;19
123. Zandt F, Prior M, Kyrios M. Repetitive behaviour in children with high functioning autism and obsessive compulsive disorder. J Autism Dev Disord. 2007;37(2)
124. Goodman WK, Price LH, Rasmussen SA, Mazure C, Delgado P, Heninger GR, et al. The Yale-Brown obsessive compulsive scale: II. Validity Arch Gen Psychiatry. 1989;46(11)
125. Goodman WK, Price LH, Rasmussen SA, Mazure C, Fleischmann RL, Hill CL, et al. The Yale-Brown obsessive compulsive scale: I. Development, use, and reliability. Arch Gen Psychiatry. 1989;46(11)
126. Hudson CC, Hall L, Harkness KL. Prevalence of depressive disorders in individuals with autism spectrum disorder: a meta-analysis. J Abnorm Child Psychol. 2019;47(1)
127. Pezzimenti F, Han GT, Vasa RA, Gotham K. Depression in youth with autism spectrum disorder. Child Adolesc Psychiatr Clin N Am. 2019;28
128. Bird G, Cook R. Mixed emotions: the contribution of alexithymia to the emotional symptoms of autism. Transl Psychiatry. 2013;3
129. Montagut-asunción M, Crespo-martín S, Pastor-cerezuela G, D'ocon-giménez A. Joint attention and its relationship with autism risk markers at 18 months of age. Children. 2022;9(4)
130. Stone WL, McMahon CR, Yoder PJ, Walden TA. Early social-communicative and cognitive development of younger siblings of children with autism spectrum disorders. Arch Pediatr Adolesc Med. 2007;161(4)
131. Naber FBA, Swinkels SHN, Buitelaar JK, Dietz C, Van Daalen E, Bakermans-Kranenburg MJ, et al. Joint attention and attachment in toddlers with autism. J Abnorm Child Psychol. 2007;35(6)
132. Johnson CP, Myers SM, Lipkin PH, Cartwright JD, Desch LW, Duby JC, et al. Identification and evaluation of children with autism spectrum disorders. Pediatrics. 2007;120
133. Zwaigenbaum L, Bauman ML, Stone WL, Yirmiya N, Estes A, Hansen RL, et al. Early identification of autism spectrum disorder: recommendations for practice and research. Pediatrics. 2015
134. Coonrod EE, Stone WL. Early concerns of parents of children with autistic and nonautistic disorders. Infants Young Child. 2004;17(3)
135. De Giacomo A, Fombonne E. Parental recognition of developmental abnormalities in autism. Eur Child Adolesc Psychiatry. 1998;7(3)
136. Reynolds AM, Malow BA. Sleep and autism spectrum disorders. Pediatr Clin N Am. 2011;58
137. Gabriels RL, Cuccaro ML, Hill DE, Ivers BJ, Goldson E. Repetitive behaviors in autism: relationships with associated clinical features. Res Dev Disabil. 2005;26(2)
138. Zwaigenbaum L, Bauman ML, Choueiri R, Kasari C, Carter A, Granpeesheh D, et al. Early intervention for children with autism spectrum disorder under 3 years of age: recommendations for practice and research. Pediatrics. 2015
139. Anderson DK, Liang JW, Lord C. Predicting young adult outcome among more and less cognitively able individuals with autism spectrum disorders. J Child Psychol Psychiatry. 2014;55(5)
140. Hyman SL, Levy SE, Myers SM, Kuo DZ, Apkon CS, Davidson LF, et al. Identification, evaluation, and management of children with autism spectrum disorder. Pediatrics. 2020;145(1)
141. Wiggins LD, Baio J, Schieve L, Lee LC, Nicholas J, Rice CE. Retention of autism spectrum diagnoses by community professionals: findings from the autism and developmental disabilities monitoring network, 2000 and 2006. J Dev Behav Pediatr. 2012;33(5)
142. Odom SL, Boyd BA, Hall LJ, Hume K. Evaluation of comprehensive treatment models for individuals with autism spectrum disorders. J Autism Dev Disord. 2010;40(4)

143. Wong C, Odom SL, Hume KA, Cox AW, Fettig A, Kucharczyk S, et al. Evidence-based practices for children, youth, and young adults with autism spectrum disorder: a comprehensive review. J Autism Dev Disord. 2015;45(7)
144. Reichow B, Hume K, Barton EE, Boyd BA. Early intensive behavioral intervention (EIBI) for young children with autism spectrum disorders (ASD). Cochrane Database Syst Rev. 2018;2018
145. Dawson G, Rogers S, Munson J, Smith M, Winter J, Greenson J, et al. Randomized, controlled trial of an intervention for toddlers with autism: the early start Denver model. Pediatrics. 2010;125(1)
146. Wieder S, Greenspan SI. Climbing the symbolic ladder in the DIR model through floor time/ interactive play. Autism. 2003;7(4)
147. Koegel RL, Kern KL. Pivotal response treatments for autism: communication, social, and academic development. Brookes Publishing Company; 2006
148. Mesibov GB, Shea V. The TEACCH program in the era of evidence-based practice. J Autism Dev Disord. 2010;40
149. Feroe AG, Uppal N, Gutiérrez-Sacristán A, Mousavi S, Greenspun P, Surati R, et al. Medication use in the management of comorbidities among individuals with autism spectrum disorder from a large nationwide insurance database. JAMA Pediatr. 2021;175(9)
150. Doyle CA, McDougle CJ. Pharmacologic treatments for the behavioral symptoms associated with autism spectrum disorders across the lifespan. Dialogues Clin Neurosci. 2012;14(3)
151. McDougle CJ, Naylor ST, Cohen DJ, Aghajanian GK, Heninger GR, Price LH. Effects of tryptophan depletion in drug-free adults with autistic disorder. Arch Gen Psychiatry. 1996;53(11):993–1000
152. Boccuto L, Chen CF, Pittman AR, Skinner CD, McCartney HJ, Jones K, et al. Decreased tryptophan metabolism in patients with autism spectrum disorders. Mol Autism. 2013;4(1)
153. Chandana SR, Behen ME, Juhász C, Muzik O, Rothermel RD, Mangner TJ, et al. Significance of abnormalities in developmental trajectory and asymmetry of cortical serotonin synthesis in autism. Int J Dev Neurosci. 2005;23(2–3)
154. McDougle CJ, Brodkin ES, Naylor ST, Carlson DC, Cohen DJ, Price LH. Sertraline in adults with pervasive developmental disorders: a prospective open-label investigation. J Clin Psychopharmacol. 1998;18(1)
155. Hollander E, Soorya L, Chaplin W, Anagnostou E, Taylor BP, Ferretti CJ, et al. A double-blind placebo-controlled trial of fluoxetine for repetitive behaviors and global severity in adult autism spectrum disorders. Am J Psychiatry. 2012;169(3)
156. Hellings JA, Kelley LA, Gabrielli WF, Kilgore E, Shah P. Sertraline response in adults with mental retardation and autistic disorder. J Clin Psychiatry. 1996;57(8)
157. Koshes RJ. Use of fluoxetine for obsessive-compulsive behavior in adults with autism [1]. Am J Psychiatry. 1997;154
158. Hossein Fatemi S, Realmuto GM, Khan L, Thuras P. Fluoxetine in treatment of adolescent patients with autism: a longitudinal open trial. J Autism Dev Disord. 1998;28(4)
159. Hollander E, Phillips A, Chaplin W, Zagursky K, Novotny S, Wasserman S, et al. A placebo controlled crossover trial of liquid fluoxetine on repetitive behaviors in childhood and adolescent autism. Neuropsychopharmacology. 2005;30(3)
160. Posey DJ, Stigler KA, Erickson CA, McDougle CJ. Antipsychotics in the treatment of autism. J Clin Invest. 2008;118
161. Barnard L, Young AH, Pearson J, Geddes J, O'Brien G. A systematic review of the use of atypical antipsychotics in autism. J Psychopharmacol. 2002;16
162. Scahill L, Aman MG, McDougle CJ, McCracken JT, Tierney E, Dziura J, et al. A prospective open trial of guanfacine in children with pervasive developmental disorders. J Child Adolesc Psychopharmacol. 2006;16(5)
163. Posey DJ, Puntney JI, Sasher TM, Kem DL, McDougle CJ. Guanfacine treatment of hyperactivity and inattention in pervasive developmental disorders: a retrospective analysis of 80 cases. J Child Adolesc Psychopharmacol. 2004;14

164. Joshi G, Wilens T, Firmin ES, Hoskova B, Biederman J. Pharmacotherapy of attention deficit/hyperactivity disorder in individuals with autism spectrum disorder: a systematic review of the literature. J Psychopharmacol. 2021;35
165. Scahill L, McCracken JT, King BH, Rockhill C, Shah B, Politte L, et al. Extended-release guanfacine for hyperactivity in children with autism spectrum disorder. Am J Psychiatry. 2015;172(12)
166. Politte LC, Scahill L, Figueroa J, McCracken JT, King B, McDougle CJ. A randomized, placebo-controlled trial of extended-release guanfacine in children with autism spectrum disorder and ADHD symptoms: an analysis of secondary outcome measures. Neuropsychopharmacology. 2018;43(8)
167. Fankhauser MP, Karumanchi VC, German ML, Yates A, Karumanchi SD. A double-blind, placebo-controlled study of the efficacy of transdermal clonidine in autism. J Clin Psychiatry. 1992;53(3)
168. Connor DF, Fletcher KE, Swanson JM. A meta-analysis of clonidine for symptoms of attention-deficit hyperactivity disorder. J Am Acad Child Adolesc Psychiatry. 1999;38(12)
169. Hirota T, Schwartz S, Correll CU. Alpha-2 agonists for attention-deficit/hyperactivity disorder in youth: a systematic review and meta-analysis of monotherapy and add-on trials to stimulant therapy. J Am Acad Child Adolesc Psychiatry. 2014;53
170. Ghanizadeh A. Atomoxetine for treating ADHD symptoms in autism: a systematic review. J Atten Disord. 2013;17
171. Azouz HG, Ghareib B, Gad HA, Elmaksoud MA. Effectiveness of atomoxetine on children with autism spectrum disorder and comorbid attention deficit hyperactivity disorder. NeuroQuantology. 2022;20(10)
172. Patra S, Nebhinani N, Viswanathan A, Kirubakaran R. Atomoxetine for attention deficit hyperactivity disorder in children and adolescents with autism: a systematic review and meta-analysis. Autism Res. 2019;12
173. Eslamzadeh M, Hebrani P, Behdani F, Moghadam MD, Panaghi L, Mirzadeh M, et al. Assessment the efficacy of atomoxetine in autism spectrum disorders: a randomized, double-blind, placebo-controlled trial. Iran J Psychiatry Behav Sci. 2018;12(2)
174. Harfterkamp M, van de Loo-Neus G, Minderaa RB, van der Gaag RJ, Escobar R, Schacht A, et al. A randomized double-blind study of atomoxetine versus placebo for attention-deficit/hyperactivity disorder symptoms in children with autism spectrum disorder. J Am Acad Child Adolesc Psychiatry. 2012;51(7):733–41
175. Cortese S, Adamo N, Del Giovane C, Mohr-Jensen C, Hayes AJ, Carucci S, et al. Comparative efficacy and tolerability of medications for attention-deficit hyperactivity disorder in children, adolescents, and adults: a systematic review and network meta-analysis. Lancet Psychiatry. 2018;5(9)
176. Research Units on Pediatric Psychopharmacology Autism Network. Randomized, controlled, crossover trial of methylphenidate in pervasive developmental disorders with hyperactivity. Arch Gen Psychiatry. 2005;62(11):1266–74
177. Deb S, Roy M, Lee R, Majid M, Limbu B, Santambrogio J, et al. Randomised controlled trials of antidepressant and anti-anxiety medications for people with autism spectrum disorder: systematic review and meta-analysis. BJPsych Open. 2021;7(6)
178. McDougle CJ, Thom RP, Ravichandran CT, Palumbo ML, Politte LC, Mullett JE, et al. A randomized double-blind, placebo-controlled pilot trial of mirtazapine for anxiety in children and adolescents with autism spectrum disorder. Neuropsychopharmacology. 2022;47(6)
179. Buitelaar JK, Van Der Gaag RJ, Van Der Hoeven J. Buspirone in the management of anxiety and irritability in children with pervasive developmental disorders: results of an open-label study. J Clin Psychiatry. 1998;59(2)
180. Ceranoglu TA, Wozniak J, Fried R, Galdo M, Hoskova B, DeLeon FM, et al. A retrospective chart review of buspirone for the treatment of anxiety in psychiatrically referred youth with high-functioning autism spectrum disorder. J Child Adolesc Psychopharmacol. 2019;29(1)

181. Gringras P, Nir T, Breddy J, Frydman-Marom A, Findling RL. Efficacy and safety of pediatric prolonged-release melatonin for insomnia in children with autism spectrum disorder. J Am Acad Child Adolesc Psychiatry. 2017;56(11)
182. Nogueira HA, de Castro CT, da Silva DCG, Pereira M. Melatonin for sleep disorders in people with autism: systematic review and meta-analysis. Prog Neuro-Psychopharmacol Biol Psychiatry. 2023;123
183. Tuchman RF, Rapin I, Shinnar S. Autistic and dysphasic children. II: Epilepsy. In: The science of mental health: Volume 2: Autism; 2013.
184. Danielsson S, Gillberg IC, Billstedt E, Gillberg C, Olsson I. Epilepsy in young adults with autism: a prospective population-based follow-up study of 120 individuals diagnosed in childhood. Epilepsia. 2005;46
185. Giovanardi Rossi P, Posar A, Parmeggiani A. Epilepsy in adolescents and young adults with autistic disorder. Brain Dev. 2000;22(2)
186. Olsson I, Steffenburg S, Gillberg C. Epilepsy in autism and autisticlike conditions: a population-based study. Arch Neurol. 1988;45(6)
187. Hara H. Autism and epilepsy: a retrospective follow-up study. Brain and Development. 2007;29(8)
188. Volkmar FR, Nelson DS. Seizure disorders in autism. J Am Acad Child Adolesc Psychiatry. 1990 Jan;29(1):127–9
189. Sansa G, Carlson C, Doyle W, Weiner HL, Bluvstein J, Barr W, et al. Medically refractory epilepsy in autism. Epilepsia. 2011;52(6)
190. Tuchman R, Alessandri M, Cuccaro M. Autism spectrum disorders and epilepsy: moving towards a comprehensive approach to treatment. Brain Dev. 2010:32
191. Besag FMC, Vasey MJ. Seizures and epilepsy in autism spectrum disorder. Psychiatr Clin N Am. 2021;44
192. Alfageh BH, Besag FMC, Gao L, Ma TT, Man KKC, Wong ICK, et al. Antipsychotic medication and risk of incident seizure in people with autism spectrum disorder: analyses with cohort and within individual study designs. J Autism Dev Disord. 2022;52(11)
193. Buie T, Campbell DB, Fuchs GJ, Furuta GT, Levy J, Van De Water J, et al. Evaluation, diagnosis, and treatment of gastrointestinal disorders in individuals with ASDs: a consensus report. Pediatrics. 2010;
194. Lefter R, Ciobica A, Timofte D, Stanciu C, Trifan A. A descriptive review on the prevalence of gastrointestinal disturbances and their multiple associations in autism spectrum disorder, vol. 56. Medicina (Lithuania); 2020
195. Wang LW, Tancredi DJ, Thomas DW. The prevalence of gastrointestinal problems in children across the United States with autism spectrum disorders from families with multiple affected members. J Dev Behav Pediatr. 2011;32(5)
196. Dargenio VN, Dargenio C, Castellaneta S, De Giacomo A, Laguardia M, Schettini F, et al. Intestinal barrier dysfunction and microbiota–gut–brain axis: Possible implications in the pathogenesis and treatment of autism spectrum disorder. Nutrients. 2023;15(7):1620.
197. Erbescu A, Papuc SM, Budisteanu M, Arghir A, Neagu M. Re-emerging concepts of immune dysregulation in autism spectrum disorders. Front Psychiatry. 2022;13
198. Thom RP, Keary CJ, Palumbo ML, Ravichandran CT, Mullett JE, Hazen EP, et al. Beyond the brain: a multi-system inflammatory subtype of autism spectrum disorder. Psychopharmacology. 2019;236(10):3045–61
199. Spann MN, Timonen-Soivio L, Suominen A, Cheslack-Postava K, McKeague IW, Sourander A, et al. Proband and familial autoimmune diseases are associated with proband diagnosis of autism spectrum disorders. J Am Acad Child Adolesc Psychiatry. 2019;58(5):496–505.
200. Edmiston E, Ashwood P, Van de Water J. Autoimmunity, autoantibodies, and autism spectrum disorder. Biol Psychiatry. 2017;81
201. Chen JA, Peñagarikano O, Belgard TG, Swarup V, Geschwind DH. The emerging picture of autism spectrum disorder: Genetics and pathology. Ann Rev Pathol: Mech Dis. 2015;10

202. Braunschweig D, Ashwood P, Krakowiak P, Hertz-Picciotto I, Hansen R, Croen LA, et al. Autism: maternally derived antibodies specific for fetal brain proteins. Neurotoxicology. 2008;29(2)
203. Braunschweig D, Duncanson P, Boyce R, Hansen R, Ashwood P, Pessah IN, et al. Behavioral correlates of maternal antibody status among children with autism. J Autism Dev Disord. 2012;42(7)
204. Braunschweig D, Krakowiak P, Duncanson P, Boyce R, Hansen RL, Ashwood P, et al. Autism-specific maternal autoantibodies recognize critical proteins in developing brain. Transl Psychiatry. 2013:3
205. Brimberg L, Sadiq A, Gregersen PK, Diamond B. Brain-reactive IgG correlates with autoimmunity in mothers of a child with an autism spectrum disorder. Mol Psychiatry. 2013;18(11)
206. Piras IS, Haapanen L, Napolioni V, Sacco R, Van de Water J, Persico AM. Anti-brain antibodies are associated with more severe cognitive and behavioral profiles in Italian children with autism spectrum disorder. Brain Behav Immun. 2014;38
207. Warren RP, Cole P, Odell JD, Pingree CB, Warren WL, White E, et al. Detection of maternal antibodies in infantile autism. J Am Acad Child Adolesc Psychiatry. 1990;29(6):873–7
208. Brown AS, Hooton J, Schaefer CA, Zhang H, Petkova E, Babulas V, et al. Elevated maternal interleukin-8 levels and risk of schizophrenia in adult offspring. Am J Psychiatry. 2004;161(5)
209. Haroon E, Raison CL, Miller AH. Psychoneuroimmunology meets neuropsychopharmacology: translational implications of the impact of inflammation on behavior. Neuropsychopharmacology. 2012;37
210. Jones KA, Thomsen C. The role of the innate immune system in psychiatric disorders. Mol Cell Neurosci. 2013;53
211. Meyer U, Feldon J. Neural basis of psychosis-related behaviour in the infection model of schizophrenia. Behav Brain Res. 2009;204(2)
212. Michel M, Schmidt MJ, Mirnics K. Immune system gene dysregulation in autism and schizophrenia. Dev Neurobiol. 2012;72(10)
213. Mou TCM, Lane MV, Ireland DDC, Verthelyi D, Tonelli LH, Clark SM. Association of complement component 4 with neuroimmune abnormalities in the subventricular zone in schizophrenia and autism spectrum disorders. Neurobiol Dis. 2022;173

Further Reading

Hazen E, McDougle CJ, editors. The Massachusetts general hospital guide to medical care in patients with autism spectrum disorder. New York, NY: Springer Publishing; 2018.
McDougle CJ, editor. Primer on autism spectrum disorder. New York, NY: Oxford University Press; 2016.
Palumbo ML, Keary CJ, McDougle CJ. Autism spectrum disorder (Chapter 7). In: McVoy M, Findling RL, editors. Clinical manual of child and adolescent psychopharmacology. 4th ed. Washington, DC: American Psychiatric Publishing, Inc.; 2023. p. 311–72.

Intellectual Disability 2

Renée M. Green and Ainsley Losh

2.1 Overview

Intellectual disability (ID) is a group of etiologically distinct conditions that are both genetically and clinically heterogeneous and is characterized by three distinct criteria. *The first criterion is significant limitations in intellectual functioning.* Intellectual functioning refers to cognitive abilities such as reasoning, problem-solving, judgment, abstract thinking, planning, practical understanding, and learning from experience [2, 3]. *The second diagnostic criterion is adaptive skills deficits.* Adaptive skills refer to how well an individual can meet community standards for personal independence and social responsibility and encompasses three domains: conceptual, social, and practical adaptive skills [3]. The conceptual domain can be thought of as the "academic" domain and involves competence in language, reading, writing, memory, math reasoning, acquisition of practical knowledge, and judgment in novel situations. The social domain involves theory of mind, empathy, social judgment, friendship abilities, and interpersonal communication skills. Last, the practical domain involves self-management across life settings including personal care, money management, job responsibilities, recreation, and self-management of behavior [2, 3]. *The third diagnostic criterion is that the onset occurs during the developmental period.* This definition is broadly consistent with both the American Association on Intellectual and Developmental Disabilities (AAIDD) and the American Psychiatric Association (APA). While nomenclature

R. M. Green (✉)
Lurie Center for Autism, Massachusetts General Hospital, Lexington, MA, USA

Department of Psychiatry, Harvard Medical School, Boston, MA, USA
e-mail: rgreen@mgh.harvard.edu

A. Losh
Lurie Center for Autism, Massachusetts General Hospital, Lexington, MA, USA
e-mail: ainsley.losh@cuanschutz.edu

R. P. Thom, C. J. McDougle (eds.), *Neuropsychiatric Care for Genetic Syndromes and Other Neurodevelopmental Disorders*,
https://doi.org/10.1007/978-3-031-76269-7_2

has evolved, the defining features of ID have not changed dramatically over the past several decades. However, one relatively new change to the diagnostic criteria involves the broadening of our conceptualization of the developmental period, which is now defined operationally as before the age of 22 years [2]. Intellectual disability is further classified by the level of severity (mild, moderate, severe, and profound) based on an individual's adaptive functioning. Historically, this had been based on intelligence quotient (IQ) scores; however, increasing recognition of the importance of identifying the level of support an individual may need and a shift toward a social-ecological model of disability have resulted in severity being defined by limitations in adaptive functioning rather than IQ [3].

Intellectual disability is often caused by a combination of various environmental and genetic factors, with most occurring during the prenatal period [4]. It can be caused by external factors such as infections, extreme malnutrition, maternal alcohol use during pregnancy, and birth complications [5]. The clinical severity of ID is broadly correlated with the presence of an identifiable causal factor, such as chromosomal imbalances and catastrophic events (e.g., perinatal asphyxia, prenatal infections, and vascular accidents) [4, 6]. While individuals with moderate to profound ID are much more likely to have an identified genetic or chromosomal abnormality, the causes of mild ID are often unknown [7, 8]. Roughly 50% of individuals with mild ID have no identifiable pre-, peri-, or postnatal cause [8]. Dominantly acting rare de novo mutations are a major cause of severe ID [5], while more complex forms of inheritance are thought to underlie milder forms of ID. There is also a strong correlation between the number of genes affected and the severity of ID.

2.1.1 Genetics of ID

Historically, it has been clinically useful to differentiate two classes of intellectual disability: syndromic and non-syndromic. Syndromic ID is when intellectual deficits are associated with a recognizable pattern of other medical comorbidities and behavioral signs (e.g., involvement of other organs and specific malformations) [4, 9] such as Down syndrome (DS) and Fragile X syndrome (FXS). Non-syndromic ID is commonly used when ID is the only feature observed in the individual. Yet, as we continue to advance our abilities to study the genetics of ID, the distinction between syndromic and non-syndromic ID has become less clear. With several forms of syndromic ID, it has been possible and useful to identify a "major gene" resulting in a specific syndromic presentation (e.g., DS, Rett syndrome, and FXS). However, this "major gene" approach to understanding the underlying genetics of ID does not appear to be an appropriate model for understanding the majority of individuals with low cognitive performance. While many single-gene causes have been identified over the past several decades, there are likely genetic modifiers, multigene involvement, or environmental factors involved that contribute to ID [10].

Cytogenetically visible chromosomal mutations can be detected in one out of seven individuals with severe cognitive impairment, with DS being the most common [6]. As new technologies advance our ability to screen for DNA copy number variations (CNVs), we are now capable of detecting small genomic regions with deletions, insertions, and duplications of segments of DNA. After the recent introduction of high-resolution array comparative genomic hybridization (CGH), it has become apparent that CNVs are an equally important cause of ID. In early research referenced by Ropers, a large cohort of individuals with "idiopathic ID," almost 15% of the sample, was found to have causative de novo deletions or duplications ranging in size between 100 kb and several megabases [6]. Numerous CNVs have recently been discovered and associated with ID and have significantly expanded the number of known microdeletion/duplication disorders [6] that previously were thought of as non-syndromic. Array CGH has also been key in revealing the functional defect causing ID in several disorders such as Pitt-Hopkins and Peters plus syndrome.

There have been several different approaches developed to study the molecular genetics of ID. Quantitative trait locus (QTL) analysis is a statistical method that links genotypic data (usually, molecular markers) with phenotypic data (e.g., ID). The goal of QTL analysis is to identify genes that predict a degree of variance in intelligence (i.e., not a single gene). These studies have largely used a "candidate gene" approach, in which prospective DNA markers are chosen based on a priori criteria [8]. This has resulted in some evidence for three classes of candidate genes: those related to synaptic transmission, brain development (e.g., cathepsin D, muscle segment homeobox 1, succinate-semialdehyde dehydrogenase, and β-synthase), and inflammatory mechanisms (e.g., insulin-like growth factor II receptor and histocompatibility complex, class II, DRβ1) [8]. In sum, it is possible and useful to identify genes associated with both syndromic and non-syndromic forms of ID as they lead to emerging avenues of research for diagnosis and treatment. However, for the majority of individuals with ID, the "major gene" approach does not emerge as an appropriate model [8].

2.2 Signs and Symptoms of Common Psychiatric Comorbidities

Historically, there was a long-held false belief that those with ID were cognitively incapable of experiencing mental illness and, therefore, protected from psychological stress. In reality, co-occurring mental health disorders are common among individuals with ID and often occur at rates higher than in the general population. A recent meta-analysis of 22 studies assessing prevalence rates of co-occurring psychiatric disorders revealed that more than a third of people with an ID meet diagnostic criteria for a co-occurring psychiatric disorder (excluding autism) [11]. Further empirical evidence has demonstrated that behavioral and psychiatric problems occur in individuals with ID at rates three to six times higher than in the general population [12]. Yet, one large factor often contributing to the under-recognition of psychiatric disorders is the challenge in applying standard diagnostic criteria, as many rely on an individual's ability to describe their internal experience in a way that may exceed the language abilities of an individual with ID. Many internalizing disorders (e.g., anxiety and depression) require a minimal level of cognitive and communicative ability to articulate and describe symptoms. As such, individuals with ID experiencing mood and/or anxiety disorders are more likely to be diagnosed with an unspecified comorbidity, reflective of this diagnostic challenge [13]. Considering the language deficits present for some individuals with ID, symptoms may need to be described by caregivers, such as an observed change from usual behavior. Further, atypical clinical presentations of psychopathology are more likely with more severe ID.

Identifying mood disorders is an important but considerable challenge, as they are not uncommon in this population. Modification of the diagnostic criteria to include more objective data is recommended. Several modified criteria have been put forth; however, all have methodological flaws [14]. Individuals with mild ID present with a fairly typical clinical presentation, which may include suicidal thoughts, and can be assessed using standard practices with only minor accommodations [15]. Depressed individuals with more severe ID have been found to exhibit symptoms such as decreased mood, crying, irritability, marked aggression, agitation, regressed behavior, stereotypies, somatic complaints, neurovegetative signs, reduced ability to think or concentrate, hypochondriacal preoccupation, and disturbed sleep patterns [14, 16]. Aggression and other behavioral problems may be symptoms of depression in individuals with more severe ID [15]. This finding supports the substitution of behavioral criteria; however, this idea remains controversial [14, 15] as some of these symptoms may be nonspecific to depression. In particular, less specific symptoms, such as irritability, could reflect several underlying nonpsychiatric causes including pain, sleep apnea, or gastroesophageal reflux disease in the context of low functional communication skills [16]. Symptoms should be assessed through both individual- and informant-reports. Yet, there are few modified informant-report questionnaires (e.g., Glasgow Depression Scale and Comprehensive Psychopathology Rating Scale) adapted for individuals with ID.

With anxiety disorders, individuals with ID may present with avoidant behaviors (particularly when they reflect a change), vague somatic complaints, sleep disorders, episodic outbursts, irritability, and brooding [17]. Additional symptoms may include agitation, screaming, crying, withdrawal, regressive/clingy behavior, or freezing [17]. Obsessional thinking and rumination may present as a repetition of the same ideas in speech. Compulsions, different from repetitive behaviors and stereotypes often observed in the ID population, more often consist of excessive rearranging, washing, and hoarding [17]. Further, numerous physical signs of anxiety including difficulty swallowing, dry mouth, flushing, sweating, palpitations, tremors, headache, pallor, fatigue, hyperventilation, muscle tension, diarrhea, increased urinary frequency, paresthesia, and insomnia may be observed [17].

Psychosis has further been shown to affect individuals with ID at rates thought to be slightly higher than the general population, with a three- to five-fold increased prevalence [18, 19]. Individuals with mild ID are likely able to discuss their symptoms although discussing a timeline or complicated sequence of events (e.g., past medication trials) may be a challenge. When differentiating psychotic symptoms from other nonpsychotic symptoms or problem behaviors, problem behaviors often have an associated benefit (e.g., attention or reaction from caregivers or peers and avoidance of something unpleasant) and follow a pattern, even if difficult to determine. In contrast, psychotic symptoms appear more arbitrarily, are internally driven, and are associated with clear changes from baseline behaviors [19]. Further, symptoms of psychosis tend to develop in late adolescence or adulthood, whereas other behaviors (e.g., stereotypies) that can be observed in ID emerge earlier during the developmental period.

2.3 Assessment

Identifying ID requires a careful assessment of intellectual functioning, adaptive behavior, and a developmental history. Individuals must present with significant limitations in intellectual and adaptive functioning, which have been defined as approximately two or more standard deviations below the mean on standardized measures of intellectual and adaptive functioning [2, 20]. Assessment must also establish that these limitations have been present during the developmental period, which has been defined by AAIDD, as before the age of 22 years [2]. Importantly, although significant impairments in intellectual functioning and adaptive behavior are often correlated, one is not causative of the other, and these two domains must be weighed equally when evaluating for ID [17]. Further, adaptive functioning, and not intellectual functioning, informs the severity level of ID, which can be specified as mild, moderate, severe, or profound. Individuals with mild ID may have some age-appropriate functioning while other skills are behind age-based expectations, such as requiring more support and practice to learn age-appropriate academic skills and demonstrating reduced social awareness, perception, or judgment (e.g., gullibility). Individuals with moderate ID typically exhibit markedly slow and more limited development of academic skills and more significant challenges with social decision-making and interactions with same-aged peers and generally require more teaching and support than individuals with mild ID to develop daily living skills. Individuals with severe ID present with limited conceptual skill development and more challenges with speech and communication than individuals with moderate ID (e.g., communicating with spoken single words or phrases and utilizing augmentative and alternative communication) and require support across all areas of daily living. Finally, individuals with profound ID generally have very limited functional communication and understanding of symbolic processes and communication and require support for all aspects of adaptive functioning, including safety and activities of daily living.

Neuropsychological evaluation, or comprehensive testing that utilizes both standardized tools and clinical assessment to evaluate individuals' core intellectual functioning, language skills, visual-spatial processing, learning and memory, and other relevant domains of functioning (e.g., behavioral functioning and internalizing problems), is the most valid and reliable approach to measuring core features of ID [21]. Instead of relying on a single measurement tool or cut point (e.g., IQ cut point), which is vulnerable to measurement error, floor effects, and threats to validity (e.g., lack of measurement invariance) [22], neuropsychological evaluation provides a comprehensive cognitive and adaptive profile that not only informs diagnosis but can also inform a profile of intervention supports. Sources of measurement error, respondent reliability, and treatment history must be considered when interpreting assessment results [2, 20] and, thus, multiple convergent data sources are critical. Providers must take a strengths-based, culturally competent, and ecological approach to neuropsychological testing that considers and values individuals' strengths and cultural, linguistic, and environmental context [23–25]. In addition to neuropsychological testing, evaluating underlying genetic contributions can provide clarity about ID subtypes and inform prognosis, common co-occurring conditions, treatment, and heritability [4, 5]. First-line genetic testing includes chromosomal microarray and specific testing for FXS [26].

Neuropsychological evaluations and genetic testing can be time- and resource-intensive for individuals, families, and systems [27] and can introduce significant service disparities [25, 28]. Pediatricians and primary care physicians serve as initial points of contact with the medical system during children's developmental period and are, therefore, well positioned to serve as first-tier identifiers of ID in their patients [29]. Though providers often screen for broader global developmental delay using tools such as the Ages and Stages Questionnaire (ASQ-III), identification of ID requires specific screening tools [30]. Indeed, emerging research supports the psychometric properties of brief screening tools for ID in clinical and community settings such as the Child and Adolescent Intellectual Disability Screening Questionnaire (CAIDS-Q), which is a brief (approximate administration time of five minutes), seven-item scale for children and adolescents that is completed by someone who knows the child well or with the child directly [29]. A tiered approach to ID assessment and diagnosis may include routine screening through pediatricians with positive screens referred for follow-up neuropsychological evaluation and genetic testing.

2.4 Psychosocial Support

Psychosocial support for individuals with ID can be effective for targeting core challenges and promoting quality of life, safety, and independence. Support needs are highly variable and specific treatment goals should be determined by the individual and their family, incorporating their values and priorities, as well as addressing any safety concerns (e.g., self-injurious behavior). Common treatment priorities include building functional communication skills to ensure that individuals are able to communicate their needs and increasing daily living skills, such as hygiene and leisure skills. It is critical that interventions are person-centered, culturally responsive, strengths-based, and minimally restrictive, prioritize relationship building between individuals, providers, and caregivers, and focus on prevention and positive responses rather than punishment procedures [31, 32].

Individuals with ID require individualized supports that include significant repetition and more opportunities to respond and receive feedback across settings and people [33]. Direct, systematic, and explicit instructions paired with visual aids, such as visual schedules and video models, can be effective for teaching new skills in deficit areas [27–30]. Interventions based on principles of behavioral learning (i.e., behavior analytic approaches), including positive reinforcement with tangible rewards, are supported as established methods for improving communication, adaptive, and pre-academic skills among young children with ID and have emerging evidence for improving academic outcomes [34–36]. Communication and adaptive skill building can also be paired with behavior analytic approaches for treating any significant unsafe behavior, such as aggression or self-injurious behavior [37, 38]. In addition to child-focused supports, caregiver training that helps caregivers develop responsive and warm parenting skills, provides psychoeducation about ID over the lifespan, and promotes caregiver wellbeing and stress management (e.g., mindfulness-based strategies) are essential intervention components for individuals with ID [32, 39].

In adults with ID, there is limited research assessing the effectiveness of psychosocial interventions in an outpatient setting. A single randomized controlled trial (RCT) has also found support for behavioral interventions (applied behavioral analysis and positive behavioral supports) for treating challenging behaviors in adults [40]. In general, the broader framework of cognitive behavioral therapy (CBT) and other treatment regimens also applies to adults with ID; however, treatment may need to be broken down into smaller goals (e.g., working on a single skill) in each session. Providers should interact directly with the adults with ID as much as possible rather than talking to family or caregivers; it will take longer to gather information, but it is important to make sure that patients experience buy-in and are engaging with what is going on from their perspective. Goal-setting should also be a routine part of therapy for adults with ID, as adults with ID do not always have the same opportunities to be involved in identifying and expressing their desires. Ultimately, the goals themselves may not vary significantly from adults without ID, including pursuing a healthy life, developing social and romantic relationships, and finding an enjoyable job, but they may face greater barriers and can be supported by family and providers if understood.

Beyond skill building across functional domains, it is imperative that psychosocial supports address emotion regulation and coping strategies, given the significant risk for co-occurring mental health challenges faced by individuals with ID [31]. Established mental health and social and emotional interventions that have been modified to address the cognitive and behavioral needs of individuals with ID show promise [41, 42]. Adaptations to traditional CBT for individuals with ID have demonstrated social validity and have emerging evidence for treating anxiety, anger, and depression among individuals with ID [41, 43]. Modified dialectical behavior therapy (DBT) that incorporates more social skill and behavioral support (e.g., tangible rewards for adaptive behaviors), paired with cognitive modification as needed, has also demonstrated promise for promoting positive outcomes among individuals with ID [42]. Hronis and colleagues (2017) provide specific recommendations for therapy adaptations based on cognitive challenges in attention (e.g., shorter and more frequent sessions), working memory (e.g., using short and simple sentences paired with visual aids), learning and memory (e.g., practice and repetition, involving caregivers), executive functioning (e.g., consistent schedule), and language and reading (e.g., visual aids) that should be considered when adapting existing evidence-based practices for individuals with ID [44]. Importantly, considering that individuals with ID are at a greater risk for sexual abuse, sexually transmitted diseases (STDs), and misinformation due to inadequate sexual education, these individualized cognitive, behavioral, and social modifications and learning supports should also be applied to sexuality interventions [45].

2.5 Biological Treatments

With regard to pharmacological treatment, current best practice guidelines advocate for a "start low and go slow" approach [46]. Further recommendations also suggest ensuring that medications have been tried for an adequate duration of time before deeming failure of a medication, outcomes should be monitored across settings, and only one medication should be changed at a time [47]. However, given the paucity of scientific evidence around treatment modifications for individuals with ID, these recommendations are based on expert consensus rather than RCTs.

In children and adolescents with ID, there is minimal data to guide the selection and use of psychotropic medications [26, 48]. Medications are typically prescribed to treat symptoms (e.g., sleep disturbances, anxiety, and disruptive behaviors) after a provider examines the underlying cause of symptoms, including medical issues, and the risk-benefit of drug use for each particular case and context [49]. Antipsychotic medications, in particular, are often prescribed off-label for youth with ID to address challenging behavior [50–52]. This practice is derived from the US Food and Drug Administration (FDA) approval of risperidone and aripiprazole for the treatment of irritability in youth with ASD [26]. However, there are limited high-quality studies examining short-term outcomes and minimal evidence of long-term effectiveness for the use of antipsychotics to treat challenging behavior among youth with ID [48]. Similar to children without ID, antipsychotic medications can be associated with side effects including weight gain, sedation, metabolic problems, and tardive dyskinesia [48, 53]. Given the limited evidence on the relative risks and benefits of the use of psychotropic medication in youth with ID, it is imperative that evidence-based psychosocial supports and environmental modifications be considered first-line interventions.

Psychopharmacological treatment for the management of behavioral problems and co-occurring psychiatric conditions in adults with ID has also become relatively common. Behavioral problems are thought of as socially unacceptable behaviors that result in distress, harm, or disadvantage to themselves or others such that intervention is required; it is the most prevalent and common indication for pharmacological treatment in individuals with ID [54]. To effectively treat behavioral problems, providers should first try to identify the underlying cause (e.g., medical, psychiatric, environmental, developmental, and skill deficits) and treat these accordingly. When the underlying etiology cannot be established, the treatment goal should be to minimize the disruption that the behavior causes to the individual. Psychopharmacologic medications used for adults with ID include antipsychotics, antidepressants, anxiolytics, mood stabilizers, and psychostimulants [55]. To date, the preponderance of medications prescribed to individuals with ID are antipsychotic medications [54]. These drugs appear to most consistently reduce symptoms of self-injury, aggression, agitation, and repetitive behaviors, with some studies reporting increased social awareness and improved sleep hygiene [56]. Limited data have also shown selective serotonin reuptake inhibitors (SSRIs) to be effective, at times, in the treatment of challenging behaviors such as aggression, self-injurious behavior, and destruction. However, overall these results are less promising and reflect smaller, noncontrolled studies [14, 57]. Importantly, psychotropic drug use among individuals with ID and challenging behavior may cause side effects, which can, in turn, negatively impact quality of life [58]. While a paucity of research exists examining the safety and efficacy of psychotropic medications in individuals with ID, these individuals may be more likely to experience side effects with standard doses of medication and may be less likely to experience therapeutic benefit [17].

While individuals with ID are at high risk for experiencing mood disorders and there is limited research on treatment, antidepressant medications are thought to be underutilized [54]. Case report-level evidence generally demonstrates that antidepressants are effective in this population. This has been further supported by a more recent retrospective study assessing the effectiveness, tolerability, and safety of SSRIs in a subset of individuals with syndromic ID (i.e., DS) [59]. Expert consensus recommends SSRIs as the first-line treatment for major depressive disorder, suicidal ideation/behavior, post traumatic stress disorder, obsessive-compulsive disorder, and other anxiety that do not meet the criteria for a DSM-5 disorder in individuals with ID, although up to 20% of individuals may experience adverse side effects [14].

2.6 Common Medical Comorbidities

Individuals with ID have higher rates of certain medical conditions and are also at elevated risk for health problems associated with inactivity [60]. In children, common medical comorbidities may be related to the underlying syndromic condition. For example, individuals with DS are susceptible to a myriad of medical conditions affecting nearly every organ system, particularly endocrine disorders, congenital heart conditions, joint and muscle disorders, and gastrointestinal disorders. Over half of all children with DS have visual impairment and/or some type of hearing loss [12]. For individuals with FXS, seizure disorders affect roughly 20% of the population and higher rates of endocrine disorders, scoliosis, joint laxity, and flat feet have been observed [12]. In general, children with ID have shown higher rates of congenital diseases, familial disorders, and acquired disorders during childhood [61] that to some degree likely reflect the genetics of some syndromic conditions. Further, pain and sleep disturbances, often the result of other underlying medical conditions, are associated with poorer quality of life in children with ID [62].

Adults with ID are at greater risk of having chronic diseases including cardiovascular and metabolic conditions compared to age-matched peers, regardless of psychiatric comorbidity [12]. Several studies have found higher rates of diabetes, obesity, high blood pressure, and hyperlipidemia [60]. There are also higher prevalence rates of dementia, seizure disorders, chronic obstructive pulmonary disease, congestive heart failure, osteoporosis, and transient ischemic attacks in individuals with ID [63]. Further, research suggests that around midlife (i.e., ~50 years), individuals with ID had higher rates of multiple comorbidities compared to those without ID [64]. Despite this, research suggests that clinicians are less likely to recommend preventive or maintenance medical care for individuals with ID, leading to undiagnosed and undertreated medical conditions and, in turn, to increased morbidity and mortality associated with cardiovascular and metabolic disorders [60]. Atypical presentation of symptoms (e.g., head banging), combined with communication and behavioral challenges often observed in more severe forms of ID, can also lead to inferior care.

These medical comorbidities, severity of cognitive deficits, and increased need for community support are associated with a reduced lifespan [65]. While better care and services have led to individuals with ID living longer lives, longevity is still reduced compared to the general population. When stratified by severity of ID, those with only mild ID and minimal need for community support seem to demonstrate life expectancies more commensurate with the general population [66, 67]. Individuals with profound ID have a reduced life expectancy, with few individuals reaching old age; this is thought to reflect associated severe neurological deficits and linked disorders [66]. Individuals with moderate and severe ID demonstrate reduced life expectancies for similar reasons [66]. Thus, life expectancy appears to diminish as the severity of ID increases.

There are few specific guidelines in the literature to help practitioners care for individuals with ID. To support both professionals and families in providing more targeted healthcare tailored to the needs of individuals with ID, the Center for Developmental Disabilities Evaluation and Research (CDDER), part of the AAIDD, developed preventive health screening guidelines for adults with ID [68]. These guidelines discuss commonly underrecognized health conditions in individuals with ID, such as gastrointestinal issues, oral disease, vision concerns, chronic recurrent infections, and respiratory disease, as well as a modified timeline for recommended preventative screenings.

Key Points to Remember

- ID is defined by cognitive and adaptive deficits that develop during the developmental period.
- ID and its severity are no longer defined by an IQ number but, more importantly, by the adaptive deficits and the resulting areas of support an individual may need.
- Individuals with ID demonstrate higher rates of psychiatric comorbidities than the general population but may go undiagnosed or untreated for longer periods of time due to diagnostic challenges and health disparities.

- Individuals with ID and psychiatric comorbidities may present differently with more behavioral symptoms, particularly as the severity of ID increases.
- Psychosocial interventions should be considered first-line treatments in addressing behavioral and psychological problems.
- Individuals with ID tend to experience side effects with standard doses of psychotropic medication and show a worse response to psychotherapeutic and psychopharmacological treatment.

References

1. Anderson LL, Larson SA, MapelLentz S, Hall-Lande J. A systematic review of U.S. studies on the prevalence of intellectual or developmental disabilities since 2000. Intellect Dev Disabil. 2019;57(5):421–38.
2. Schalock RL, Luckasson R, Tassé MJ, editors. Intellectual disability: definition, diagnosis, classification, and systems of support. 12th ed. American Association of Intellectual and Developmental Disabilities; 2021.
3. Association AP. Diagnostic and statistical manual of mental disorders, text revision Dsm-5-tr. 5th ed. Washington, DC: Amer Psychiatric Pub Inc.; 2022. p. 1142.
4. Chiurazzi P, Pirozzi F. Advances in understanding—genetic basis of intellectual disability. F1000Research. 2016;5. F1000 Faculty Rev-599.
5. Vissers LELM, Gilissen C, Veltman JA. Genetic studies in intellectual disability and related disorders. Nat Rev Genet. 2016;17(1):9–18.
6. Ropers HH. Genetics of intellectual disability. Curr Opin Genet Dev. 2008;18(3):241–50.
7. Hodapp RM, Dykens EM. Mental retardation. In: Child psychopathology. New York, NY: The Guilford Press; 1996. p. 362–89.
8. Iarocci G, Petrill SA. Behavioral genetics, genomics, intelligence, and mental retardation. In: Burack JA, Hodapp RM, Iarocci G, Zigler E, editors. The Oxford handbook of intellectual disability and development. Oxford University Press; 2011. https://doi.org/10.1093/oxfordhb/9780195305012.013.0002. [cited 2023 Feb 11].
9. Hill WD, Davies G, Liewald DC, Payton A, McNeil CJ, Whalley LJ, et al. Examining non-syndromic autosomal recessive intellectual disability (NS-ARID) genes for an enriched association with intelligence differences. Intelligence. 2016;54:80–9.
10. Kaufman L, Ayub M, Vincent JB. The genetic basis of non-syndromic intellectual disability: a review. J Neurodev Disord. 2010;2(4):182–209.
11. Mazza MG, Rossetti A, Crespi G, Clerici M. Prevalence of co-occurring psychiatric disorders in adults and adolescents with intellectual disability: a systematic review and meta-analysis. J Appl Res Intellect Disabil. 2020;33(2):126–38.
12. Gentile JP, Gillig PM. Psychiatry of intellectual disability: a practical manual. Oxford, Hoboken, NJ: Wiley-Blackwell; 2012. p. 394.
13. El Mrayyan N, Eberhard J, Ahlstrom G. The occurrence of comorbidities with affective and anxiety disorders among older people with intellectual disability compared with the general population: a register study. BMC Psychiatry. 2019;19(1):166.
14. Janowsky DS, Davis JM. Diagnosis and treatment of depression in patients with mental retardation. Curr Psychiatry Rep. 2005;7(6):421–8.
15. Hurley AD. Mood disorders in intellectual disability. Curr Opin Psychiatry. 2006;19(5):465.
16. Morrison AK, Weston C. Mood disorders. In: Psychiatry of intellectual disability. John Wiley & Sons, Ltd.; 2012. p. 125–45. https://doi.org/10.1002/9781119945925.ch7. [cited 2023 Mar 23].

17. Blankenship KM. Anxiety disorders. In: Psychiatry of intellectual disability. John Wiley & Sons, Ltd; 2012. p. 146–60. https://doi.org/10.1002/9781119945925.ch8. [cited 2023 Mar 24].
18. Cooper SA, Smiley E, Morrison J, Allan L, Williamson A, Finlayson J, et al. Psychosis and adults with intellectual disabilities. Soc Psychiatry Psychiatr Epidemiol. 2007;42(7):530–6.
19. Cowan A. Psychotic disorders. In: Psychotic disorders. John Wiley & Sons, Ltd; 2012. p. 161–90. https://doi.org/10.1002/9781119945925.ch9. [cited 2023 Apr 14].
20. Tassé MJ, Luckasson R, Schalock RL. The relation between intellectual functioning and adaptive behavior in the diagnosis of intellectual disability. Intellect Dev Disabil. 2016;54(6):381–90.
21. Greenspan S, Woods GW. Intellectual disability as a disorder of reasoning and judgement: the gradual move away from intelligence quotient-ceilings. Curr Opin Psychiatry. 2014;27(2):110.
22. Wicherts JM. The importance of measurement invariance in neurocognitive ability testing. Clin Neuropsychol. 2016;30(7):1006–16.
23. Byrd DA, Rivera Mindt MM, Clark US, Clarke Y, Thames AD, Gammada EZ, et al. Creating an antiracist psychology by addressing professional complicity in psychological assessment. Psychol Assess. 2021;33:279–85.
24. D'Amato RC, Crepeau-Hobson F, Huang LV, Geil M. Ecological neuropsychology: an alternative to the deficit model for conceptualizing and serving students with learning disabilities. Neuropsychol Rev. 2005;15(2):97–103.
25. Rivera Mindt M, Byrd D, Saez P, Manly J. Increasing culturally competent neuropsychological services for ethnic minority populations: a call to action. Clin Neuropsychol. 2010;24(3):429–53.
26. Siegel M, McGuire K, Veenstra-VanderWeele J, Stratigos K, King B, Bellonci C, et al. Practice Parameter for the assessment and treatment of psychiatric disorders in children and adolescents with intellectual disability (intellectual developmental disorder). J Am Acad Child Adolesc Psychiatry. 2020;59(4):468–96.
27. Ryan JJ, Glass LA, Brown CN. Administration time estimates for Wechsler Intelligence Scale for Children-IV subtests, composites, and short forms. J Clin Psychol. 2007;63(4):309–18.
28. Suther S, Kiros GE. Barriers to the use of genetic testing: a study of racial and ethnic disparities. Genet Med. 2009;11(9):655–62.
29. McKenzie K, Murray G, Murray A, Delahunty L, Hutton L, Murray K, et al. Child and adolescent intellectual disability screening questionnaire to identify children with intellectual disability. Dev Med Child Neurol. 2019;61(4):444–50.
30. Riou EM, Ghosh S, Francoeur E, Shevell MI. Global developmental delay and its relationship to cognitive skills. Dev Med Child Neurol. 2009;51(8):600–6.
31. Griffith GM, Hutchinson L, Hastings RP. "I'm not a patient, I'm a person": the experiences of individuals with intellectual disabilities and challenging behavior—a thematic synthesis of qualitative studies. Clin Psychol Sci Pract. 2013;20:469–88.
32. Man J, Kangas M. Best practice principles when working with individuals with intellectual disability and comorbid mental health concerns. Qual Health Res. 2020;30(4):560–71.
33. Courtade GR, Test DW, Cook BG. Evidence-based practices for learners with severe intellectual disability. Res Pract Pers Sev Disabil. 2014;39(4):305–18.
34. Adibsereshki N, Abkenar SJ, Ashoori M, Mirzamani M. The effectiveness of using reinforcements in the classroom on the academic achievement of students with intellectual disabilities. J Intellect Disabil. 2015;19(1):83–93.
35. Eldevik S, Jahr E, Eikeseth S, Hastings RP, Hughes CJ. Cognitive and adaptive behavior outcomes of behavioral intervention for young children with intellectual disability. Behav Modif. 2010;34(1):16–34.
36. Ho H, Perry A, Koudys J. A systematic review of behaviour analytic interventions for young children with intellectual disabilities. J Intellect Disabil Res. 2021;65(1):11–31.
37. Didden R, Korzilius H, van Oorsouw W, Sturmey P. Behavioral treatment of challenging behaviors in individuals with mild mental retardation: meta-analysis of single-subject research. Bodfish J, editor. Am J Ment Retard. 2006;111(4):290–8.

38. Heyvaert M, Saenen L, Campbell JM, Maes B, Onghena P. Efficacy of behavioral interventions for reducing problem behavior in persons with autism: an updated quantitative synthesis of single-subject research. Res Dev Disabil. 2014;35(10):2463–76.
39. Crnic KA, Neece CL, McIntyre LL, Blacher J, Baker BL. Intellectual disability and developmental risk: promoting intervention to improve child and family well-being. Child Dev. 2017;88(2):436–45.
40. Hassiotis A, Robotham D, Canagasabey A, Romeo R, Langridge D, Blizard R, et al. Randomized, single-blind, controlled trial of a specialist behavior therapy team for challenging behavior in adults with intellectual disabilities. Am J Psychiatry. 2009;166(11):1278–85.
41. Blakeley-Smith A, Meyer AT, Boles RE, Reaven J. Group cognitive behavioural treatment for anxiety in autistic adolescents with intellectual disability: a pilot and feasibility study. J Appl Res Intellect Disabil. 2021;34(3):777–88.
42. Brown JF, Brown MZ, Dibiasio P. Treating individuals with intellectual disabilities and challenging behaviors with adapted dialectical behavior therapy. J Ment Health Res Intellect Disabil. 2013;6(4):280–303.
43. Vereenooghe L, Langdon PE. Psychological therapies for people with intellectual disabilities: a systematic review and meta-analysis. Res Dev Disabil. 2013;34(11):4085–102.
44. Hronis A, Roberts R, Roberts L, Kneebone I. Cognitive behavioural therapy for children and adolescents with intellectual disability and anxiety: a therapist manual. Discov Psychol. 2022;2(1):24.
45. McDaniels B, Fleming A. Sexuality education and intellectual disability: time to address the challenge. Sex Disabil. 2016;34(2):215–25.
46. Sullivan WF, Berg JM, Bradley E, Cheetham T, Denton R, Heng J, et al. Primary care of adults with developmental disabilities: Canadian consensus guidelines. Can Fam Physician. 2011;57(5):541–53.
47. Kishore MT, Udipi GA, Seshadri SP. Clinical Practice Guidelines for Assessment and Management of intellectual disability. Indian J Psychiatry. 2019;61(Suppl. 2):194–210.
48. McQuire C, Hassiotis A, Harrison B, Pilling S. Pharmacological interventions for challenging behaviour in children with intellectual disabilities: a systematic review and meta-analysis. BMC Psychiatry. 2015;15(1):303.
49. Molina-Ruiz RM, Martín-Carballeda J, Asensio-Moreno I, Montañés-Rada F. A guide to psychopharmacological treatment of patients with intellectual disability in psychiatry. Int J Psychiatry Med. 2017;52(2):176–89.
50. Haw C, Stubbs J. A survey of off-label prescribing for inpatients with mild intellectual disability and mental illness. J Intellect Disabil Res. 2005;49(11):858–64.
51. Olfson M, Crystal S, Huang C, Gerhard T. Trends in antipsychotic drug use by very young, privately insured children. J Am Acad Child Adolesc Psychiatry. 2010;49(1):13–23.
52. Tsiouris JA. Pharmacotherapy for aggressive behaviours in persons with intellectual disabilities: treatment or mistreatment? J Intellect Disabil Res. 2010;54(1):1–16.
53. Iasevoli F, Barone A, Buonaguro EF, Vellucci L, de Bartolomeis A. Safety and tolerability of antipsychotic agents in neurodevelopmental disorders: a systematic review. Expert Opin Drug Saf. 2020;19(11):1419–44.
54. Manetta CT, Gentile JP. Psychotropic medications. In: Psychiatry of intellectual disability. John Wiley & Sons, Ltd; 2012. p. 250–77. https://doi.org/10.1002/9781119945925.ch12.
55. Deb S, Kwok H, Bertelli M, Salvador-Carulla L, Bradley E, Torr J, et al. International guide to prescribing psychotropic medication for the management of problem behaviours in adults with intellectual disabilities. World Psychiatry. 2009;8(3):181–6.
56. Aman MG, Madrid A. Atypical antipsychotics in persons with developmental disabilities. Ment Retard Dev Disabil Res Rev. 1999;5(4):253–63.
57. Janowsky DS, Shetty M, Barnhill J, Elamir B, Davis JM. Serotonergic antidepressant effects on aggressive, self-injurious and destructive/disruptive behaviours in intellectually disabled adults: a retrospective, open-label, naturalistic trial. Int J Neuropsychopharmacol. 2005;8(1):37–48.

58. Scheifes A, Walraven S, Stolker JJ, Nijman HLI, Egberts TCG, Heerdink ER. Adverse events and the relation with quality of life in adults with intellectual disability and challenging behaviour using psychotropic drugs. Res Dev Disabil. 2016;49–50:13–21.
59. Thom RP, Palumbo ML, Thompson C, McDougle CJ, Ravichandran CT. Selective serotonin reuptake inhibitors for the treatment of depression in adults with down syndrome: a preliminary retrospective chart review study. Brain Sci. 2021;11(9):1216.
60. Stanish HI, Temple VA, Frey GC. Health-promoting physical activity of adults with mental retardation. Ment Retard Dev Disabil Res Rev. 2006;12(1):13–21.
61. Markovic-Jovanovic SR, Milovanovic JD, Jovanovic AN, Zivkovic JB, Balovic AD, Nickovic V, et al. Comorbidities in children with intellectual disabilities. Birth Defects Res. 2020;112(1):54–61.
62. Reddihough D, Leonard H, Jacoby P, Kim R, Epstein A, Murphy N, et al. Comorbidities and quality of life in children with intellectual disability. Child Care Health Dev. 2021;47(5):654–66.
63. McDermott S, Moran R, Platt T, Dasari S. Variation in health conditions among groups of adults with disabilities in primary care. J Community Health. 2006;31(3):147–59.
64. van den Bemd M, Schalk B, Bischoff E, Cuypers M, Leusink GL. Chronic disease prevalence and patterns of comorbidities in people with intellectual disabilities. Eur J Pub Health. 2021;31(Suppl. 3).
65. Chaney RH, Eyman RK. Patterns of mortality over 60 years among persons with mental retardation in a residential facility. Ment Retard. 2000;38(3):289–93.
66. Patja K, Iivanainen M, Vesala H, Oksanen H, Ruoppila I. Life expectancy of people with intellectual disability: a 35-year follow-up study. J Intellect Disabil Res. 2000;44(5):591–9.
67. Sutherland G, Couch MA, Iacono T. Health issues for adults with developmental disability. Res Dev Disabil. 2002;23(6):422–45.
68. Preventative Health recommendations for adults with intellectual disability [Brochure]. Massachusetts Department of Developmental Services; 2019.

Further Reading

Gentile JP, Gillig PM. Psychiatry of intellectual disability: a practical manual. Wiley-Blackwell. 2012.

Massachusetts Department of Developmental Services. Preventive health recommendations for adults with intellectual disability: guidelines for community practitioners; 2019.

Schalock RL, Luckasson R, Tasse MJ. An overview of intellectual disability: definition, diagnosis, classification, and systems of supports (12th ed.). Am J Intellect Dev Disabil. 2021;126(6):439–42. https://doi.org/10.1352/1944-7558-126.6.439.

World Psychiatry Association. Clinical Bulletin of the Developmental Disabilities Division. International guide to prescribing psychotropic medication for the management of problem behaviours in adults with intellectual disabilities; 2010.

3 Williams Syndrome

Ana Fish, Barbara R. Pober, and Robyn P. Thom

3.1 Overview

Williams syndrome (WS, also known as Williams–Beuren syndrome) is a relatively rare, multisystem neurodevelopmental disorder. Individuals with WS are at risk for a broad array of medical and psychiatric problems, accompanied by mild-to-moderate intellectual disability (ID).

The earliest reports of WS were published in the 1960s. They focused on children and emphasized the presence of cardiovascular disease, a distinct facial appearance, cognitive disability, and an over-friendly personality [1, 2]. Since then, much has been learned about the medical and psychiatric features of WS across the lifespan, as well as the underlying genetic mechanism.

3.1.1 Epidemiology

Williams syndrome is a pan-ethnic disorder without gender or racial predilection and occurs worldwide. Only a single systematic study estimates the prevalence of WS; it indicates a WS prevalence of 1 in 7500 births [3].

Parents and providers often inquire about life expectancy, but to date, no study on this topic exists. Sudden death mortality due to the cardiovascular problems of WS is reported to be 25–100 fold higher than comparably aged individuals in the

A. Fish
Cambridge Health Alliance, Cambridge, MA, USA

B. R. Pober
Massachusetts General Hospital, Boston, MA, USA

R. P. Thom (✉)
Lurie Center for Autism, Lexington, MA, USA
e-mail: RTHOM@MGH.HARVARD.EDU

R. P. Thom, C. J. McDougle (eds.), *Neuropsychiatric Care for Genetic Syndromes and Other Neurodevelopmental Disorders*,
https://doi.org/10.1007/978-3-031-76269-7_3

general population [4]. Non-cardiovascular causes of death are occasionally listed in small series of older adults and include but are not limited to diabetes, malignancy, and renal failure [5]. However, one of the authors of this chapter (BRP) follows many older adults in their 60s and 70s, indicating that longevity is possible.

3.2 Signs and Symptoms of Psychiatric Comorbidities

Individuals with WS experience high rates of psychiatric symptoms, most commonly inattention, hyperactivity, anxiety, and sleep problems [6]. Somewhat less commonly reported are depressive disorders (3–25%), obsessive-compulsive disorder (2–5%), and psychotic symptoms (5–6%) [7–9]. These psychiatric symptoms have a significant impact on quality of life, and clinicians should be aware of their prevalence and presentation in this population.

3.2.1 Anxiety

In a meta-analysis conducted by Royston and colleagues (n = 391, age range: 4–55 years), the prevalence of anxiety disorders in individuals with WS was compared to those in the general population and individuals with ID [10]. Individuals with WS had considerably higher rates of anxiety disorders (48%) compared to the estimated rate in the child ID population (12%) and the lower rates reported in the general population. Common anxiety disorders in WS include specific phobias (30–54%), generalized anxiety disorder (12–25%), and agoraphobia (24%) [7–9]. However, the prevalence of social anxiety disorder in individuals with WS remains unclear [6].

Common triggers for anxiety in this population include unpleasant sensory phenomena such as loud or unexpected noises, unanticipated changes in the environment or schedule, and negative emotions in others [6, 11]. Some phobias experienced by individuals with WS may be related to some of the phenotypic characteristics of the syndrome. For example, a heightened sensitivity to auditory stimuli and frequent hospitalizations or health issues may lead to fears of loud noises and blood/injury, respectively [8, 10].

The clinical presentation of anxiety in individuals with WS is broad, and untreated anxiety can lead to angry or emotional outbursts [6, 9]. Parents report a diverse range of behaviors associated with anxiety, including verbalizing anxious feelings, seeking reassurance, crying, seeking proximity to their caretakers, repetitive behaviors, and pacing. Other observable symptoms of anxiety in individuals with WS include repetitive body movements such as rocking or bouncing and skin picking [6, 9].

Children with WS frequently worry about a variety of upcoming events, but once the event has occurred, their worry dissipates [9]. This anticipatory worry is perseverative and can also pertain to enjoyable events. These symptoms may lie at the intersection of worry and obsessiveness, and some parents resist using the term "worry" to describe their child's anticipatory anxiety [9]. In fact, although anticipatory anxiety can be impairing and take up a significant amount of time, it may not meet the full criteria for generalized anxiety disorder or any other anxiety disorder based on the Diagnostic and Statistical Manual of Mental Disorders, Fifth Edition, Text Revision (DSM-5-TR) criteria. As such, standardized assessment tools for diagnosing anxiety disorders in individuals with WS should be used with caution [9].

3.2.2 Attention-Deficit/Hyperactivity Disorder (ADHD)

Individuals with WS are also at an increased risk for ADHD. A prospective study that used a structured clinical interview to evaluate psychiatric disorders in 119 children with WS between the ages of 4 and 16 years found that 64.7% met the DSM-IV criteria for ADHD [9]. This rate is significantly higher than the prevalence rate of ADHD in comparably aged children in the general population, which ranges from 3–7%.

The predominantly inattentive presentation of ADHD was the most common subtype [9]. Finally, ADHD symptoms may persist into adulthood in individuals with WS [12]. A cross-sectional study of 70 adults with WS (aged 19–39 years) reported a high prevalence of distractibility (69%) and excessive chatter (83%). Their caregivers also reported that adults with WS often lost concentration easily and required considerable supervision to remain on task [12].

3.2.3 Sleep Disorders

Sleep problems are a well-documented concern among individuals with WS, affecting 36–57% of children [13]. Research has consistently documented sleep disturbances across the lifespan in WS, with significant sleep problems already present in children as young as 18 months of age [14]. High levels of daytime drowsiness are commonly reported in adolescents and young adults, with as many as 34% meeting criteria for excessive daytime sleepiness [15].

A parent-completed questionnaire study that included 64 school-aged children with WS found that 97% of school-aged children with WS experienced sleep problems such as night waking, bedtime resistance, high levels of sleep anxiety, and increased sleep latency [16]. Sleep abnormalities have also been observed using actigraphy in a small study that included 24 school-aged children with WS [17]. Finally, studies utilizing polysomnography have indicated that children with WS spend more time awake following sleep onset than typically developing children [18]. It has been speculated that abnormal levels of sleep-related hormones, specifically melatonin and cortisol, may be a contributing factor to the sleep disturbances experienced by those with WS [13, 19].

In clinical practice, sleep apnea (primarily obstructive sleep apnea [OSA] but sometimes mixed OSA and central apnea) is observed in adults with WS. No study has yet been published on sleep apnea frequency, but several risk factors (hypotonia, micrognathia, and obesity) are common in WS. A subset of individuals with WS are able to tolerate a positive pressure treatment like continuous positive airway pressure (CPAP), but many are not. Accordingly, untreated sleep apnea may persist, or alternate interventions may need to be considered.

3.2.4 Less Common Disorders

The prevalence and manifestation of depression in youth and adults with WS have been relatively under-investigated. Two small studies indicate a point prevalence of depression of 10–11% in adults with WS [20, 21]. Although limited data is available on the prevalence of major depressive disorder (MDD) in individuals with WS, the point prevalence of 11% is higher than the estimated rates of MDD in the general population of 5.1% [22].

Functional neurological symptom disorder (FNSD), which is also referred to as conversion disorder, is a neurobehavioral condition characterized by one or more symptoms of altered voluntary motor or sensory function that cannot be attributed to any recognized neurological disorder. While there is limited research on FNSD in individuals with WS, a case series has been reported in the literature [23]. Functional neurological symptom disorder may be more common in individuals with WS than previously recognized, and further studies are needed to explore the prevalence, clinical manifestations, risk factors, and management of FNSD in this population [23].

3.3 Assessment

3.3.1 Genetics and Diagnostic Testing

A giant leap forward in the understanding of WS occurred in 1993. Using fluorescence in situ hybridization (FISH), deletion of an elastin gene on the long arm of one copy of chromosome 7 was demonstrated in persons with WS [24], confirming that WS is a genetic disorder. We now know that the vast majority of persons with WS have a 1.5–1.8 megabase deletion at chromosome 7q11.23. This deletion leads to having only one copy (instead of the normal two) of a stretch of 26–28 genes [25]. This results in reduced gene product, which in turn, is responsible for the features of WS. For instance, having only a single copy of the elastin gene is the primary driver of the cardiovascular pathology that typifies WS. As another example, there is considerable human and mouse model evidence that the deletion of a copy of GTF2I and a related gene, GTF2IRD1, contributes to the neurodevelopmental phenotype [25]. Finally, a small (not yet quantified) percent of persons with WS have an atypically sized microdeletion, either smaller or larger than typical, which can result in milder and more severe phenotypes, respectively.

The diagnosis of WS is most commonly established using specialized genetic testing (fluorescent in situ hybridization [FISH] or chromosomal microarray [CMA]) since routine chromosome analysis does not detect WS [25]. Fluorescent in situ hybridization and CMA can also be applied to a fetal tissue sample obtained by amniocentesis or chorionic villus sampling (CVS). These tests, however, are not routinely offered as part of standard prenatal testing. In the not too distant future, prenatal screening for WS might become feasible due to advances in noninvasive prenatal testing (NIPT) technology. Should NIPT become widely available and sufficiently sensitive to detect WS, the prevalence of WS might decline due to pregnancy terminations.

3.4 Psychosocial Treatments

A comprehensive, developmentally appropriate, and individually tailored approach to psychosocial treatments is a cornerstone of the care of persons with WS. Components of psychosocial interventions that are commonly utilized and helpful to many include special education services, optimizing the educational/vocational environment, and adapting evidence-based psychological and behavioral approaches to address specific treatment goals. For example, adapted social skills training and cognitive behavioral therapy (CBT) may be of benefit for improved social relationships and anxiety, respectively. Early research seeking to adapt evidence-based therapies to better suit the WS neuropsychiatric profile is discussed further in this section.

3.4.1 Social Skills Training

Although individuals with WS typically have high social interest, this is often accompanied by social skill deficits and unsatisfactory personal relationships. Social skills training programs have been developed to teach social skills to the autism spectrum disorder (ASD) population [26]; however, these commercially available programs may not effectively address the unique social difficulties experienced by adults with WS. In response to this, Fisher and colleagues developed a WS social skills training program that targets conversation skills and relationship building and can be delivered through virtual care [27].

3.4.2 Exposure Therapy

Exposure therapy, which involves gradual and systematic exposure to feared stimuli, is a key component of evidence-based treatment for anxiety in the general population. Klein-Tasman and colleagues have modified exposure therapy by infusing a playful and humor-based approach for children with WS. A case series describes nine children with WS, aged 4 through 10 years, who participated in several sessions of therapy over a 2- or 3-day period [28]. Examples of some of the phobic stimuli addressed included fears of motorcycles, hand dryers, blood pressure cuffs, and blenders. This intervention resulted in decreased fear, anxiety, and emotion dysregulation for many of the participants.

3.4.3 Cognitive Behavioral Therapy

While CBT is a first-line treatment for anxiety in the general population, there is currently a lack of CBT treatment manuals available for anxiety in adults with WS and ID. To investigate the acceptability and initial effectiveness of adapting commonly used, evidence-based CBT principles in adults with WS, Thom et al. developed a modified CBT curriculum for adults with WS including psychoeducation, relaxation training, and cognitive skills [29]. This program was piloted in a group-based, telehealth format with four adults with WS. Remarkably, all four participants experienced a significant decrease in their clinician-rated anxiety rating scale score. Key adaptations to traditional CBT included incorporating a caregiver as a therapy partner, utilizing simplified language, delivering therapy at a slower pace, and simplifying CBT concepts [30].

3.5 Biological Treatments

Despite the frequency of co-occurring behavioral symptoms in individuals with WS, few reports on pharmacological intervention have been published. The safe use of psychiatric medications in individuals with WS requires the consideration of medical comorbidities, contraindications, adverse effects, and monitoring parameters. A review of commonly used psychotropic medications and a discussion of their relative effectiveness and safety profile in WS was published in 2021 [6].

3.5.1 Anxiety

Buspirone, a 5-HT$_{1A}$ receptor partial agonist and D_3/D_4 antagonist, has shown promise for the treatment of anxiety in individuals with WS. A retrospective chart review study including 24 individuals with WS (aged 7–47 years) who received treatment with buspirone for anxiety demonstrated a response rate of approximately 70% [31]. Buspirone was also observed to be generally well-tolerated and safe. The most common side effect was nausea (13%), and more than 80% of patients remained on buspirone at the time of their most recent clinical visit. An open-label trial of buspirone for anxiety in this population is currently underway.

While selective serotonin reuptake inhibitors (SSRIs) and serotonin norepinephrine reuptake inhibitors (SNRIs) are typically well-tolerated medications, there is limited data on their efficacy and tolerability in individuals with WS. Green et al. (2012) conducted a longitudinal study involving 21 children with WS and an anxiety disorder, of which five were treated with an SSRI [32]. Two of the five children treated with SSRIs no longer met the criteria for an anxiety disorder at follow-up, and four of five children were rated as "much improved" after treatment with an SSRI. It should be noted that the efficacy and tolerability of SSRIs have been studied more extensively in youth with ASD, another neurodevelopmental condition. Selective serotonin reuptake inhibitors have been associated with low efficacy and high rates of adverse effects including insomnia, motor hyperactivity, agitation, and aggression in youth with ASD [33]. Furthermore, SSRIs and SNRIs have potential adverse effects relevant to the WS population, such as weight gain, QTc interval prolongation, increased falls/fracture risk, and mildly increased blood pressure (SNRIs only) [34–38].

3.5.2 Attention-Deficit/Hyperactivity Disorder

Despite the high prevalence of inattention and distractibility, particularly in children with WS, evidence-based treatments for ADHD in this population remain limited. A retrospective cohort study of 38 youth with WS (mean age 13.1 years) who had been treated with methylphenidate (0.3–0.5 mg/kg) reported a 72% response rate [32]. Notably, sadness (61%), which was described as striking and dramatic, was a common side effect. Considering the high prevalence of cardiovascular pathology in individuals with WS, collaboration with the patient's cardiologist is recommended prior to and during a trial of methylphenidate. Further research, both on stimulant medications, such as methylphenidate, and non-stimulant alternatives, such as alpha-$_2$ agonists and atomoxetine, are needed. Based on clinical observation (RPT), inattention is a target symptom that may be particularly challenging to treat pharmacologically.

3.5.3 Sleep Disorders

Sleep disturbances are common in individuals with WS, and pharmacologic treatments are often used to improve sleep quality. Two parent survey studies have been conducted on pharmacologic treatments for sleep disorders in children with WS. The first survey of 513 parents reported that 25% of children had taken a medication for impaired sleep, with melatonin being the most common (67%), followed by diphenhydramine (29%), and then quetiapine (8%) [39]. In this survey, 91% of those who had taken melatonin found it "helpful" or "somewhat helpful," with adverse effects reported by only 6% of the participants [39]. In another survey assessing 28 families of children with WS (mean age 4.7 years), five children were treated with clonazepam (0.25–0.75 mg nightly), a benzodiazepine, with a positive clinical response described as fewer and shorter awakenings according to parent report and confirmed with polysomnography [18]. It should be noted, however, that benzodiazepines are not commonly used in clinical practice for sleep disorders due to the potential for dependence, tolerance, and impaired cognitive function.

3.5.4 Depression

There is limited literature on the use of pharmacotherapy for MDD in individuals with WS. Only one report of the pharmacologic treatment of MDD in WS has been published, which included a case series of three adult patients with WS (aged 24, 25, and 26 years) who had MDD with psychotic features. All three individuals responded to treatment with a combination of a second-generation antipsychotic (SGA) and an antidepressant [40]. Based on clinical experience (RPT), SNRIs (e.g., duloxetine) appear to be generally effective and well-tolerated for depressive disorders in adults with WS; however, systematic research is needed.

3.5.5 Body-Focused Repetitive Behaviors

Finally, some individuals with WS experience problematic body-focused repetitive behaviors such as skin picking, hair pulling, or hair cutting. The use of N-acetylcysteine may be helpful in some cases [41].

3.6 Medical Features of Williams Syndrome

There is a lengthy list of potential medical problems that can occur in persons with WS; importantly, the extent and severity of these problems can vary greatly, leading to wide phenotypic variability across individuals. Some problems are more common at certain ages (e.g., in young childhood and in adulthood), but even comparably aged individuals can have dissimilar sets of problems. It is important to mention that no single individual with WS develops all of the conditions on the potential problem list.

The most prevalent and impactful medical problems for a psychiatrist to be aware of involve the cardiovascular, gastrointestinal, and endocrine systems. A snapshot of typical problems that can be seen in several other systems such as the ocular, ear-nose-throat (ENT), and neurological systems is provided in Table 3.1.

I. **Cardiovascular Disease**: Key cardiovascular features of WS include an increased frequency of vasculopathy, hypertension, rhythm disturbances, valve involvement, anesthesia-related complications, and sudden death.
   - Vasculopathy: Vascular stenoses of medium and large-sized arteries are among the most distinctive and common features of WS, occurring in at least 75% of patients. Characteristically involved locations are supravalvular aortic stenosis (SVAS), branch or peripheral pulmonary stenosis, and descending aorta stenosis, though the involvement of renal, mesenteric, coronary, and intracranial arteries is well-documented. The extent and distribution of narrowing range from clinically insignificant to sufficiently severe to be incompatible with life. Management consists of lifelong cardiology monitoring with intervention to enlarge significantly narrowed regions surgically or by dilation/stenting, depending on the nature and location of the narrowing [42, 43].

Table 3.1 Select medical features of Williams syndrome

Additional systems medically involved in WS	Common manifestations	Notes
Auditory/ENT	Frequent ear infections, hyperacusis, hearing loss	
Dental	Small, abnormally-shaped teeth and/or absent teeth, malocclusion, limited ability to independently maintain dental hygiene	
Genitourinary	Urinary frequency, enuresis, bladder diverticula, structural renal anomaly, nephrocalcinosis	
Musculoskeletal	Joint laxity (except joint tightness at hamstrings and heel cords), scoliosis, diminished bone mineral density	
Neurological	Mixed hypotonia (central) and hypertonia (extremities), brisk but symmetric deep tendon reflexes (DTRs), clonus, poor balance, "benign essential" tremor, Chiari type 1 malformation	Chiari type 1 usually asymptomatic and detected incidentally
Ophthalmology	Strabismus, refractive errors, cataract, narrow-angle glaucoma	
Skin and Hair	Hernias, premature graying of hair	
Stature	Short stature, early and blunted pubertal growth spurt	WS growth curves should be used during childhood

– Hypertension: The estimated lifetime frequency of high blood pressure in WS is approximately 50% with possible childhood onset. General population cutoffs are used to define hypertension, but some questions exist about the validity of these cutoffs since WS arteries are stiffer than normal. Given the high prevalence of anxiety in WS, particularly in medical settings, initial "office" readings tend to be elevated. Because of this, serial blood pressure measurements at home or at school, or 24-hour ambulatory blood pressure monitoring, may be more informative. In terms of antihypertensive medication, there is no consensus on the preferred class of drug. Screening for renal artery stenosis should be considered before commencing angiotensin receptor blockers [44].
– Sudden death with or without anesthesia: There are numerous reports of sudden death, particularly in young children with WS, often, but not always, associated with anesthesia. Various cardiac risk factors have been identified or hypothesized (e.g., obstruction of coronary ostia, right ventricular and left ventricular outflow obstruction, prolonged QTc interval, and decreased heart rate variability). To minimize the sudden death risk attributed to anesthesia, guidelines for patient risk stratification and periprocedural anesthesia management have been published [45, 46].

- Rhythm disturbances: It is prudent to obtain a cardiology consult and electrocardiogram (EKG) when considering the administration of a potentially rhythm-altering medication because several types of rhythm disturbances, including but not limited to arrhythmias, prolonged QTc interval, and decreased heart rate variability, are common at baseline.
  (i) Arrhythmias: There is increasing documentation of arrhythmias in patients with WS. A recent study of 74 children and young adults with WS who wore a 24-h ambulatory EKG monitoring device on one or more occasions documented arrhythmias in nine out of 74 subjects (12%) [47]. The most common abnormalities were atrial arrhythmias (such as atrial tachycardia) though others, including ventricular rhythm abnormalities, were also observed. Risk factors for an arrhythmia included intermittent ectopic atrial rhythm on baseline EKG, older age, and syncope, but not the severity of cardiac disease [48].
  (ii) Prolonged QTc interval: Several investigators have reported prolonged QTc interval in a subset of persons with WS [47, 49–51]. The impact of this finding, particularly on the increased rate of sudden death in WS, continues to be investigated. Tachycardia, a consistent finding in WS across the lifespan, appears to have a small contributory effect to QTc prolongation, but additional, as of yet unidentified, factors likely exist. Therefore, it is prudent to minimize the use of QTc interval-prolonging medications or institute close EKG monitoring if these medications offer important therapeutic benefits. Genetic long QTc syndromes (e.g., LQT1 OMIM 192500 and LQT2 OMIM 613688) and prolonged QTc interval observed in WS appear to be distinct. The former is known to be caused by various ion channel mutations, while no ion channel gene is deleted in the WS microdeletion.
  (iii) Heart rate variability: Decreased heart rate variability (along with increased heart rate and increased frequency of premature ventricular contractions) was recently reported in WS compared to controls [52]. Investigators speculate this is due to autonomic dysregulation and that it could be a risk factor for sudden death in WS.
- Valve involvement: Valvar involvement, such as prolapse or regurgitation of the mitral valve, is reported to affect approximately 20% of persons with WS [53]. The extent of involvement is often mild, but valve replacement surgery has been reported [54].

II. **Gastrointestinal Problems**: Gastrointestinal abnormalities are common throughout the lifespan in WS. The most prevalent conditions are constipation and gastroesophageal reflux disorder (GERD) [55]. "Lifestyle" factors such as low roughage diet, limited fluid intake, limited physical activity, and hypotonia can contribute to constipation, though it is possible that abnormalities in the enteric nervous system could also contribute. Persons with WS appear to be particularly vulnerable to the consequences of chronic constipation and are at risk for developing rectal prolapse, hemorrhoids, and early-onset diverticular disease including diverticulitis [56, 57]. Recurring bouts of abdominal pain are frequently endorsed. At times, an etiology is identifiable; accordingly, symptoms should not be labeled as "functional" or secondary to anxiety without an appropriate medical assessment and workup. Feeding difficulties, particularly textured food intolerance, commonly complicate the transition to solid foods in young childhood. Many adults report the persistence of distinct food preferences; this can result in a limited food repertoire as well as a decreased ability to swallow a "pill" or comply with unpalatable-tasting medication.

III. **Weight**: Growth curves specific for WS, aged 0–20 years old, exist and demonstrate that smaller than typical size, in terms of weight as well as height, is common, especially in childhood [58, 59]. While ~10% of adults with WS remain underweight (BMI <18.5 kilograms/meter^2), many, if not the majority, become either overweight (BMI 25–<30 kilograms/meter^2) or obese (BMI $\geq$ 30 kg/m^2) [60–62], similar to the US general population. Among women with WS who gain excess weight, it often accumulates in a pear-shaped distribution consistent with a diagnosis of lipedema [63]. There are likely multiple reasons for having either a low or high BMI, including background genetics, medications, lifestyle factors, and eating disorders.

IV. **Endocrine Abnormalities**: Endocrine disturbances involving homeostasis of glucose, thyroid hormone, and calcium level are well-described.

   (i) Prediabetes and diabetes: A number of studies show that the majority of adolescents and adults with WS have impaired glucose regulation, most often prediabetes but sometimes "silent diabetes" [64]. The primary risk factor for this glucose dysregulation is the genetic perturbation (e.g., chromosome 7 microdeletion) responsible for WS, though additional modifiable risk factors are obesity and unhealthy lifestyle. Of note, the hemoglobin A1c level is less sensitive in diagnosing impaired glucose regulation in WS than in the general population.

   (ii) Subclinical hypothyroidism (elevated TSH [thyroid stimulating hormone] accompanied by normal free thyroxine [T4] or total T4) is observed in as many as one-third of the WS population and is often associated with thyroid lobe hypoplasia. In contrast, actual hypothyroidism is less common, possibly in the 3–5% range, and autoimmune thyroid disease is very uncommon [65–67]. Though TSH elevation in subclinical hypothyroidism is often mild, decisions about further workup and thyroid hormone supplementation should involve an endocrinologist.

(iii) Hypercalcemia was long considered the "hallmark" endocrine abnormality in WS. Due to the widespread availability of laboratory testing, we now know that clinically significant hypercalcemia is not as prevalent as previously thought and, furthermore, is not restricted to young childhood. Data from a full age-range cohort indicated a 6% frequency of "actionable" hypercalcemia [plasma Ca level 0.5 mg/dL above pediatric-adjusted norms], with a peak frequency of 10% in toddlers [68]. Infantile hypercalcemia commonly develops in the setting of failure to thrive or an acute dehydrating illness, while in adults medical problems such as parathyroid adenoma are often the trigger. There are a range of treatment options from laboratory monitoring escalating up to bisphosphonate infusion.

(iv) Pubertal development in girls and boys with WS starts, on average, 1 or 2 years earlier compared to the general population [64, 67]. This is likely due to normal but "early" activation of the hypothalamic-pituitary axis. No data on menopause exists, though parents anecdotally relay it also occurs "early."

A snapshot of select other medical features that often complicate WS is provided below in Table 3.1 [55, 56, 69].

Key Points to Remember

- Williams syndrome is a genetic disorder caused by a 1.5–1.8 megabase deletion at chromosome 7q11.23.
- Medical comorbidities in WS include but are not limited to vasculopathy and hypertension, arrhythmia (including prolonged QTc interval), sudden death, obesity in adults, and prediabetes/diabetes.
- The most common psychiatric comorbidities are ADHD, anxiety disorders, and sleep problems.
- Adapted social skills training and cognitive behavioral therapy may be of benefit for improved social relationships and anxiety, respectively.
- The use of psychopharmacology in individuals with WS should take into account the available effectiveness data as well as the individual's medical comorbidities.
- Emerging data support the safety and effectiveness of buspirone for anxiety in WS.

Photographs of Individuals with the Syndrome

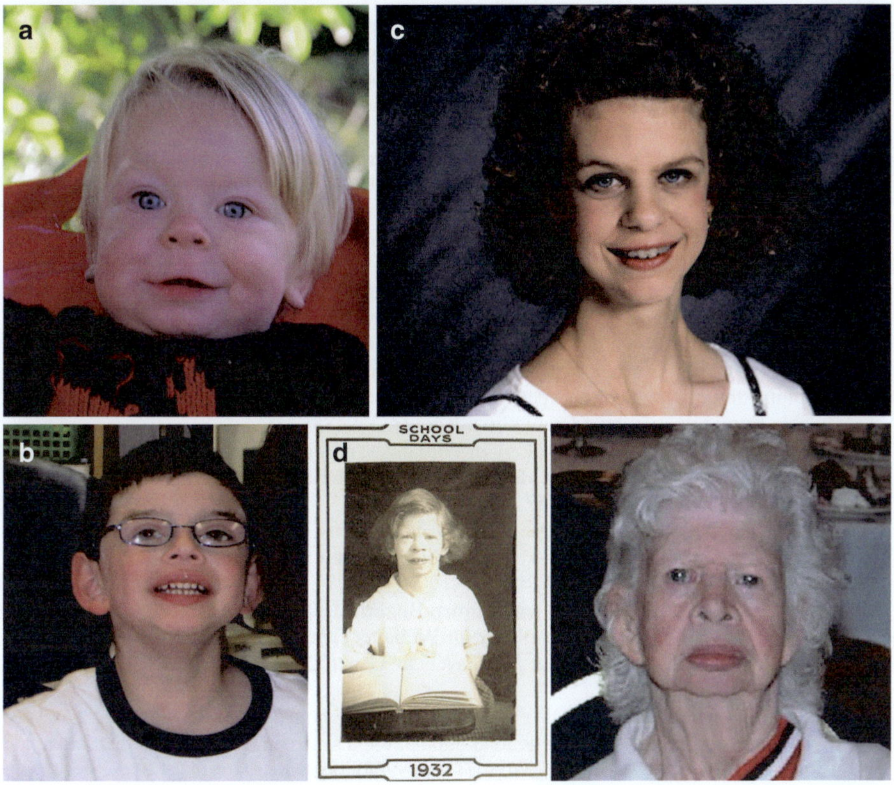

Patients with Williams syndrome: Four unrelated patients with Williams syndrome are shown in Panels **a**-**d**. The young child (Panel **a**) has a flat nasal bridge, upturned nasal tip, long philtrum, mild periorbital puffiness, full cheeks, and a delicate chin. The school-age child (Panel **b**) has full lips, a wide mouth, and mildly increased interdental spacing. The young adult (Panel **c**) has a prominent nose and nasal tip, a wide mouth, and a full lower lip. Panel **d** shows a patient at 12 years of age (left) and at 83 years of age (right). From N Engl J Med, Pober BR, Williams-Beuren syndrome, 362, 239-252, Copyright © 2010. Massachusetts Medical Society. Reprinted with permission

References

1. Williams JC, Barratt-Boyes BG, Lowe JB. Supravalvular aortic stenosis. Circulation. 1961;24:1311–8. Available from: https://pubmed.ncbi.nlm.nih.gov/14007182/
2. Beuren AJ, Apitz J, Harmjanz D. Supravalvular aortic stenosis in association with mental retardation and a certain facial appearance. Circulation. 1962;26:1235–40. Available from: https://pubmed.ncbi.nlm.nih.gov/13967885/
3. Strømme P, Bjømstad PG, Ramstad K. Prevalence estimation of Williams syndrome. J Child Neurol. 2002;17(4):269–71. Available from: http://www.ncbi.nlm.nih.gov/pubmed/12088082
4. Wessel A, Gravenhorst V, Buchhorn R, Gosch A, Partsch CJ, Pankau R. Risk of sudden death in the Williams-Beuren syndrome. Am J Med Genet A. 2004;127A(3):234–7. Available from: https://pubmed.ncbi.nlm.nih.gov/15150772/
5. Sauna-aho O, Bjelogrlic-Laakso N, Sirén A, Kangasmäki V, Arvio M. Cognition in adults with Williams syndrome—a 20-year follow-up study. Mol Genet. Genomic Med. 2019;7(6) Available from: https://pubmed.ncbi.nlm.nih.gov/31033253/
6. Thom RP, Pober BR, McDougle CJ. Psychopharmacology of Williams syndrome: safety, tolerability, and effectiveness. Expert opinion on drug safety. Taylor and Francis Ltd.; 2021. Available from: https://pubmed.ncbi.nlm.nih.gov/33369485/
7. Dodd HF, Porter MA. Psychopathology in Williams syndrome: the effect of individual differences across the life span. J Ment Health Res Intellect Disabil. 2009;2(2):89–109. Available from: 10.1080/19315860902725867
8. Dykens EM. Anxiety, fears, and phobias in persons with Williams syndrome. Dev Neuropsychol. 2003;23(1–2):291–316. Available from: http://www.tandfonline.com/doi/abs/10.1080/87565641.2003.9651896
9. Leyfer OT, Woodruff-Borden J, Klein-Tasman BP, Fricke JS, Mervis CB. Prevalence of psychiatric disorders in 4 to 16-year-olds with Williams syndrome. Am J Med Genet Part B, Neuropsychiatr Genet Off Publ Int Soc Psychiatr Genet. 2006;141B(6):615–22. https://doi.org/10.1002/ajmg.b.30344.
10. Royston R, Howlin P, Waite J, Oliver C. Anxiety disorders in Williams syndrome contrasted with intellectual disability and the general population: a systematic review and meta-analysis. J Autism Dev Disord. 2017;47(12):3765–77. https://doi.org/10.1007/s10803-016-2909-z.
11. Royston R, Oliver C, Howlin P, Waite J. Anxiety characteristics in individuals with Williams syndrome. J Appl Res Intellect Disabil. 2021;34(4):1098–107. Available from: https://pubmed.ncbi.nlm.nih.gov/33561900/
12. Davies M, Udwin O, Howlin P. Adults with Williams syndrome: preliminary study of social, emotional and behavioural difficulties. Br J Psychiatry. 1998;172:273–6. Available from: https://pubmed.ncbi.nlm.nih.gov/9614479/
13. Santoro SD, Giacheti CM, Rossi NF, Campos LMG, Pinato L. Correlations between behavior, memory, sleep-wake and melatonin in Williams-Beuren syndrome. Physiol Behav. 2016;159:14–9. Available from: https://pubmed.ncbi.nlm.nih.gov/26976740/
14. Gwilliam K, Joyce A, Dimitriou D. Early manifestation of sleep problems in toddlers with Williams Syndrome using a mixed method longitudinal approach. Res Dev Disabil. 2020:104. Available from: https://pubmed.ncbi.nlm.nih.gov/32505082/
15. Goldman SE, Malow BA, Newman KD, Roof E, Dykens EM. Sleep patterns and daytime sleepiness in adolescents and young adults with Williams syndrome. J Intellect Disabil Res. 2009;53(2):182–8. Available from: https://pubmed.ncbi.nlm.nih.gov/19067782/
16. Annaz D, Hill CM, Ashworth A, Holley S, Karmiloff-Smith A. Characterisation of sleep problems in children with Williams syndrome. Res Dev Disabil. 2011;32(1):164–9. Available from: http://www.ncbi.nlm.nih.gov/pubmed/20940094
17. Ashworth A, Hill CM, Karmiloff-Smith A, Dimitriou D. Cross syndrome comparison of sleep problems in children with Down syndrome and Williams syndrome. Res Dev Disabil. 2013;34(5):1572–80. Available from: https://pubmed.ncbi.nlm.nih.gov/23475007/

18. Arens R, Wright B, Elliott J, Zhao H, Wang PP, Brown LW, et al. Periodic limb movement in sleep in children with Williams syndrome. J Pediatr. 1998;133(5):670–4. Available from: http://www.ncbi.nlm.nih.gov/pubmed/9821427
19. Sniecinska-Cooper AM, Iles RK, Butler SA, Jones H, Bayford R, Dimitriou D. Abnormal secretion of melatonin and cortisol in relation to sleep disturbances in children with Williams syndrome. Sleep Med. 2015;16(1):94–100. Available from: https://pubmed.ncbi.nlm.nih.gov/25441742/
20. Stinton C, Tomlinson K, Estes Z. Examining reports of mental health in adults with Williams syndrome. Res Dev Disabil. 2012;33(1):144–52. Available from: https://pubmed.ncbi.nlm.nih.gov/22093659/
21. Cherniske EM, Carpenter TO, Klaiman C, Young E, Bregman J, Insogna K, et al. Multisystem study of 20 older adults with Williams syndrome. Am J Med Genet A. 2004;131(3):255–64. Available from: https://pubmed.ncbi.nlm.nih.gov/15534874/
22. Kessler RC, Sampson NA, Berglund P, Gruber MJ, Al-Hamzawi A, Andrade L, et al. Anxious and non-anxious major depressive disorder in the World Health Organization World Mental Health Surveys. Epidemiol Psychiatr Sci. 2015;24(3):210–26. Available from: /pmc/articles/PMC5129607/?report=abstract
23. Thom RP, Balaj K, Keary CJ, Pober BR, McDougle CJ. Functional neurological symptom disorder in Williams syndrome: Case series and review of relevant literature. J Acad Consult Psychiatry. 2022;63(2):170–9. Available from: https://pubmed.ncbi.nlm.nih.gov/34619410/
24. Ewart AK, Morris CA, Atkinson D, Jin W, Sternes K, Spallone P, et al. Hemizygosity at the elastin locus in a developmental disorder. Williams syndrome Nat Genet. 1993;5(1):11–6. Available from: http://www.ncbi.nlm.nih.gov/pubmed/7693128
25. Kozel BA, Barak B, Kim CA, Mervis CB, Osborne LR, Porter M, et al. Williams syndrome. Nat Rev Dis Primers. 2021:7. Available from: https://pubmed.ncbi.nlm.nih.gov/34140529/
26. Soares EE, Bausback K, Beard CL, Higinbotham M, Bunge EL, Gengoux GW. Social skills training for autism spectrum disorder: a meta-analysis of in-person and technological interventions. J Technol Behav Sci. 2021;6(1):166–80. Available from: https://pubmed.ncbi.nlm.nih.gov/33225056/
27. Fisher MH, Kammes RR, Black RS, Houck K, Cwiakala K. A distance-delivered social skills program for young adults with Williams syndrome: evaluating feasibility and preliminary efficacy. J Autism Dev Disord. 2022;52(12):5162–76. Available from: https://pubmed.ncbi.nlm.nih.gov/35575839/
28. Klein-Tasman B, Young B, Levine K, Rivera K, Mieciela E, Yund BD, French S. Acceptability and effectiveness of humor- and play-infused exposure therapy for fears in Williams syndrome. Evidence-Based Pract Child Adolesc Ment Heal. 2022;7(1):94–111.
29. Thom R, Pineda J, Nowinski L, Birtwell K, Hooker J, McGuire J, et al. A virtually delivered adapted cognitive behavioral therapy group for adults with Williams syndrome and anxiety. Cogn Behav Pract. 2022;
30. Pineda J, Nowinski L, Birtwell K, Hooker J, McGuire J, McDougle C, et al. Clinical challenges and solutions in adapting cognitive behavioral therapy for anxiety in adults with intellectual disability. J Cogn Psychother.
31. Shin E, Renzi D, Canales C, Ravichandran C, McDougle CJ, Thom RP. Buspirone for the treatment of anxiety in Williams syndrome: a retrospective chart review study. Expert Opin Pharmacother. 2024;25(1):113–20. Available from: https://pubmed.ncbi.nlm.nih.gov/38247447/
32. Green T, Avda S, Dotan I, Zarchi O, Basel-Vanagaite L, Zalsman G, et al. Phenotypic psychiatric characterization of children with Williams syndrome and response of those with ADHD to methylphenidate treatment. Am J Med Genet Part B Neuropsychiatr Genet. 2012:159. B(1):13–20. Available from: https://pubmed.ncbi.nlm.nih.gov/22052570/
33. McDougle C, Kresch L, Posey D. Repetitive thoughts and behavior in pervasive developmental disorders: treatment with serotonin reuptake inhibitors. J Autism Dev Disord. 2000;30(5):427–35. Available from: http://www.ncbi.nlm.nih.gov/pubmed/11098879

34. Beach SR, Celano CM, Sugrue AM, Adams C, Ackerman MJ, Noseworthy PA, et al. QT prolongation, Torsades de Pointes, and psychotropic medications: A 5-year update. Psychosomatics. 2018;59(2):105–22. Available from: http://www.ncbi.nlm.nih.gov/pubmed/29275963
35. Burcu M, Zito JM, Safer DJ, Magder LS, Dos Reis S, Shaya FT, et al. Association of antidepressant medications with incident type 2 diabetes among medicaid-insured youths. JAMA Pediatr. 2017;171(12):1200–7.
36. Kumar M, Bajpai R, Shaik AR, Srivastava S, Vohora D. Alliance between selective serotonin reuptake inhibitors and fracture risk: an updated systematic review and meta-analysis. European Journal of Clinical Pharmacology Springer. 2020; Available from: https://pubmed.ncbi.nlm.nih.gov/32556910/
37. Wang CY, Fu SH, Wang CL, Chen PJ, Wu FLL, Hsiao FY. Serotonergic antidepressant use and the risk of fracture: a population-based nested case–control study. Osteoporos Int. 2016;27(1):57–63. Available from: https://pubmed.ncbi.nlm.nih.gov/26126579/
38. Zhong Z, Wang L, Wen X, Liu Y, Fan Y, Liu Z. A meta-analysis of effects of selective serotonin reuptake inhibitors on blood pressure in depression treatment: Outcomes from placebo and serotonin and noradrenaline reuptake inhibitor controlled trials. Neuropsychiatr Dis Treat 2017;13:2781–96. Available from: /pmc/articles/PMC5683798/?report=abstract.
39. Martens MA, Seyfer DL, Andridge RR, Coury DL. Use and effectiveness of sleep medications by parent report in individuals with Williams syndrome. J Dev Behav Pediatr. 2017;38(9):765–71. Available from: https://pubmed.ncbi.nlm.nih.gov/28937452/
40. Valdes F, Keary CJ, Mullett JE, Palumbo ML, Waxler JL, Pober BR, et al. Major depressive disorder with psychotic features in Williams Syndrome: a case series. J Autism Dev Disord. 2018;48(3):947–52. Available from: https://pubmed.ncbi.nlm.nih.gov/29164439/
41. Carroll H, McDougle C, Thom R. N-acetylcysteine for trichotemnomania in an adult female with Williams syndrome. J Clin Psychopharmacol2. 2024;44(3):321–3.
42. Collins RT. Cardiovascular disease in Williams syndrome. Curr Opin Pediatr. 2018;30(5):609–15. Available from: http://www.ncbi.nlm.nih.gov/pubmed/30045083
43. Del Pasqua A, Rinelli G, Toscano A, Iacobelli R, Digilio C, Marino B, et al. New findings concerning cardiovascular manifestations emerging from long-term follow-up of 150 patients with the Williams-Beuren-Beuren syndrome. Cardiol Young. 2009;19(6):563–7. Available from: https://pubmed.ncbi.nlm.nih.gov/19941695/
44. Sivasubramanian R, Meyers KE. Hypertension in children and adolescents with Turner syndrome (TS), Neurofibromatosis 1 (NF1), and Williams Syndrome (WS). Curr Hypertens Rep. 2021;23(4). Available from: https://pubmed.ncbi.nlm.nih.gov/33779870/
45. Staudt GE, Eagle SS. Anesthetic considerations for patients with Williams syndrome. Journal of Cardiothoracic and Vascular Anesthesia. W.B. Saunders; 2020. Available from: https://pubmed.ncbi.nlm.nih.gov/32127269/
46. Abu-Sultaneh S, Gondim MJ, Alexy RD, Mastropietro CW. Sudden cardiac death associated with cardiac catheterization in Williams syndrome: a case report and review of literature. Cardiol Young. 2019;29(4):457–61. Available from: https://pubmed.ncbi.nlm.nih.gov/30950363/
47. Deitch AM, Giacone HM, Chubb H, Algaze CA, Lechich KMM, Collins RT. Arrhythmias in Williams syndrome. Am J Cardiol. 2023;195:91–7. Available from: https://pubmed.ncbi.nlm.nih.gov/37037070/
48. Ramphul K, Pekyi-Boateng PK, Verma R, Sombans S, Frimpong SK, Ayirebi-Acquah E, et al. Investigating cardiac arrhythmias among patients with Williams syndrome in the United States: an analysis using the 2016 to 2020 national inpatient sample. Am J Cardiol. 2023;200:250. Available from: https://pubmed.ncbi.nlm.nih.gov/37393156/
49. Collins RT, Aziz PF, Gleason MM, Kaplan PB, Shah MJ. Abnormalities of cardiac repolarization in Williams syndrome. Am J Cardiol. 2010;106(7):1029–33. Available from: http://www.ncbi.nlm.nih.gov/pubmed/20854969
50. Brink BD, Feinn R, Kozel BA, Billington CJ, Liu D, Yu E, et al. Frequency of QTc interval Prolongation in Children and Adults with Williams syndrome. Pediatr Cardiol. 2022;43(7):1559–67. Available from: https://pubmed.ncbi.nlm.nih.gov/35366065/

51. Algaze CA, Deitch AM, Chubb H, Aziz PF, Collins RT. Importance of formula-specific centile thresholds for evaluation of heart rate-corrected QT prolongation in Williams syndrome. Am J Cardiol. 2022;183:99–104. Available from: https://pubmed.ncbi.nlm.nih.gov/36114024/
52. Levin MD, Cathey BM, Smith K, Osgood S, Raja N, Fu YP, et al. Heart rate variability analysis may identify individuals with Williams-Beuren syndrome at risk of sudden death. JACC Clin Electrophysiol. 2023;9(3):359–70. Available from: https://pubmed.ncbi.nlm.nih.gov/36752464/
53. Collins RT, Kaplan P, Somes GW, Rome JJ. Long-term outcomes of patients with cardiovascular abnormalities and Williams syndrome. Am J Cardiol. 2010;105(6):874–8. Available from: https://pubmed.ncbi.nlm.nih.gov/20211336/
54. Cha SG, Song MK, Lee SY, Kim GB, Kwak JG, Kim WH, et al. Long-term cardiovascular outcome of Williams syndrome. Congenit Heart Dis. 2019;14(5):684–90. Available from: https://pubmed.ncbi.nlm.nih.gov/31166070/
55. Morris CA, Braddock SR, Chen E, Trotter TL, Berry SA, Burke LW, et al. Health care supervision for children with Williams syndrome. Pediatrics. 2020;145(2) Available from: https://pubmed.ncbi.nlm.nih.gov/31964759/
56. Cherniske EM, Carpenter TO, Klaiman C, Young E, Bregman J, Insogna K, et al. Multisystem study of 20 older adults with Williams syndrome. Am J Med Genet. 2004;131A(3):255–64. Available from: http://www.ncbi.nlm.nih.gov/pubmed/15534874
57. Partsch CJ, Siebert R, Caliebe A, Gosch A, Wessel A, Pankau R. Sigmoid diverticulitis in patients with Williams-Beuren syndrome: relatively high prevalence and high complication rate in young adults with the syndrome. Am J Med Genet A. 2005;137(1):52–4. Available from: https://pubmed.ncbi.nlm.nih.gov/16007633/
58. Martin NDT, Smith WR, Cole TJ, Preece MA. New height, weight and head circumference charts for British children with Williams syndrome. Arch Dis Child. 2007;92(7):598–601. Available from: https://pubmed.ncbi.nlm.nih.gov/17301110/
59. Morris CA, Demsey SA, Leonard CO, Dilts C, Blackburn BL. Natural history of Williams syndrome: physical characteristics. J Pediatr. 1988;113(2):318–26.
60. Renzi D, Stanley T, Waxler J, Lee H, Pober B, Nordstrom M. Body mass index variation in adults with Williams syndrome: associations with predicted dietary intake and food behaviors. Food. Nutr Res. 2023:67. Available from: https://pubmed.ncbi.nlm.nih.gov/37441515/
61. Masserini B, Bedeschi MF, Bianchi V, Scuvera G, Beck-Peccoz P, Lalatta F, et al. Prevalence of diabetes and pre-diabetes in a cohort of Italian young adults with Williams syndrome. Am J Med Genet A. 2013;161(4):817–21. Available from: https://pubmed.ncbi.nlm.nih.gov/23495209/
62. Nordstrøm M, Paus B, Andersen LF, Kolset SO. Dietary aspects related to health and obesity in Williams syndrome, Down syndrome, and Prader-Willi syndrome. Food. Nutr Res. 2015:59. Available from: https://pubmed.ncbi.nlm.nih.gov/25653019/
63. Waxler JL, Guardino C, Feinn RS, Lee H, Pober BR, Stanley TL. Altered body composition, lipedema, and decreased bone density in individuals with Williams syndrome: a preliminary report. Eur J Med Genet. 2017;60(5):250–6. Available from: https://pubmed.ncbi.nlm.nih.gov/28254647/
64. Stanley TL, Leong A, Pober BR. Growth, body composition, and endocrine issues in Williams syndrome. Curr Opin Endocrinol Diabetes Obes. 2021;28(1):64–74. Available from: https://pubmed.ncbi.nlm.nih.gov/33165016/
65. Cambiaso P, Orazi C, Digilio MC, Loche S, Capolino R, Tozzi A, et al. Thyroid morphology and subclinical hypothyroidism in children and adolescents with Williams syndrome. J Pediatr. 2007;150(1):62–5. Available from: https://pubmed.ncbi.nlm.nih.gov/17188616/
66. Palacios-Verdú MG, Segura-Puimedon M, Borralleras C, Flores R, Del CM, Campuzano V, et al. Metabolic abnormalities in Williams-Beuren syndrome. J Med Genet. 2015;52(4):248–55. Available from: https://pubmed.ncbi.nlm.nih.gov/25663682/
67. Kim Y-M, Cho JH, Kang E, Kim G-H, Seo E-J, Lee BH, et al. Endocrine dysfunctions in children with Williams-Beuren syndrome. Ann Pediatr Endocrinol Metab. 2016;21(1):15–20. https://doi.org/10.6065/apem.2016.21.1.15.

68. Sindhar S, Lugo M, Levin MD, Danback JR, Brink BD, Yu E, et al. Hypercalcemia in patients with Williams-Beuren syndrome. J Pediatr. 2016;178:254–60. Available from: https://pubmed.ncbi.nlm.nih.gov/27574996/
69. Management of Williams syndrome a clinical guideline.

Further Reading

Kozel BA, Barak B, Kim CA, Mervis CB, Osborne LR, Porter M, Pober BR. Williams syndrome. Nat Rev. Dis Primers. 2021;7(1):42. https://doi.org/10.1038/s41572-021-00276-z.

Morris CA, et al. Health care supervision for children with Williams syndrome. Pediatrics. 2020;145(2):e20193761.

Pober BR. Williams-Beuren syndrome. N Engl J Med. 2010;362(3):239–52. https://doi.org/10.1056/NEJMra0903074. Erratum in: N Engl J Med. 2010 Jun 3;362(22):2142

Thom RP. Psychiatric and behavioral manifestations of Williams syndrome. Curr Opin Psychiatry. 2024;37(2):65–70. https://doi.org/10.1097/YCO.0000000000000914.

Thom RP, Pober BR, McDougle CJ. Psychopharmacology of Williams syndrome: safety, tolerability, and effectiveness. Expert Opin Drug Saf. 2021;20(3):293–306. https://doi.org/10.1080/14740338.2021.1867535.

4 Down Syndrome

Michelle L. Palumbo, Stephanie Santoro, and Yamini Howe

4.1 Overview of the Neurodevelopmental Disorder

Down syndrome (DS) is a common chromosomal cause of intellectual disability, with an estimated population prevalence in the USA of 6.7 per 10,000. Due to improved childhood survival rates, the population prevalence of DS has increased over time. The life expectancy of individuals with DS has also improved from an estimated mean of 26 years in 1950 to 53 years in 2010 among individuals living in the USA [1].

A partial or complete trisomy of the 21st chromosome causes DS. The most common cause (95% of cases) is a full additional 21st chromosome (free trisomy) due to a nondisjunction error during maternal meiosis of oocytes. Less commonly (~5%), the extra chromosomal material is the result of an unbalanced translocation. Rarely (~2%), mosaic DS can occur, such that some cells in an individual's body may have an extra chromosome 21, while others do not, leading to a variable presentation of symptoms [2, 3].

If a prenatal genetic diagnosis is not made, a diagnosis of DS can be made after birth based on a physical examination. Common features such as generalized low muscle tone, up-slanting of the palpebral fissures, flattening of the nasal bridge, the presence of nuchal folds, and a single palmar crease are commonly appreciable at

M. L. Palumbo (✉)
Massachusetts General Hospital for Children, Lexington, MA, USA
e-mail: mlpalumbo@mgh.harvard.edu

S. Santoro
Massachusetts General Hospital, Boston, MA, USA
e-mail: SSantoro3@mgh.harvard.edu

Y. Howe
Cortica, Burlington, MA, USA
e-mail: yhowe@corticacare.com

R. P. Thom, C. J. McDougle (eds.), *Neuropsychiatric Care for Genetic Syndromes and Other Neurodevelopmental Disorders*,
https://doi.org/10.1007/978-3-031-76269-7_4

birth. When a clinical diagnosis of DS is suspected, confirmatory genetic testing is recommended [4].

Some medical conditions are more common among individuals with DS than the general population, including hearing and vision abnormalities, congenital heart disease, frequent ear infections and respiratory illnesses, feeding difficulties and gastrointestinal atresias, thyroid conditions, and autoimmune diseases. These issues will be further discussed in subsequent sections.

4.2 Signs and Symptoms of Most Common Psychiatric Comorbidities

Approximately 13–38% of children and 25–38% of adults with DS experience psychiatric disorders [5]. Externalizing behaviors such as attention-deficit/hyperactivity disorder (ADHD) are more common in children with DS, while internalizing disorders such as depression become more common with increased age [6]. This section will review the presentation of the more common psychiatric conditions in people with DS.

4.2.1 ADHD

The prevalence rate of ADHD in DS ranges from 6.1 to 44% [7]. The clinical presentation of ADHD in children with DS is similar to ADHD in the general population including excessive activity, impulsivity, and difficulties with sustaining attention. Studies of ADHD in DS suggest that the inattentive subtype is more common than the hyperactive/impulsive subtype; however, the hyperactive/impulsive subtype more commonly presents to clinical care. When evaluating and treating ADHD, it is important to consider medical comorbidities common in people with DS, including sleep apnea, thyroid disorders, cognitive impairment, and hearing and visual difficulties, which may mimic or influence ADHD symptoms and potentially change treatment [8], For example, if sleep apnea is suspected and confirmed by a sleep study, then a trial of treatment for sleep apnea, i.e., CPAP (continuous positive airway pressure), may be warranted prior to starting medication for ADHD.

4.2.2 Autism Spectrum Disorder (ASD)

Estimates of the prevalence of co-occurring ASD and DS are variable, ranging from 5% to 39% [9]. More recent estimates range between 7% and 10% [10]. The diagnosis of ASD is often delayed in children with DS, with an average diagnosis of ASD between the ages of 6 and 16 years. This is likely due to diagnostic overshadowing; for example, the language delays and intellectual disability common to DS can overshadow a diagnosis of ASD. Individuals with autism and DS tend to have a lower IQ, unusual or excessive stereotypies, social withdrawal, anxiety, and higher levels of inappropriate speech than individuals with DS alone. Some predictors for ASD in individuals with DS include seizures (infantile spasms and myoclonic), early hypothyroidism, brain injury post cardiac surgery, and a family history of ASD or ASD traits [10].

4.2.3 Depression

Prevalence rates of depression in people with DS have been reported to be between 6% and 18%, with a generally accepted central lifetime estimate of approximately 10% [11]. In a large population-based, case-control study of 6,078 individuals with DS, people with DS had a 1.27-times greater likelihood of developing depression [12]. The presentation of depression in DS is similar to that seen in adults without DS. Additional symptoms of depression in people with DS can include a loss of self-care skills, social withdrawal, somatic complaints, aggression, and decreased speech. Individuals with DS may have more challenges expressing feelings of worthlessness, hopelessness, guilt, and suicidal ideation due to baseline cognitive and/or expressive language limitations. When evaluating individuals with DS and depressive symptoms, it is essential to be aware of the overlap between symptoms of depression and dementia. Depression can look similar to dementia in people with DS [13]. Not all patients with DS develop dementia. Clinicians should consider the risks versus benefits of treating a presumed patient with DS and dementia, particularly in younger adults (i.e., under the age of 40 years) and/or when depressive symptoms precede or co-occur with cognitive changes.

4.2.4 Anxiety

Earlier literature suggested that the prevalence of anxiety in individuals with DS was lower compared to that observed in the general population [14]. More recent studies have estimated the prevalence of anxiety in DS to be approximately 9% [12]. Due to difficulties with expressive language and intellectual limitations, individuals with DS may be unable to self-report anxiety symptoms [15]. Based on clinical experience, common anxiety symptoms in a person with DS include pacing, elopement, nail biting, skin picking, repetitive questions and behaviors, increased self-talk, avoidance, sleep disturbance, tantrums, and meltdowns. Another challenge with diagnosing individuals with DS with anxiety is that anxiety may be so longstanding that the family and caregivers have adapted their lives to accommodate it, thus lessening the affected individual's anxiety. In these cases, anxiety significantly impacts both the individual's quality of life as well as their family's.

4.2.5 Obsessive-Compulsive Disorder (OCD)

Individuals with DS have a 20-times increased likelihood of being diagnosed with obsessive-compulsive disorder (OCD) compared to the general population [12]. However, OCD may be overdiagnosed in individuals with DS due to the overlap in features of OCD and the commonly observed repetitive behaviors in individuals with DS [16, 17]. Examples of repetitive behaviors commonly observed in individuals with DS include twirling objects and following daily routines. These repetitive behaviors may increase during periods of distress, fear, and anxiety. Based on our clinical experience, repetitive behaviors as a manifestation of anxiety are more common than true OCD in DS. Case reports of OCD in individuals with DS consist of cases with predominantly compulsive behaviors such as repetitively walking out the front door and entering through the back door, excessive orderliness, and repetitively wearing the same garment. None of the described behaviors included more classic symptoms of OCD, such as hand washing or checking [18]. One phenomenon clinicians may encounter is obsessional slowness, which some clinicians consider to be on the OCD spectrum, and is characterized by the individual spending an extraordinary amount of time on basic routines to the point of dysfunction [19].

4.2.6 Bipolar Disorder

The prevalence of bipolar disorder in individuals with DS is largely unknown. In a cohort of 6,078 individuals with DS, individuals with DS had a lower likelihood of bipolar 1 disorder than those without DS [12]. Individuals with DS and bipolar disorder can present with episodic hyperactivity, irritability, euphoria, noisiness, pressured speech, mood lability, and sleep changes. From a clinical standpoint, clinicians are more likely to encounter individuals with depression than bipolar disorder but should be vigilant for periods of mania that could develop after the initial major depressive episode [20].

4.2.7 Regression

Cases of regression in DS were first described as catatonic psychosis by Rollin in 1946. In that manuscript, Rollin described individuals with DS who experienced "sudden and dramatic" alterations in behavior and regression in acquired skills starting at the age of 11–14 years. There has been a renewed interest in this phenomenon over the past 20 years. This phenomenon has been given many names, including DS disintegrative disorder, unexplained regression in DS, new-onset autistic regression, acute regression of DS, and catatonia of DS. This clinical entity is characterized by a rapid decline in functioning, which often entails significant deterioration or loss of daily living skills, language changes, and neuropsychiatric changes, including mood, behavioral, and personality changes and motor slowing [21]. At this time, the etiology of adolescent regression in DS is not known, although psychological stressors and immune dysregulation have been proposed as potential causes [22].

4.2.8 Catatonia

Catatonia in people with DS presents similarly to people without DS, with motor symptoms, alterations in posture, and behavioral changes. Catatonia can occur in school-aged children as well as adults with DS. Catatonia in people with DS is more likely to occur in individuals with other comorbid conditions, including hypothyroidism and ASD, as well as after exposure to stressful life events [23].

4.2.9 Psychosis

Psychosis has been reported to occur more often in individuals with DS than in typically developing individuals as well as those with other intellectual disabilities. Symptoms of psychosis and DS are similar to those seen in typically developing individuals and can include auditory and visual hallucinations, delusions, decreased language, and withdrawal. Clinicians need to consider the individual's developmental age and cognitive abilities when evaluating for psychosis. It is not uncommon for individuals with intellectual disabilities to have a blurred line between reality and fantasy, similar to that observed in young, typically developing children. In addition, many individuals with DS engage in self-talk, which may appear as if the individual is responding to internal stimuli [24]. While distinguishing between self-talk and responding to internal stimuli can be a challenge, typically the context of nonpsychotic self-talk has some basis in reality, such as talking to themselves about their day or repeating lines from favorite shows.

4.2.10 Alzheimer's Disease

Much research has been dedicated to the relationship between DS and early-onset Alzheimer's disease (AD), which is related to amyloid precursor protein overproduction [2]. Clinical symptoms appear after 40 years of age, and 77% of individuals with DS aged 60–69 years and up to 100% of those aged >70 years will develop cognitive decline [2]. Dementia is the proximal cause of death in 70% of older adults with DS [25]. Initial symptoms of dementia often include a decline in episodic memory, attention, and executive function, which then proceed to include declines in visuospatial ability, verbal fluency, motor coordination, and planning [25]. It is recommended that screening for dementia begin at the age of 40 years for all adults with DS [26].

4.3 Assessment

The genetic confirmation of DS can be established through several means. Prenatal screening of DS through noninvasive prenatal screening (NIPS) is available. In the case of a positive NIPS, expectant mothers should be offered confirmatory prenatal diagnostic testing through amniocentesis or chorionic villus sampling (CVS). It is essential to understand that NIPS is a screening rather than a diagnostic test. After birth, DS can be diagnosed through routine chromosome analysis, which will demonstrate the additional chromosomal material. It is important to know that chromosome analysis of an expanded cell count, typically 50 cells, may be needed to detect mosaicism. Additionally, although chromosomal microarray, which analyzes the ratio of chromosome complement (or fluorescence in situ hybridization (FISH) test), would detect the additional chromosome material from chromosome 21 in DS, neither chromosomal microarray nor FISH describes the relationship of this material to other chromosomes. In other words, a chromosomal microarray and FISH test cannot distinguish between free trisomy 21 and translocation trisomy 21. The distinction between free trisomy 21 and translocation trisomy 21 has potential implications for recurrence risk counseling for parents. It would lead one to offer testing to parents to evaluate for a balanced translocation if the infant is found to have translocation trisomy 21 [27].Therefore, the "gold standard" diagnostic test is *routine chromosome analysis*, which can be performed prenatally (on amniocytes or CVS) or after birth (on infant's peripheral blood or cord blood) and can both detect trisomy 21 as well as distinguish between free trisomy and translocations.

In some instances, one might want to proceed with additional genetic testing beyond chromosome analysis in patients with DS. For example, in those with DS and co-occurring ASD, one might follow the tiered workup for ASD as outlined by the American College of Medical Genetics [2].

4.4 Psychosocial Treatment

Non-pharmacological treatments for developmental, behavioral, and psychiatric co-occurring conditions with DS are varied. In early childhood, cognitive, language, and fine and gross motor delays are best treated with developmental therapy, speech-language therapy (ST), physical therapy (PT), and occupational therapy (OT). In the USA, these interventions are generally provided by Early Intervention or Birth-to-Three programs.

After the age of 3 years, interventions for DS include educational interventions (in the USA, generally provided as part of an Individualized Education Program or IEP), behavioral therapies, and psychotherapeutic strategies. Educational interventions are varied and are generally similar to teaching others with intellectual disabilities. However, many people with DS have relative adaptive skill strengths compared to their intellectual abilities. Positive behavior supports and Applied Behavioral Analysis (ABA)-based interventions are helpful for individuals with DS with or without co-occurring ASD. Additional outpatient rehabilitative services

(ST, PT, and OT) on an ongoing basis outside of school may also be required. Access to ongoing comprehensive medical care and adequate community, recreational, and social services also play a role in preventing and treating mental health concerns for individuals with DS.

For psychiatric conditions, psychotherapy can be beneficial. Cognitive behavioral therapy (CBT) has, in general, some evidence for use in individuals with intellectual disabilities and co-occurring anxious or depressive symptoms. There are no studies or reports of CBT specifically for individuals with DS at this time.

4.5 Biological Treatments

4.5.1 ADHD

Treatment studies for ADHD in DS are limited. In a retrospective study by Roche et al. [28] including 21 individuals with DS, 76% demonstrated improved concentration and hyperactivity with methylphenidate (MPH). Symptoms of oppositional defiant disorder also improved in a subset of patients with MPH treatment. Of note, this study also included subjects with ASD; these subjects demonstrated improvement in concentration, decreased hyperactivity, and oppositional behavior. The average dose for individuals who responded to MPH was 0.82 mg/kg/day. Reported side effects included loss of appetite (29%), dose-related worsening of tics (14%), apathy (14%), and insomnia (19%). Rebound effects were noticed in 19%. The authors of this study do not further define what they considered to be rebound effects. Of note, 43% of subjects in the study experienced no adverse events. Considering the higher rate of congenital heart disease in individuals with DS, it is vital to be aware of the presence of or a history of congenital heart disease when considering ADHD treatments. In patients with congenital heart disease, getting a baseline EKG and consulting with the patient's cardiologist is recommended [28]. An open-label trial of guanfacine for ADHD included 23 subjects with DS with an age range of 4–12 years. The Aberrant Behavioral Checklist, irritability (ABC–I) and hyperactivity (ABC-H) subscales, and total ABC score decreased with treatment. Side effects reported included nighttime sedation and asymptomatic low blood pressure [29]. Finally, a case report of a 7-year-old female with DS and comorbid ADHD described a favorable response to extended-release methylphenidate [30], albeit accompanied by a significant increase in repetitive and compulsive behaviors. The addition of aripiprazole 3 mg daily resulted in the resolution of the compulsive symptoms.

4.5.2 Autism Spectrum Disorder

There are currently no FDA-approved treatments for the core symptoms of ASD. At this time, risperidone and aripiprazole are only approved for autistic-related irritability. Of note, studies that contributed to these FDA approvals did not include subjects with DS. In 2008, Capone and colleagues published findings of an open-label trial of risperidone for behavioral symptoms in children with DS. Twenty-three subjects participated in this study. The total daily dose of risperidone ranged from 0.25 to 1.5 mg per day, and the duration of treatment was for up to 13 weeks. The scores on multiple ABC subscales decreased significantly. Side effects included increased appetite, weight gain (1.0–6.8 kg), excessive daytime sedation, and extra-pyramidal symptoms [31]. In 2016, Bacanli and colleagues [32] published a case of a 6-year-old male with DS and ASD treated with 5 mg of aripiprazole for behavioral symptoms, including hyperactivity, provoked aggression, and self-injurious behavior. Improvements in the irritability, hyperactivity, and lethargy subscales of the ABC were observed. Side effects included sedation and a 0.2-kg weight gain.

4.5.3 Depression

Before 2021, the literature on the treatment of depression in DS existed in small case reports in which most of the patients were treated with tricyclic antidepressants (TCAs), which are no longer considered first-line in the treatment of major depressive disorder. In 2021, Thom et al. reported findings of a retrospective chart review of 11 adults with DS (mean age 46 years). All patients in this study completed at least a 12-week course of a selective serotonin reuptake inhibitor. Nine out of the 11 (82%) patients were considered treatment responders. Approximately 36% experienced adverse reactions, most commonly daytime sedation and anger. In this study, eight were on fluoxetine, two were on sertraline, and one was on escitalopram [11].

4.5.4 Anxiety

Evidence for the treatment of anxiety in people with DS is limited to a case series consisting of one adolescent and two young adults with DS. Improvement was seen with buspirone (dose range 10–22.5 mg/day). All three patients tolerated buspirone and had no adverse events [15].

4.5.5 Bipolar Disorder

Evidence for treating bipolar disorder is limited to case reports. The described cases were treated with various medications, including typical antipsychotics, carbamazepine, and lithium. Given the propensity for obesity, medications that have a lower tendency for weight gain are preferred in patients with DS [20].

4.5.6 Catatonia

For catatonia in people with DS, high doses of benzodiazepines such as lorazepam are considered the first line of treatment. If lorazepam is ineffective, electroconvulsive therapy (ECT) is regarded as the next best step [20]. Other pharmacological agents that have shown some promise in treating catatonia in people with DS include quinidine and dextromethorphan [23].

4.5.7 Regression

Among those with regression, emerging evidence suggests that intravenous immunoglobulin (IVIg) and ECT may be effective for some; psychiatric medications were used in some patients who had resolution of regression symptoms [33, 34]. Of course, each individual with DS is unique and may have different medical and behavioral features that change throughout their lifespan. Therefore, tailoring treatment to an individual is always necessary.

4.5.8 Alzheimer's Disease

Currently, there are no approved drugs for treating dementia in persons with DS. Furthermore, a Cochrane review published in 2015 concluded that insufficient evidence exists to determine whether medications approved for treating sporadic Alzheimer's dementia are effective in treating cognitive decline in persons with DS [25].

4.6 Common Medical Comorbidities that Affect Psychopharmacologic Treatment

DS is associated with a unique profile of co-occurring medical conditions; several conditions are more likely to occur in DS, such as congenital heart disease [2, 3]. However, some diseases, such as solid tumors, are less common in individuals with DS [35]. To address the unique medical care needs of individuals with DS, guidance from the American Academy of Pediatrics (AAP) has been published, with the most recent update in 2022 [36]. Evidence-based guidance has also been published for adults with DS [26].

We now focus on select co-occurring medical conditions for psychiatrists to be aware of. Medical comorbidities can manifest as behavioral symptoms or contribute to worsening maladaptive behaviors in individuals with DS; clinicians need to be mindful of these common medical comorbidities when generating a differential diagnosis of comorbid psychiatric disorders and before initiating psychoactive drug treatment [20].

4.6.1 Congenital Heart Disease (CHD)

Congenital heart disease (CHD) is one of the co-occurring medical diagnoses associated with DS [37, 38]. Among patients with DS, the presence of CHD is a known contributor to morbidity and mortality [31]. Reviewing the existing literature, Santoro and Steffensen found that the prevalence of CHD in DS ranged from 20% to 58% in 18 studies; in later decades, the reported prevalence appeared constant, around 40–50% [39]. Freeman et al. reported the prevalence of CHD at 44%, including stillbirths; of these, atrioventricular septal defects are most common (45%), followed by ventricular septal defect (35%), secundum atrial septal defect (8%), tetralogy of Fallot (4%), and patent ductus arteriosus (7%) [40]. Adults with DS are at risk for valvular heart disease [26].

4.6.2 Obstructive Sleep Apnea

More than half (50–79%) of those with DS have obstructive sleep apnea (OSA) [36], with prevalence increasing through the lifespan. Obstructive sleep apnea can be silent/asymptomatic, and referral to a pediatric sleep laboratory for a sleep study or polysomnogram for all children with DS between ages 3 and 4 years is now recommended [36]. Obstructive sleep apnea can also cause symptoms such as heavy breathing, snoring, uncommon sleep positions, frequent night awakening, daytime sleepiness, apneic pauses, and behavior problems [36]. In patients with DS who have OSA, medications that increase appetite and are associated with weight gain (e.g., atypical antipsychotics and some mood stabilizers including valproic acid and lithium) should be avoided whenever possible [20].

4.6.3 Thyroid Disease

Approximately 50% of people with DS have Hashimoto's hypothyroidism, with prevalence increasing over the lifespan; 1 or 2% of infants with DS have congenital hypothyroidism [36]. Dry skin and hair thinning may be symptoms of hypothyroidism; it is recommended that thyroid function labs are checked at 6 months of age and then annually [36]. Similarly, for those diagnosed with hypothyroidism, the physician prescribing levothyroxine for treatment will typically follow thyroid function lab values often to ensure appropriate dosage to replace thyroid hormone and normalize lab values. Hypothyroidism, including untreated or insufficiently treated thyroid disease, should be ruled out before beginning antidepressant medication in a patient with DS presenting with depression [20].

4.6.4 Hearing

Hearing impairment is common in DS; 75–84% of individuals with DS may have conductive hearing loss [4, 36]. Hearing loss may fluctuate over time and occurs across the lifespan, but normal or nearly normal hearing can be achieved with otolaryngologic and audiologic interventions [4]. In general, hearing loss is a risk factor for delayed expressive language, challenges with articulation, and subsequent cognitive and psychosocial outcomes [41]. Prasher et al. found that adults with DS and a co-occurring hearing impairment had significantly more maladaptive behaviors than adults without hearing loss [42]. As such, excluding contributing hearing loss when treating behavior concerns in patients with DS is important.

4.6.5 Vision

Visual problems, including nystagmus, glaucoma, cataracts, strabismus, keratoconus, and refractive errors, are seen in 57% of people with DS [4]. Vision impairments in children and adults with DS can result in adverse cognitive outcomes and impact social behavior [41]. As such, it is important to exclude contributing vision issues when treating behavior concerns in patients with DS.

Key Points to Remember

- Down syndrome is the most common chromosomal cause of intellectual disability.
- People with Down syndrome have an increased risk of medical comorbidities including congenital heart defects, gastrointestinal diseases, and endocrine abnormalities.
- People with Down syndrome have an elevated risk for psychiatric disorders.
- It is essential for clinicians to be aware and vigilant for medical comorbidities as these may affect symptoms and treatment management.
- Dementia and depression in people with Down syndrome can look similar. Depression is more likely in a young adult (under the age of 40 years) and/or when symptoms of depression precede or accompany cognitive changes.
- Individuals with Down syndrome have a high tendency toward obesity. Therefore, weight-neutral psychotropic medications are generally preferred.

Photographs of Individuals with the Syndrome

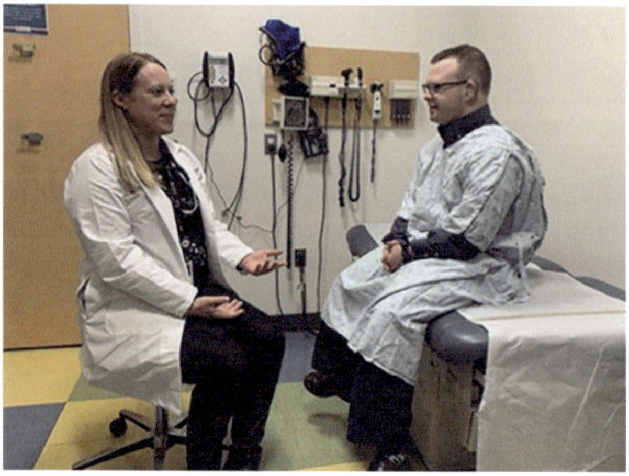

References

1. de Graaf G, Buckley F, Skotko BG. Estimation of the number of people with Down syndrome in the United States. Genet Med. 2017;19(4):439–47.
2. Antonarakis SE, Skotko BG, Rafii MS, Strydom A, Pape SE, Bianchi DW, et al. Down syndrome. Nat Rev Dis Primer. 2020;6(1):9.
3. Bull MJ, Committee on Genetics. Health supervision for children with Down syndrome. Pediatrics. 2011;128(2):393–406.
4. Bull MJ. Down syndrome. N Engl J Med. 2020;382(24):2344–52.
5. McCarthy J, Boyd J. Psychopathology and young people with Down's syndrome: childhood predictors and adult outcome of disorder. J Intellect Disabil Res. 2001;45(Pt 2):99–105.
6. Dykens EM. Psychiatric and behavioral disorders in persons with Down syndrome. Ment Retard Dev Disabil Res Rev. 2007;13(3):272–8.
7. Ekstein S, Glick B, Weill M, Kay B, Berger I. Down syndrome and attention-deficit/hyperactivity disorder (ADHD). J Child Neurol. 2011;26(10):1290–5.
8. Esbensen AJ, Vincent LB, Epstein JN, Kamimura-Nishimura K, Wiley S, Angkustsiri K, et al. Co-occurring medical and behavioural conditions in children with Down syndrome with or without ADHD symptom presentation. J Intellect Disabil Res. 2022;66(3):282–96.
9. Spinazzi NA, Velasco AB, Wodecki DJ, Patel L. Autism spectrum disorder in Down syndrome: experiences from caregivers. J Autism Dev Disord. 2023.
10. Vicari S, Pontillo M, Armando M. Neurodevelopmental and psychiatric issues in Down's syndrome: assessment and intervention. Psychiatr Genet. 2013;23(3):95–107.
11. Thom RP, Palumbo ML, Thompson C, McDougle CJ, Ravichandran CT. Selective serotonin reuptake inhibitors for the treatment of depression in adults with Down syndrome: a preliminary retrospective chart review study. Brain Sci. 2021;11(9):1216.
12. Rivelli A, Fitzpatrick V, Chaudhari S, Chicoine L, Jia G, Rzhetsky A, et al. Prevalence of mental health conditions among 6078 individuals with Down syndrome in the United States. J Patient-Centered Res Rev. 2022;9(1):58–63.
13. Cooper SA, Collacott RA. Clinical features and diagnostic criteria of depression in Down's syndrome. Br J Psychiatry J Ment Sci. 1994;165(3):399–403.

14. Alexander M, Petri H, Ding Y, Wandel C, Khwaja O, Foskett N. Morbidity and medication in a large population of individuals with Down syndrome compared to the general population. Dev Med Child Neurol. 2016;58(3):246–54.
15. Howe YJ, Thom RP, Notson EE, McDougle CJ, Palumbo ML. Buspirone for the treatment of generalized anxiety disorder in Down syndrome: 3 cases. J Dev Behav Pediatr. 2022;43(1):38–43.
16. Evans DW, Kleinpeter FL, Slane MM, Boomer KB. Adaptive and maladaptive correlates of repetitive behavior and restricted interests in persons with Down syndrome and developmentally-matched typical children: a two-year longitudinal sequential design. PLoS One. 2014;9(4):e93951.
17. Glenn S. Repetitive behaviours and restricted interests in individuals with Down syndrome—one way of managing their world? Brain Sci. 2017;7(6):66.
18. Prasher VP, Day S. Brief report: obsessive-compulsive disorder in adults with Down's Syndrome. J Autism Dev Disord. 1995;25(4):453–8.
19. Charlot L, Fox S, Friedlander R. Obsessional slowness in Down's syndrome. J Intellect Disabil Res. 2002;46(Pt 6):517–24.
20. Palumbo ML, McDougle CJ. Pharmacotherapy of Down syndrome. Expert Opin Pharmacother. 2018;19(17):1875–89.
21. Santoro J, Filippink R, Baumer N, Bulova P, Handen B. Down syndrome regression disorder: updates and therapeutic advances. Curr Opin Psychiatry. 2023;36(2):96–103.
22. Rosso M, Fremion E, Santoro SL, Oreskovic NM, Chitnis T, Skotko BG, et al. Down syndrome disintegrative disorder: a clinical regression syndrome of increasing importance. Pediatrics. 2020;145(6):e20192939.
23. Santoro JD, Pagarkar D, Chu DT, Rosso M, Paulsen KC, Levitt P, et al. Neurologic complications of Down syndrome: a systematic review. J Neurol. 2021;268(12):4495–509.
24. Dykens EM, Shah B, Davis B, Baker C, Fife T, Fitzpatrick J. Psychiatric disorders in adolescents and young adults with Down syndrome and other intellectual disabilities. J Neurodev Disord. 2015;7(1):9.
25. Fortea J, Zaman SH, Hartley S, Rafii MS, Head E, Carmona-Iragui M. Alzheimer's disease associated with Down syndrome: a genetic form of dementia. Lancet Neurol. 2021;20(11):930–42.
26. Tsou AY, Bulova P, Capone G, Chicoine B, Gelaro B, Harville TO, et al. Medical care of adults with Down syndrome: a clinical guideline. JAMA. 2020;324(15):1543–56.
27. Sheets KB, Crissman BG, Feist CD, Sell SL, Johnson LR, Donahue KC, et al. Practice guidelines for communicating a prenatal or postnatal diagnosis of Down syndrome: recommendations of the national society of genetic counselors. J Genet Couns. 2011;20(5):432–41.
28. Roche M, Mircher C, Toulas J, Prioux E, Conte M, Ravel A, et al. Efficacy and safety of methylphenidate on attention deficit hyperactivity disorder in children with Down syndrome. J Intellect Disabil Res. 2021;65(8):795–800.
29. Capone GT, Brecher L, Bay M. Guanfacine use in children with Down syndrome and comorbid attention-deficit hyperactivity disorder (ADHD) with disruptive behaviors. J Child Neurol. 2016;31(8):957–64.
30. Sertdemir M, Akça ÖF. Aripiprazole treatment of compulsive behaviors associated with methylphenidate in a child with Down syndrome. J Clin Psychopharmacol. 2018;38(2):159–61.
31. Capone GT, Goyal P, Grados M, Smith B, Kammann H. Risperidone use in children with Down syndrome, severe intellectual disability, and comorbid autistic spectrum disorders: a naturalistic study. J Dev Behav Pediatr. 2008;29(2):106–16.
32. Bacanli A. Aripiprazole use in children diagnosed with Down syndrome and comorbid autism spectrum disorders. J Child Adolesc Psychopharmacol. 2016;26(3):306–8.
33. Santoro SL, Baumer NT, Cornacchia M, Franklin C, Hart SJ, Haugen K, et al. Unexplained regression in Down syndrome: Management of 51 patients in an international patient database. Am J Med Genet A. 2022;188(10):3049–62.
34. Santoro JD, Partridge R, Tanna R, Pagarkar D, Khoshnood M, Rehmani M, et al. Evidence of neuroinflammation and immunotherapy responsiveness in individuals with Down syndrome regression disorder. J Neurodev Disord. 2022;14(1):35.

35. Hasle H, Clemmensen IH, Mikkelsen M. Risks of leukaemia and solid tumours in individuals with Down's syndrome. Lancet Lond Engl. 2000;355(9199):165–9.
36. Bull MJ, Trotter T, Santoro SL, Christensen C, Grout RW, Council on Genetics, et al. Health supervision for children and adolescents with Down syndrome. Pediatrics. 2022;149(5):e2022057010.
37. Lin AE, Santoro S, High FA, Goldenberg P, Gutmark-Little I. Congenital heart defects associated with aneuploidy syndromes: new insights into familiar associations. Am J Med Genet C Semin Med Genet. 2020;184(1):53–63.
38. Versacci P, Di Carlo D, Digilio MC, Marino B. Cardiovascular disease in Down syndrome. Curr Opin Pediatr. 2018;30(5):616–22.
39. Santoro SL, Steffensen EH. Congenital heart disease in Down syndrome—a review of temporal changes. J Congenit Cardiol. 2021;5(1):1.
40. Freeman SB, Taft LF, Dooley KJ, Allran K, Sherman SL, Hassold TJ, et al. Population-based study of congenital heart defects in Down syndrome. Am J Med Genet. 1998;80(3):213–7.
41. Schworer EK, Ahmed A, Hogenkamp L, Moore S, Esbensen AJ. Associations among co-occurring medical conditions and cognition, language, and behavior in Down syndrome. Res Dev Disabil. 2022;126:104236.
42. Prasher VP. Screening of hearing impairment and associated effects on adaptive behaviour in adults with Down syndrome. Br J Dev Disabil. 1995;41(81):126–32.

Further Reading

Bull MJ. Committee on Genetics. Health supervision for children with Down syndrome. Pediatrics. 2011;128(2):393–406.

Bull MJ. Down syndrome. N Engl J Med. 2020;382(24):2344–52.

Palumbo ML, McDougle CJ. Pharmacotherapy of Down syndrome. Expert Opin Pharmacother. 2018;19(17):1875–89.

Angelman Syndrome

5

Christopher J. Keary, Nicole Simon, and Amanda Tourjee

5.1 General Overview

Angelman syndrome (AS) is a neurodevelopmental disorder that results in severe-to-profound intellectual disability (ID), gross and fine motor deficits, minimal expressive language, epilepsy, and a behavioral profile notable for strong social affinity and hyperexcitability. The disorder is named after Dr. Harry Angelman whose original paper describing three children with common behavioral and motor features as well as facial dysmorphology led to the identification of the syndrome [1]. More recent efforts have sought to develop criteria encompassing the most salient clinical features of AS to aid in its recognition [2]. The following features are universally seen in patients with AS: severe developmental delay with resulting functional challenges, speech impairment that differentially affects expressive language compared to receptive, movement disorder with gait ataxia, and behavioral features including frequent laughter/smiling, excitability, hand waving, and hypermotor behaviors. While the majority of patients with AS are nonverbal, a minority may have a small number of intelligible words, and a scant few demonstrate the use of multi-word phrases. Receptive language abilities are also delayed, but strong skills are demonstrated in terms of recognized vocabulary [3]. Microcephaly and epilepsy occur in more than 80% of cases. Common but not universal features include facial dysmorphology such as flat occiput, occipital groove, protruding tongue, and prognathism (underbite), hypopigmented skin, light hair and eye color, and wide mouth/wide-spaced teeth. Additional features include feeding challenges, drooling and mouthing behaviors, strabismus, scoliosis, constipation, and disordered sleep. Electroencephalographic (EEG) studies have traditionally played a

C. J. Keary (✉) · N. Simon · A. Tourjee
Angelman Syndrome Program, Lurie Center for Autism, Massachusetts General Hospital for Children, Boston, MA, USA
e-mail: CKEARY@MGH.HARVARD.EDU

R. P. Thom, C. J. McDougle (eds.), *Neuropsychiatric Care for Genetic Syndromes and Other Neurodevelopmental Disorders*,
https://doi.org/10.1007/978-3-031-76269-7_5

major role in the identification of AS, as abnormalities in delta power and rhythmicity are typically seen regardless of wakefulness or seizure status [4].

Angelman syndrome is caused by insufficient expression of ubiquitin-protein ligase E3A (UBE3A), which is from the *UBE3A* gene on the maternal copy of chromosome 15 [5]. The preferential expression of *UBE3A* from the maternal allele is due to *UBE3A* being paternally imprinted and, therefore, silenced. Haploinsufficiency of the *UBE3A* gene can come about through multiple different molecular mechanisms. These include deletion of the maternal 15q11.2–13.1 region (representing about three-quarters of cases), paternal uniparental disomy (UPD), mutation of the maternal *UBE3A* gene, and imprinting center defects. While all patients share some common features such as ID and impaired expressive language, patients with deletions in the 15q11.2–13.1 region generally demonstrate more severe motor impairment and seizures [6]. The understanding of the genetic underpinnings of the syndrome has aided in early recognition and diagnosis, with more recent studies suggesting prevalence rates in the 1:20,000–1:50,000 range [7, 8].

It is still being understood how deficient *UBE3A* expression translates to the phenotypic features of AS. UBE3A is responsible for ubiquitination, a cellular process that marks proteins for degradation and removal [9]. It also has a regulatory role for multiple other genes involved in nervous system development [10]. Postmortem studies in patients with AS demonstrate abnormal neuronal distribution and arborization [11]. Mouse models of AS wherein the *UBE3A* gene has been inactivated, show phenotypic features similar to those seen in humans, including epilepsy, cognitive impairment, and ataxic gait [12]. Murine research has demonstrated that the long noncoding antisense transcript at the *UBE3A* locus (UBE3A-ATS) differentially prevents expression of the paternal chromosome [13]. Efforts to block the expression of UBE3A-ATS are the focus of current research aimed toward therapeutics that may restore the expression of *UBE3A* in patients with AS. Additional important research efforts seek to characterize the nature of the cognitive, neurologic, and behavioral challenges in this population, including a National Institutes of Health-funded study assessing the natural course of the syndrome across the lifespan [14–16].

5.2 Signs and Symptoms of Common Psychiatric Comorbidities

While clinical evaluation should focus on the caregivers' chief complaint, the clinician should also screen for hyperactivity/inattention, aggression/self-injury, anxiety, impairing repetitive behaviors, and disordered sleep, as these are the most common behavioral concerns in patients with AS [17].

Hyperactivity is one of the most consistently reported behavioral concerns in patients with AS. Some of the first case series describing patients across the age range included descriptions of hyperactivity [18–20] that was a frequent area of clinical concern. Hypermotoric behavior represented a common enough feature of the condition that it is now considered one of the consensus criteria of clinical features [2]. One of the first studies to formally assess behavioral concerns in a large group of patients with AS demonstrated elevated scores on standardized measures of hyperactivity [21]. Another study found higher levels of hyperactivity among subjects with AS compared to groups with general developmental disability [22]. Data from the natural history study in AS represents some of the strongest evidence for the clinical impact of hyperactivity. Sadhwani and colleagues' 2019 analysis of 301 individuals with AS reported concerns with hyperactivity and short attention span by 65% and 87% of caregivers, respectively [17]. Hyperactivity was associated with higher cognitive functioning as well as increased parental stress. This study found worsening hyperactivity with age, although other studies reported decreased hyperactivity with age [21, 23].

The recognition of hyperactivity in a clinical interview is often aided by the clear appearance of hypermotoric behavior in the office environment. Patients may not be able to tolerate even short interviews without exploration of the office, and caregivers often come prepared for appointments with behavioral supports such as preferred leisure activities or the use of seatbelts and shoulder straps on a wheelchair. Caregivers may report concerns regarding their child's constant need to move or explore, resulting in inadvertent property destruction or risk of injury. Therapists and teachers may note the need for constant movement breaks or that distractibility limits therapeutic and/or educational progress. Behavioral programs that incentivize on-task work may be of limited benefit because of the need for constant movement. Such behaviors may be worse during unstructured time, particularly in the summer, reflecting the patient's inability to sustain their attention on preferred leisure activities. Frequently patients require a prolonged summer school program to avoid behavioral worsening.

Aggressive and self-injurious behavior (SIB) also represent some of the most common behavioral concerns expressed by caregivers [17, 24, 25]. Biting, hair pulling, forceful grabs, or head banging, frequently directed toward parents, siblings, school peers, or teachers are common. Such behaviors can have a wide range of antecedents and precipitating factors that may be unrelated to irritable mood or intent to harm others. For example, such behaviors may occur during periods of apparent excitement or social interactions, with the aim of seeking or maintaining a preferred caregiver's attention [26]. Such behaviors may alternatively indicate hunger, pain, or tiredness and the clinician should also evaluate for co-occurring medical conditions that may be causing discomfort. Unrecognized medical illnesses, particularly constipation, dysmenorrhea, gastroesophageal reflux disease (GERD), dental problems, scoliosis, or postictal confusion/sedation, can easily be missed in patients with AS. The high rate of stereotypy in patients with AS suggests a strong preference for certain types of sensory input (particularly chewing, for example). Biting or other unsafe behaviors may be driven by patients' unique sensory needs rather than a clear external trigger. Finally, such behaviors may occur in response to non-preferred demands, indicating an attempt to communicate frustration or escape a caregiver's demand.

Anxiety is another possible precipitant for aggression or SIB. Caregiver reports have identified these challenging behaviors as a response to potential anxiety-provoking stimuli such as separation, crowds, new environments, strangers, or a fear of falling [25, 27]. These studies found that aggression was a common behavioral manifestation of distress in response to these situations. Loud vocalizations, fearful facial expressions, tremulousness, and crying were also common. Another notable behavior seen in such circumstances was gagging, vomiting, or swallowing, raising the need to carefully distinguish between symptoms of anxiety and gastroenterological conditions.

Given the range of potential precipitating factors of aggression and SIB, the evaluator should assess for antecedents and consequences in order to understand the behaviors and develop a treatment plan. Clinicians should assess for common precipitants that might suggest anxiety (crowds, novelty, or anticipated separation), poor frustration tolerance (denied access to preferred activity), desire for attention (patient delight when caregiver attention follows the behavior), or even hyperactivity (boredom and lack of structure). Signs of adrenergic excess such as sweating, tremulousness, and nausea may also suggest anxiety, though clinicians should attempt to distinguish these from conditions such as GERD. It is not unusual for behaviors to have different triggers depending on the situation or for the same behaviors to be more impactful in adolescence, compared to earlier in life.

Repetitive behaviors and restricted/highly focused interests are also commonly reported in patients with AS. These behaviors can include repetitive chewing/mouthing [2] and body-focused stereotypies such as an obsessional fixation with specific hand and body movements [28]. Repetitive chewing and mouthing can damage teeth, result in calluses on fingers, or damage fingernails and toenails. Clinicians should consider whether stereotyped behaviors are truly impairing before they consider developing a treatment plan. It is important to assess whether behaviors exacerbate distractibility or impair progress in various therapies. The co-occurrence of pica, defined as compulsive swallowing of nonfood items, can be dangerous and should be identified. If present, patients require close individual supervision in schools, day programs, and other settings because, if an item is swallowed, it may require urgent medical attention.

Finally, disordered sleep is seen in the majority of patients with AS, with some studies reporting estimates as high as 80% [29–31]. The most common sleep issues include difficulty initiating sleep, frequent nighttime awakening, and reduced total sleep time [15, 32]. While these challenges are most prevalent in children, it is not uncommon for sleep disorders to persist into adulthood [33, 34]. Caregivers may become accustomed to persistently disordered sleep patterns in their loved ones with AS and may not raise the behavior as a main concern. Therefore, clinicians should ask about sleep patterns as part of the behavioral assessment since poor sleep complicates the care of patients with AS and can contribute to caregiver stress [35].

5.3 Assessment

The development of a treatment plan should begin with confirming the diagnosis of AS. A definitive diagnosis can be made in the vast majority of cases through genetic testing, which may begin with a chromosomal microarray (CMA). This testing detects clinically significant deletions or duplications and will identify the ~70% of patients who inherited their AS through a deletion on the maternal chromosome 15 that includes the *UBE3A* gene. DNA methylation tests and UBE3A sequencing tests may be performed next if the concern is still high for AS. DNA methylation testing in the 15q11.2–13.1 region allows for the identification of the imprinting status of each chromosome, which will diagnose AS in patients with UPD and imprinting center defects. Finally, a specific *UBE3A* sequence analysis will identify small mutations in *UBE3A* or the imprinting center that are too small to be identified by other methods.

Once the diagnosis is confirmed, an assessment of behavioral concerns should include identifying common antecedents and consequences in order to ascertain the function of challenging behaviors. Gathering observations from multiple informants who work with the patient in different environments can be illuminating. An absence of external antecedents should prompt the evaluator to consider if pain or discomfort due to an underlying medical condition (for instance, constipation, dysmenorrhea, or GERD) may be contributing. Similarly, behavioral problems can occur in response to medication changes, which may indicate the presence of side effects that the patient can't communicate. Changes in or the loss of daytime routine and structure can be the precipitating factor for problematic behaviors, as can changes in staff who work with the patient.

The development of a treatment plan for behavioral concerns should include recommendations for skill-based therapies (speech, physical, and occupational), behavioral treatments/plans, contributing comorbid medical issues, and the use of psychiatric medications. Communication between the different members of a treatment team can be essential. For instance, behavioral therapists may work with speech therapists to choose an icon on an augmentative and alternative communication (AAC) device to seek attention to replace disruptive and attention-seeking behavior. Therapists should be kept apprised of medication changes to give feedback on their effects, and medical specialists should communicate to avoid multiple medication changes at once. Finally, parents and caregivers must be included as active participants in the development of treatment plans to leverage their experience and expertise in understanding their loved ones with AS.

5.4 Psychosocial Treatments

5.4.1 Role and Evidence Base for Behavioral Therapy in Angelman Syndrome

Behavioral therapies, such as Applied Behavior Analysis (ABA), play an important role in the understanding and treatment of behavioral concerns in AS. Applied Behavioral Analysis is a discipline in which behavioral principles are applied in real-world settings such as schools and homes with the goal of improving socially important issues such as behaviors, communication, and learning [36]. Key features of an ABA-based approach include the objective measurement of behavior through data collection, analysis of the function of the behavior, and the systematic use of procedures based on scientifically established principles of behavior, such as reinforcement and punishment [37]. The Individuals with Disabilities Education Act (IDEA, 1997/2004) requires that a functional behavioral assessment (FBA), the standard behavioral assessment used in ABA, be completed before developing a behavior plan for any child with a disability. Children with AS and problematic behavior are, therefore, entitled to an FBA that informs a behavior plan.

In the past 50 years, a substantial scientific evidence base supporting ABA as a treatment for children and adults with ID and related disorders has developed (e.g., [38–42]). Specifically, ABA-based procedures have been shown to be effective in reducing problematic behaviors and developing adaptive skills. However, few research studies have specifically examined the effects of ABA therapy on individuals with AS. Despite small sample sizes, the studies that have been published are promising and indicate the need for further research [26, 43–47].

5.4.1.1 Skill Development

Given the high prevalence of ID within AS, it is important to highlight the value of using ABA to teach a variety of skills. The effect of educational approaches using ABA principles on the neurological development of four children ages 3.1–9.2 years with AS was evaluated using pre- and post-standardized measures of cognitive, adaptive, and language functioning [43]. The approaches were used for one year. The control group included other children with AS matched by chronological age, gender, and molecular diagnostic subtype. Results showed improvement for the treatment group in receptive language and fine motor movements that remained at the nonsignificant level compared to controls, likely owing to the small sample size. The use of the ABA teaching methodology, discrete trial training (DTT), to teach functional skills to three children ages 3.1–6.9 years with AS has also been reported [44]. Discrete trial training is one of several teaching techniques within ABA that uses a structured teaching approach to break skills down into smaller components. Functional skills included following one-step directions, requesting preferred items, self-help skills, and play and leisure skills. Parents viewed this teaching methodology and its outcomes favorably.

Self-help skills vary amongst individuals with AS. Regarding toileting into adulthood, only about a third of individuals (including adults) remain dry during the daytime and fewer overnight [15, 19]. One study found that the use of a modified Azrin-Foxx toilet training procedure was successful in six children ages 6–19 years with AS and ID [45]. This toileting procedure is based on the principles of ABA. The initial procedure includes drinking fluids every 30 min, scheduled toileting every 30 min until elimination occurs, and the use of edible and social reinforcers every 5 min for remaining dry and/or for elimination. When accidents occur, the participant is prompted to change clothing and clean the soiled area, toys are removed from the bathroom, and there are no reinforcers for remaining dry for the next hour. While the typical procedures were modified, all six participants showed improvement in toileting skills and maintained those skills over the next 2.5 years. For example, some of the participants showed signs of self-initiating toilet use, and all of the participants needed less assistance while dressing.

5.4.1.2 Social Interest and Functional Analysis (FA)

Since children with AS often have a strong social interest, an effective methodology to teach social skills is particularly relevant and needed. In the absence of learning appropriate social interactions, an individual with AS may use challenging behavior to elicit attention. One study found the use of an ABA-based procedure, discrimination training, successful in teaching three boys with AS how to appropriately initiate social interactions with others [46].

A study including 12 children with aggression and AS hypothesized that an experimental functional analysis (FA) would find that the aggressive behavior was attention-maintained [26]. Experimental FA is recommended for use in ABA when an FBA does not yield conclusive results about the hypothesized function of the behavior. An FBA relies on indirect assessment and observation tools. In an FA, environmental variables are systematically manipulated in an attempt to demonstrate the function of the behavior or turn the behavior on or off. Results of the experimental FA indicated that behavior was maintained by attention in only one of the 12 children. However, the results might be misleading as the authors noted that the pattern of increased aggression in the high social contact condition paired with positive affect might indicate that the aggression serves to maintain and initiate social contact (attention-maintained).

The social nature of individuals with AS is a strength that can be leveraged to build strong relationships with caregivers, which can help increase motivation and quality of life. Social reinforcers (high-fives, smiles, praise, etc.) should be embedded throughout the day to create a positive environment and assist with skill development. Additionally, pictures, videos, and sensory interventions can all serve as reinforcers for individuals with AS.

5.4.1.3 Functional Communication Training (FCT)

A few studies have found that Functional Communication Training (FCT) can help to reduce challenging behaviors in individuals with AS [47]. In FCT, an intervention widely used in ABA, challenging behavior is replaced by a functionally equivalent communicative response [48]. For example, if the challenging behavior is escape-motivated, the individual may be taught to say "break," sign "break," or touch a break symbol instead of engaging in the challenging behavior. The individual is then granted a brief escape from an undesirable task. Because the consequence (escape from a non-preferred task) is the same, the behavior of communicating the need for a break replaces the challenging behavior. In one study, FA was used to identify the function of challenging behavior in three individuals with AS. In all three children, challenging behavior decreased because of FCT [47].

In conclusion, the limited but promising research on the use of ABA in AS, in conjunction with the vast amount of research on the success of ABA within the ID population as a treatment for problematic behaviors, suggests this approach should be a key aspect of addressing behavioral concerns and developing skills in children and adults with AS.

5.4.2 Additional Non-Pharmacological Interventions

5.4.2.1 Hyperactivity

Non-pharmacologic interventions for hyperactivity involve a balance between accommodations that reduce attentional demands and support the need for physical movement and incentives that increase motivation for sustained attention. Many school-based supports include scheduling more frequent movement breaks, reward systems for sustaining attention using the concepts of ABA described above, and even a 1:1 staff member to allow inclusion while minimizing classroom disruption. While general distractibility is common, patients with AS may be particularly sensitive to distraction from social interaction. Thus, schools must find the balance between offering inclusion time among peers and individual time to allow for making progress in therapies. Hyperactivity often persists into adulthood, emphasizing the need for physical activity in the day programs that serve adults with AS. Finally, all staff members working with patients with AS should be aware of the risk of falls due to the combination of hyperactivity, ataxia, and still-emerging ambulation skills. Wheelchairs can play an important role in containing hypermotoric behavior, even among those who can ambulate independently. This may allow for greater community involvement in a safe way.

5.4.2.2 Aggression/Self-Injurious Behavior

The beginning of any treatment plan for aggression and SIB includes an examination of the antecedents and consequences of such behaviors in order to understand their function. Functional behavioral assessments, as described above, aid in this process and allow for focused treatment ideas based on the function of the behavior. Augmentative and alternative communication devices or strategies can provide the opportunity for functional communication, allowing the patient to voice pain or hunger. Systematic redirection of the patient to use communication strategies to "take a break" or request social interaction can replace disruptive or attention-seeking behaviors that seem to "come out of the blue." It is common for AAC specialists and behavioral therapists to need to work together to develop a behavioral treatment plan when seeking to direct patients to use communication rather than challenging behavior. For aggression/SIB that occurs in response to non-preferred demands or limit setting, patients may respond to a consistent "first this, then that" reward system. Such programs can be implemented formally as part of a behavioral plan under the guidance of a specialist such as a Board-Certified Behavioral Analyst (BCBA). It is easy for well-meaning teachers, family, and staff to inadvertently reinforce unsafe behaviors, particularly when behaviors are attention-seeking and cannot be safely ignored. Expert behavioral consultation helps support and empower teaching staff and caregivers to respond consistently and safely to these behaviors. Finally, overexcitability can play a major role in impulsive aggression in AS. Occupational therapists can play an important role in identifying sensory experiences that might be leading to excitability and calming sensory strategies (for instance, weighted blankets).

5.4.2.3 Repetitive Behaviors

Treatment approaches for repetitive behaviors in patients with AS, when necessary, include occupational therapy and using systems of reinforcement through behavioral techniques. Repetitive behaviors often include stereotypies which are reinforced by preferred sensory input rather than external stimuli or circumstances. High rates of sensory-seeking behaviors as well as hyper- or hyporesponsive sensory processing have been identified in populations with AS [49]. Occupational therapy can include an assessment of patients' sensory processing and allow for the identification of alternative methods to get preferred sensory input. Chewy tubes, weighted blankets, and hand fidgets may all serve to replace other sensory-seeking behaviors that cause hygiene or safety issues. Instituting new sensory interventions may require a reward system or the use of a timer to increase tolerance for the initially less preferred sensory item.

5.4.2.4 Sleep Disorders

There is an important role for environmental and behavioral treatments in addressing sleep disorders in AS. Environmental interventions include white noise machines, consistent bedtimes, cool temperatures, and heavy curtains. Enclosed beds with a camera in the room for monitoring can both prevent unsafe nighttime wandering and monitor for medical issues such as seizures that may also be disrupting sleep. Behavioral treatments seek to reduce the pattern wherein a caregiver's presence becomes a necessary "sleep-onset association." When this becomes the case, it can worsen mid-cycle awakenings wherein patients become hypervigilant to the presence of caregivers, which may promote wakefulness during lighter stages of sleep. Behavioral interventions seek to support the patient in tolerating increasing durations of time alone in bed at the time of sleep-onset.

A recent 26-week trial in two 18-year-olds with AS compared behavioral treatment techniques to a control group [50]. Outcome measures included questionnaires, sleep diaries, actigraphy, and videosomnography [50]. Important components of the treatment program included education on normal sleep and sleep problems as well as treatment recommendations from and routine meetings with a behavioral therapist. Recommended techniques included bedtime fading, gradual extinction, and gradual distancing [51]. Improvements were seen in total sleep time, sleep-onset latency, and both the number and duration of awakenings after sleep-onset compared to the control group. These data indicate that once the contribution from co-occurring medical issues has been ruled out, the first-line treatment for sleep disturbance in AS should be behavioral [33, 52].

5.5 Biological Treatments

5.5.1 Hyperactivity/Impulsivity

Pharmacologic interventions for hyperactivity in AS are drawn predominantly from research in individuals with autism spectrum disorder (ASD), with little in the way of research specific to AS. Among neurotypical patients with attention-deficit/hyperactivity disorder (ADHD), stimulant medications are the first-line treatment for hyperactivity and inattention [53]. A recent case series suggests a need for caution with such medications in patients with AS due to poor tolerability of stimulants [54]. Adverse events seen in double-blind, placebo-controlled trials of stimulants in children with ASD include irritability, appetite suppression, difficulty falling asleep, and emotional outbursts [55]. Guanfacine is a non-stimulant medication with Food and Drug Administration (FDA) approval for the treatment of ADHD in children aged 6–17 years. It has the benefit of improved tolerability in studies of children with ASD where hyperactivity was the target of treatment [56]. Guanfacine is, therefore, a superior first-line treatment for hyperactivity in AS, though clinicians should watch for constipation or fatigue as side effects. Other non-stimulant medications, including atomoxetine and clonidine, have also demonstrated improvements in hyperactivity in some patients with ASD ([57, 58], respectively) and may also be considered. Viloxazine is a newer norepinephrine reuptake inhibitor that received FDA approval for the treatment of ADHD in children aged 6–17 years. The ability to administer this medication without swallowing the capsule whole, as is needed with atomoxetine, offers ease of administration in AS; however, no trials have yet assessed its benefit or safety in patients with AS.

5.5.2 Aggression and Self-Injurious Behavior

Anxiety in patients with AS has been identified as a frequent area of concern for caregivers [29], and parents have reported aggression as the most common behavioral manifestation of suspected anxiety in patients with AS [25]. Therefore, treatments effective for anxiety are a common starting point for pharmacotherapy for aggressive behaviors in AS. In a case series of three adult patients with AS secondary to a maternal deletion of chromosome 15 q11–13, buspirone at a dosage of 2.5–10 mg given twice daily significantly reduced symptoms associated with anxiety, specifically SIB and aggression [59]. Buspirone is a serotonin $(5\text{-HT})_{1A}$ receptor partial agonist with an FDA indication for the treatment of generalized anxiety disorder in adults [60]. A recent analysis failed to show significant improvement in anxiety in neurotypical children [61]. Mirtazapine is a tetracyclic antidepressant, which is FDA-approved for use in adults with major depressive disorder. In a chart review of eight pediatric patients with AS, mirtazapine was reported to have a positive effect on behavior including a reduction in aggressive behaviors [62]. Clonazepam and short-term use of lorazepam have FDA indications for the treatment of anxiety disorders. Selective serotonin reuptake inhibitors (SSRIs) and other serotonergic medications are often first-line treatments for anxiety disorders in the neurotypical population; however, they have not yet been formally studied in AS. Results from studies of their use in children with ASD to target anxiety or repetitive behaviors have largely been negative [63–66], with some studies showing relatively high rates of behavioral activation and other side effects [67].

In addition to treatments effective for anxiety, clinicians may also consider pharmacological interventions helpful for irritability. Much of the pharmacological treatment of irritability in patients with AS in clinical practice is drawn from studies of medications used to treat irritability in patients with ASD. Propranolol is a beta blocker, primarily used as a treatment for hypertension, that has been studied for the treatment of irritability in various populations. A retrospective case series of patients with ASD (age range 11–32 years) who were prescribed propranolol for aggression and self-injury found that 39 out of 46 (84.7%) patients showed improvement on the Clinical Global Impressions Improvement (CGI-I) subscale [68]. Similarly, case studies in patients with ASD have found improvement in oppositional behavior with guanfacine [69] and aggression/irritability with clonidine [70]. Long-acting guanfacine and clonidine both carry FDA indications for the treatment of ADHD and may be specifically considered when hyperactivity or impulsivity is thought to be a contributing factor to aggression. Finally, two antipsychotic medications, risperidone and aripiprazole, have an FDA indication for the treatment of "irritability associated with ASD" in children and adolescents. No studies have examined their use for irritability in patients with AS. Potential side effects seen among patients with ASD include increased appetite, weight gain, constipation, fatigue, metabolic syndrome, and tardive dyskinesia. Antiepileptic drugs such as topiramate or gabapentin are commonly considered in clinical practice for the treatment of aggression in AS. The antiepileptic drugs such as valproic acid, carbamazepine, and oxcarbazepine should be used with significant caution as they can worsen seizures and motor function in AS [71].

5.5.3 Sleep Disorders

Both medical and behavioral issues should be considered when addressing sleep disturbance in children with AS. Low iron has been previously known to cause periodic leg movements during sleep, which may contribute to sleep difficulties in children with AS [72, 73]. A retrospective study of children with AS and disturbed patterns of sleep found that a significant portion of them had low iron and experienced improvement in sleep with iron replacement therapy [73]. Medical comorbidities such as epilepsy, GERD, and constipation are felt to likely impact sleep in patients with AS [32, 74]. These medical comorbidities should be evaluated for and, if present, addressed prior to treating sleep disturbance with medications.

One of the few double-blind, placebo-controlled trials of medications for sleep in AS was a trial of melatonin used for sleep disturbance in children [75]. Dosing was 5 mg of immediate release melatonin in children 6 years and older and 2.5 mg in children under 6 years of age. Children receiving melatonin were found to have decreased sleep-onset latency and increased total sleep time when compared to children receiving placebo. Studies of long-acting melatonin have been done in patients with ASD and have demonstrated not just decreased sleep-onset latency but also longer sleep duration at dosages between 2 and 10 mg per day [76, 77]. Using a long-acting formulation may be considered in patients with AS with interrupted mid-cycle sleep.

In a retrospective study of caregivers of patients with AS, participants were asked to rate the effectiveness and tolerability of medications used for sleep disturbance in their loved ones with AS [78]. The three most commonly prescribed medications were melatonin, clonidine, and trazodone with good tolerability and substantial numbers of caregivers reporting good effectiveness for each of these three medications. A separate retrospective chart review examined the use of mirtazapine, a noradrenergic and specific serotonergic antidepressant with antihistamine effects, for sleep disturbance among eight patients ages 3–16 years old with AS [62]. Seven out of eight of the patients reported improvements such as increased total sleep time, decreased nocturnal awakenings, and decreased time to fall asleep. Dosages between 3.75 and 30 mg nightly were used and side effects included increased appetite and weight gain. Other medications with anticonvulsant activity such as gabapentin or pregabalin, the antipsychotic medication quetiapine, and medications in the benzodiazepine class are also commonly used in clinical practice and may be considered for the treatment of sleep disturbance in AS, though additional trials are required to fully determine their efficacy, safety, and tolerability.

5.6 Common Medical Comorbidities

Epilepsy represents the most common comorbid medical condition in AS and contributes substantially to the medical care needs of these patients [79]. Epilepsy is most common, and often most severe, among patients with maternal deletion mechanisms of inheritance [80]. Seizure frequency often, but not always, improves in adolescence and adulthood. The treatment of epilepsy can be complicated, with most patients requiring multiple trials of different anticonvulsant medications and a significant portion of patients experiencing status epilepticus [81]. Patients can develop a wide range of seizure types including generalized tonic-clonic, atonic, absence, and myoclonic. Clinicians should be alert to the development of nonconvulsive status epilepticus (NCSE), which may present with mental status changes and skill regression without convulsions or symptoms more clearly indicative of a seizure. One study noted that features of NCSE can include eye rolling, eye fluttering, head nodding, somnolence, or motor regression and such episodes can be triggered by infection [82]. The behavioral consequences of epilepsy can be difficult to distinguish from myoclonus and tremor, which are also common neurologic features in AS and highlight the need for close collaboration with neurologists.

Gastrointestinal concerns are also common in AS and include constipation and GERD [83]. The cause of constipation is often multifactorial and can be exacerbated by a lack of mobility or medications prescribed for seizures or behavioral concerns. Ensuring regular physical activity as well as adequate fluid and fiber intake are important aspects of treatment, though many individuals with AS require the use of oral medications or suppositories [84]. Gastroesophageal reflux disease can present with coughing, repetitive swallowing, vomiting, regurgitating food during sleep, or signs of pain that occur after meals. While vomiting is reported by caregivers as a possible behavioral feature of anxiety [25], it is important to rule out GERD with the consideration of a trial of a proton pump inhibitor or H_2 receptor antagonist medication.

Orthopedic concerns in AS should be considered, including in adults, as they can be a frequent cause of pain and resultant behavioral changes. Hip dysplasia, subluxated or pronated ankles, and/or contractures can all complicate the development of independent ambulation [84]. The risk for scoliosis increases with age in patients with AS and warrants standard screening at checkups and a referral to orthopedics, if present [85]. The development of obesity in adulthood combined with decreased stamina can result in worsening motor function with time and warrants ongoing physical therapy.

Finally, ophthalmic and dental issues should be considered in the assessment of medical comorbidities. Ophthalmic concerns in AS include strabismus, exotropia, and astigmatism [86]. Intolerance of wearing glasses is a common challenge in AS, making it difficult to correct refractive errors. Clinicians may have to take into account vision challenges when considering AAC interventions for speech limitations. Similarly, tooth brushing can be difficult to implement, as can tolerance of dental examinations. Repetitive chewing and mouthing of objects can result in damage to the enamel and warrant the development of behavioral plans that institute soft chewy tubes. Dental pain should be considered in patients with acute behavioral changes, and many patients will require premedication or anesthesia for a thorough dental examination.

Key Points to Remember

- Angelman syndrome (AS) is a neurodevelopmental disorder characterized by intellectual disability, limited expressive language, sleep disorder, epilepsy, gross and fine motor impairment, and behavioral challenges.
- Speech therapy, occupational therapy, and applied behavioral analysis can all have a role in reducing challenging behaviors including aggression, self-injury, and hyperactivity.

- Treatments for anxiety including buspirone, mirtazapine, clonazepam, and propranolol may reduce aggressive behaviors, and atypical antipsychotics may be considered in severe cases.
- Alpha-$_2$ agonist medications such as guanfacine are superior first-line treatments for hyperactivity in patients with AS based on case reports of substantial behavioral worsening with stimulant medications.
- Behavioral therapy can be effective for the treatment of sleep disorders in AS by addressing the anxiety that arises with separation at bedtime.

Photographs of Individuals with the Syndrome

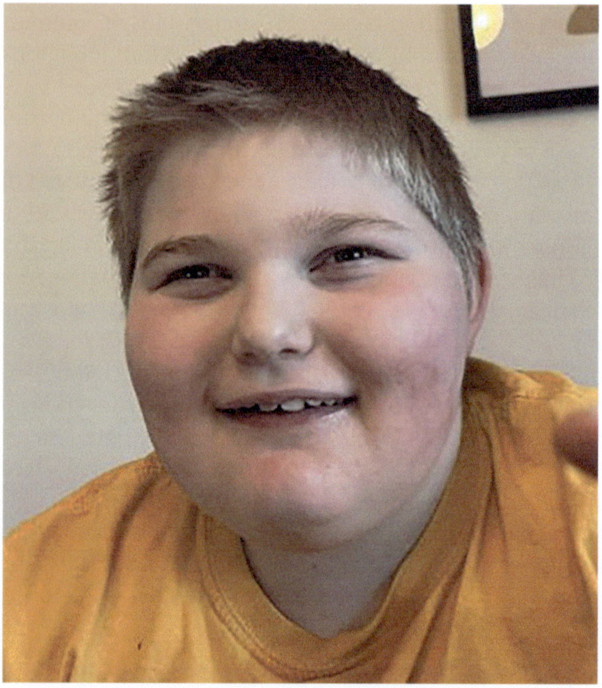

References

1. Angelman H. "Puppet" children. A report on three cases. Dev Med Child Neurol. 1965;7:681–8.
2. Williams CA, Beaudet AL, Clayton-Smith J, et al. Angelman syndrome 2005: updated consensus for diagnostic criteria. Am J Med Genet A. 2006;140:413–8.
3. Gentile JK, Tan W-H, Horowitz LT, Bacino CA, Skinner SA, Barbieri-Welge R, et al. A neurodevelopmental survey of Angelman syndrome with genotype-phenotype correlations. J Dev Behav Pediatr. 2010;31(7):592–601.

4. Sidorov MS, Deck GM, Dolatshahi M, Thibert RL, Bird LM, Chui CJ, Philpot BD. Delta rhythmicity is a reliable EEG biomarker in Angelman syndrome: a parallel mouse and human analysis. J Neurodev Disord. 2017;8:9–17.
5. Kishino T, Lalande M, Wagstaff J. UBE3A/E6-AP mutations cause Angelman syndrome. Nat Genet. 1997;15(1):70–3.
6. Minassian BA, DeLorey TM, Olsen RW, et al. Angelman syndrome: correlations between epilepsy phenotypes and genotypes. Ann Neurol. 1998;43:485–93.
7. Oiglane-Shlik E, Talvik T, Zordania R, et al. Prevalence of Angelman syndrome and Prader-Willi syndrome in Estonian children: Sister syndromes not equally represented. Am J Med Genet A. 2006;140:1936–43.
8. Luk HM, Lo IF. Angelman syndrome in Hong Kong Chinese: a 20 years' experience. Eur J Med Genet. 2016;59:315–9.
9. Jiang YH, Beaudet AL. Human disorders of ubiquitination and proteasomal degradation. Curr Opin Pediatr. 2004;16(4):419–26.
10. Low KS, Chen D. Genome-wide gene expression profiling of the Angelman syndrome mice with Ube3a mutation. Eur J Hum Genet. 2010;18:1228–35.
11. Kyriakides T, Hallam LA, Hockey A, Silberstein P, Kakulas BA. Angelman's syndrome: a neuropathological study. Acta Neuropathol. 1992;83:675–8.
12. Jiang YH, Armstrong D, Albrecht U, et al. Mutation of the Angelman ubiquitin ligase in mice causes increased cytoplasmic p53 and deficits of contextual learning and long-term potentiation. Neuron. 1998;21(4):799–811.
13. Meng L, Person RE, Huang W, et al. Truncation of Ube3a-ATS unsilences paternal Ube3a and ameliorates behavioral defects in the Angelman syndrome mouse model. PLoS Genet. 2013;9:e1004039.
14. Sadhwani A, Wheeler A, Gwaltney A, et al. Developmental skills of individuals with Angelman syndrome assessed using the Bayley-III. J Autism Dev Disord. 2023;53(2):720–37.
15. Larson AM, Shinnick JE, Shaaya EA, et al. Angelman syndrome in adulthood. Am J Med Genet A. 2015;167A:331–44.
16. Cassater D, Bustamante M, Sach-Peltason L, et al. Clinical characterization of epilepsy in children with Angelman syndrome. Pediatr Neurol. 2021;124:42–50.
17. Sadhwani A, Willen JM, LaVallee N, et al. Maladaptive behaviors in individuals with Angelman syndrome. Am J Med Genet A. 2019;179(6):983–92.
18. Zori RT, Hendrickson J, Woolven S, et al. Angelman syndrome: clinical profile. J Child Neurol. 1992;7:270–80.
19. Clayton-Smith J, Laan L. Angelman syndrome: a review of clinical and genetic aspects. J Med Genet. 2003;40:87–95.
20. Buntinx IM, Hennekam RCM, Brouwer OF, et al. Clinical profile of Angelman syndrome at different ages. Am J Med Genet. 1995;56:176–83.
21. Clarke DJ, Marston G. Problem behaviors associated with 15q-Angelman syndrome. Am J Ment Retard. 2000;105(1):25–31.
22. Barry RJ, Leitner RP, Clarke AR, et al. Behavioral aspects of Angelman syndrome: a case control study. Am J Med Genet. 2005;132:8–12.
23. Wheeler AC, Sacco P, Cabo R. Unmet clinical needs and burden in Angelman syndrome: a review of the literature. Orphanet J Rare Dis. 2017;12(1):164.
24. Arron K, Oliver C, Moss J, et al. The prevalence and phenomenology of self-injurious and aggressive behavior in genetic syndromes. J Intellect Disabil Res. 2011;55(2):109–20.
25. Keary CJ, Mullett JE, Nowinski L, et al. Parent description of anxiety in Angelman syndrome. J Autism Dev Disord. 2021;52(8):3612–25.
26. Strachan R, Shaw R, Burrow C, et al. Experimental functional analysis of aggression in children with Angelman syndrome. Res Dev Disab. 2009;30:1095–106.
27. Wheeler AC, Okoniewski KC, Wylie A, et al. Anxiety-associated and separation distress-associated behaviours in Angelman syndrome. J Intellect Disabil Res. 2019;63(10):1234–47.
28. Moss J, Oliver C, Arron K, et al. The prevalence and phenomenology of repetitive behavior in genetic syndromes. J Autism Dev Disord. 2009;39:572–88.

29. Clayton-Smith J. Angelman syndrome: evolution of the phenotype in adolescents and adults. Dev Med Child Neurol. 2001;43(7):476–80.
30. Sueri C, Ferlazzo E, Elia M, et al. Epilepsy and sleep disorders improve in adolescents and adults with Angelman syndrome: a multicenter study on 46 patients. Epilepsy Behav. 2017;75:225–9.
31. Veatch OL, Malow BA, Lee HS, et al. Evaluating sleep disturbances in children with rare genetic neurodevelopmental syndromes. Pediatr Neurol. 2021;123:30–7.
32. Conant KD, Thibert RL, Thiele EA. Epilepsy and the sleep–wake patterns found in Angelman syndrome. Epilepsia. 2009;50(11):2497–500.
33. Pelc K, Cheron G, Boyd SG, et al. Are there distinctive sleep problems in Angelman syndrome? Sleep Med. 2008;9(4):434–41.
34. Bruni O, Ferri R, D'Agostino G, et al. Sleep disturbances in Angelman syndrome: a questionnaire study. Brain Dev. 2004;26:233–40.
35. Griffith GM, Hastings RP, Oliver C, et al. Psychological well-being in parents of children with Angelman, Cornelia de Lange and Cri du Chat syndromes. J Intellect Disabil Res. 2011;55(4):397–410.
36. Baer D, Wolf M, Risley T. Some current dimensions of applied behavior analysis. J Appl Behav Anal. 1968;1:91–7.
37. Hanley GP, Iwata BA, McCord BE. Functional analysis of problem behavior: a review. J Appl Behav Anal. 2003;36:147–85.
38. Borrero CSW, Vollmer TR. Experimental analysis and treatment of multiply controlled problem behavior: a systemic replication and extension. J Appl Behav Anal. 2006;39:375–9.
39. Brosnan J, Healy O. A review of behavioral interventions for the treatment of aggression in individuals with developmental disabilities. Res Dev Disabil. 2011;32:437–46.
40. McGee SK, Ellis J. Extinction effects during the assessment of multiple problem behaviors. J Appl Behav Anal. 2000;33:313–6.
41. Hassiotis A, Robotham D, Canagasabey A, Romeo R, Langridge D, Blizard R, King M. Randomized, single-blind, controlled trial of a specialist behavior therapy team for challenging behavior in adults with intellectual disabilities. Am J Psychiatry. 2009;166:1278–85.
42. Roscoe EM, Iwata BA, Goh HL. A comparison of noncontingent reinforcement and sensory extinction as treatment for self-injurious behavior. J Appl Behav Anal. 1998;31:635–46.
43. Summers J. Neurodevelopmental outcomes in children with Angelman syndrome after 1 year of behavioural intervention. Dev Neurorehabil. 2012;15:239–52.
44. Summers JA, Szatmari P. Using discrete trial instruction to teach children with Angelman syndrome. Focus Aut Other Dev Disabil. 2009;24(4):216–22.
45. Didden R, Sikkema PE, Bosman ITM, Duker PC. Use of a modified Azrin–Foxx toilet training procedure with individuals with Angelman syndrome. J Appl Res Intellect Disabil. 2008;14:64–70.
46. Fichtner C, Tiger J. Teaching discriminated social approaches to individuals with Angelman syndrome. J Appl Behav Anal. 2015;
47. Radstaake M, Didden R, Lang R, et al. Functional analysis and functional communication training in the classroom for three children with Angelman syndrome. J Dev Phys Disabil. 2013;25:49–63.
48. Carr EG, Durand V. Reducing behavior problems through functional communication training. J Appl Behav Anal. 1985;18:111–26.
49. Heald M, Adams D, Oliver C. Profiles of atypical sensory processing in Angelman, Cornelia de Lange and Fragile X syndromes. J Intellect Disabil Res. 2020;64(2):117–30.
50. Bindels-de Heus KG, Hooven-Radstaake MT, Legerstee JS, et al. Sleep problems in children with Angelman syndrome: the effect of a behavioral intervention program. Res Dev Disabil. 2023;135:104444.
51. Spruyt K, Curfs LM. Non-pharmacological management of problematic sleeping in children with developmental disabilities. Dev Med Child Neurol. 2015;57(2):120–36.
52. Summers JA, Allison DB, Lynch PS, Sandler L. Behaviour problems in Angelman syndrome. J Intellect Disabil Res. 1995;39:97–106.

53. Wolraich ML, Hagan JF Jr, Allan C, et al. Clinical practice guidelines for the diagnosis, evaluation and treatment of attention-deficit/hyperactivity disorder in children and adolescents. Pediatrics. 2019;144(4):e20192528.
54. Keary CJ, Thom RP, McDougle CJ. Stimulant intolerance in children with Angelman syndrome with hyperactivity: a case series. Psychiatr Genet. 2022;32(2):80–6.
55. Research Units on Pediatric Psychopharmacology Autism Network. Randomized, controlled, crossover trial of methylphenidate in pervasive developmental disorders with hyperactivity. Arch Gen Psychiatry. 2005;62(11):1266–74.
56. Scahill L, McCracken JT, King BH, et al. Extended-release guanfacine for hyperactivity in children with autism spectrum disorder. Am J Psychiatry. 2015;172(12):1197–206.
57. Harfterkamp M, Loo-Neus G, Minderaa RB, et al. A randomized double-blind study of atomoxetine versus placebo for attention-deficit/hyperactivity disorder symptoms in children with autism spectrum disorder. J Am Acad Child Adolesc Psychiatry. 2012;51(7):733–41.
58. Fankhauser MP, Karumanchi VC, German ML, et al. A double-blind, placebo-controlled study of the efficacy of transdermal clonidine in autism. J Clin Psychiatry. 1992;53(3):77–82.
59. Balaj K, Nowinski L, Walsh B, Mullett J, Palumbo ML, Thibert RL, et al. Buspirone for the treatment of anxiety-related symptoms in Angelman syndrome: a case series. Psychiatr Genet. 2019;29(2):51–6.
60. Riddle MA, Bernstein GA, Cook EH, et al. Anxiolytics, adrenergic agents, and naltrexone. J Am Acad Child Adolesc Psychiatry. 1999;38(5):546–56.
61. Strawn JR, Mills JA, Cornwall GJ, Mossman SA, Varney ST, Keeshin BR, et al. Buspirone in children and adolescents with anxiety: a review and Bayesian analysis of abandoned randomized controlled trials. J Child Adolesc Psychopharmacol. 2018;28(1):2–9.
62. Hanzlik E, Klinger SA, Carson R, et al. Mirtazapine for sleep disturbance in Angelman syndrome: a retrospective chart review of 8 pediatric cases. J Clin Sleep Med. 2020;16(4):591–5.
63. Hollander E, Phillips A, Chaplin W, Zagursky K, Novotny S, Wasserman S, Iyengar R. A placebo controlled crossover trial of liquid fluoxetine on repetitive behaviors in childhood and adolescent autism. Neuropsychopharmacology. 2005;30(3):582–9.
64. Bishop JR, Najjar F, Rubin LH, Guter SJ, Owley T, Mosconi MW, et al. Escitalopram pharmacogenetics: CYP2C19 relationships with dosing and clinical outcomes in autism spectrum disorder. Pharmacogenet Genomics. 2015;25(11):548.
65. Coleman DM, Adams JB, Anderson AL, Frye RE. Rating of the effectiveness of 26 psychiatric and seizure medications for autism spectrum disorder: results of a national survey. J Child Adolesc Psychopharmacol. 2019;29(2):107–23.
66. Simonoff E, Mowlem F, Pearson O, Anagnostou E, Donnelly C, Hollander E, et al. Citalopram did not significantly improve anxiety in children with autism spectrum disorder undergoing treatment for core symptoms: secondary analysis of a trial to reduce repetitive behaviors. J Child Adolesc Psychopharmacol. 2022;32(4):233–41.
67. King BH, Hollander E, Sikich L, McCracken JT, Scahill L, Bregman JD, et al. Lack of efficacy of citalopram in children with autism spectrum disorders and high levels of repetitive behavior: Citalopram ineffective in children with autism. Arch Gen Psychiatry. 2009;66(6):583–90.
68. London EB, Yoo JH, Fethke ED, Zimmerman-Bier B. The safety and effectiveness of high-dose propranolol as a treatment for challenging behaviors in individuals with autism spectrum disorders. J Clin Psychopharmacol. 2020;40(2):122–9.
69. Politte LC, Scahill L, Figueroa J, McCracken JT, Kind B, McDougle CJ. A randomized, placebo-controlled trial of extended-release guanfacine in children with autism spectrum disorder and ADHD symptoms: an analysis of secondary outcome measures. Neuropsychopharmacology. 2018;43(8):1772–8.
70. Ming X, Gordon E, Kang N, Wagner GC. Use of clonidine in children with autism spectrum disorders. Brain Dev. 2008;30(7):454–60.
71. Valente KD, Koiffmann CP, Fridman C, et al. Epilepsy in patients with Angelman syndrome caused by deletion of the chromosome 15q11-13. Arch Neurol. 2006;63:122–8.

72. Miano S, Bruni O, Elia M, Musumeci SA, Verrillo E, Ferri R. Sleep breathing and periodic leg movement pattern in Angelman syndrome: a polysomnographic study. Clin Neurophysiol. 2005;116(11):2685–92.
73. Ryan CS, Edlund W, Mandrekar J, Wong-Kisiel LC, Gavrilova RH, Kotagal S. Iron deficiency and its role in sleep disruption in patients with Angelman syndrome. J Child Neurol. 2020;35(14):963–9.
74. Bindels-de Heus KG, Mous SE, ten Hooven-Radstaake M, van Iperen-Kolk BM, Navis C, Rietman AB, et al. An overview of health issues and development in a large clinical cohort of children with Angelman syndrome. Am J Med Genet A. 2020;182(1):53–63.
75. Braam W, Didden R, Smits MG, et al. Melatonin for chronic insomnia in Angelman syndrome: a randomized placebo-controlled trial. J Child Neurol. 2008;23(6):649–54.
76. Gringras P, Nir T, Breddy J, Frydman-Marom A, Findling RL. Efficacy and safety of pediatric prolonged-release melatonin for insomnia in children with autism spectrum disorder. J Am Acad Child Adolesc Psychiatry. 2017;56(11):948–57.
77. Maras A, Schroder CM, Malow BA, Findling RL, Breddy J, Nir T, et al. Long-term efficacy and safety of pediatric prolonged-release melatonin for insomnia in children with autism spectrum disorder. J Child Adolesc Psychopharmacol. 2018;28(10):699–710.
78. Pereira JA, Ravichandran CT, Mullett J, et al. Characterization of sleep habits and medication outcomes for sleep disturbance in children and adults with Angelman syndrome. Am J Med Genet A. 2020;182(8):1913–22.
79. Willgoss T, Cassater D, Connor S, et al. Measuring what matters to individuals with Angelman syndrome and their families: development of a patient-centered disease concept model. Child Psychiatry Hum Dev. 2021;52(4):654–68.
80. Lossie AC, Whitney MM, Amidon D, et al. Distinct phenotypes distinguish the molecular classes of Angelman syndrome. J Med Genet. 2001;38:834–45.
81. Thibert RL, Larson AM, Hsieh DT, et al. Neurologic manifestations of Angelman syndrome. Pediatr Neurol. 2013;48:271–9.
82. Worden L, Grocott O, Tourjee A, et al. Diazepam for outpatient treatment of nonconvulsive status epilepticus in pediatric patients with Angelman syndrome. Epilepsy Behav. 2018;82:74–80.
83. Glassman LW, Grocott OR, Kunz PA, et al. Prevalence of gastrointestinal symptoms in Angelman syndrome. Am J Med Genet A. 2017;173(10):2703–9.
84. Duis J, Bindels-de Heus GCB, Valstar MJ, et al. A multidisciplinary approach and consensus statement to establish standards of care for Angelman syndrome. Mol Genet Genomic Med. 2022;10:e1843.
85. Grieco JC, Gouelle A, Weeber EJ. Identification of spatiotemporal gait parameters and pressure-related characteristics in children with Angelman syndrome: a pilot study. J Appl Res Intellect Disabil. 2018;31(6):1219–24.
86. Dickinson AJ, Fielder AR, Young ID, Duckett DP. Ocular findings in Angelman's (happy puppet) syndrome. Ophthalmic Paediatr Genet. 1990;11(1):1–6.

Further Reading

Bindels-de Heus KG, Hooven-Radstaake MT, Legerstee JS, et al. Sleep problems in children with Angelman syndrome: the effect of a behavioral intervention program. Res Dev Disabil. 2023;135:104444.

Sadhwani A, Willen JM, LaVallee N, et al. Maladaptive behaviors in individuals with Angelman syndrome. Am J Med Genet A. 2019;179(6):983–92. This trial presents findings from the Natural History study of Angelman Syndrome reporting the prevalence of challenging behaviors and how they change into adolescence and adulthood

Williams CA, Driscoll DJ, Dagli AI. Clinical and genetic aspects of Angelman syndrome. Genet Med. 2010;12(7):385–95. A summary of the genetics of Angelman Syndrome as well as clinical features

6 Prader-Willi Syndrome

Julia Katz

6.1 Overview

Prader-Willi syndrome (PWS) is a neurodevelopmental genetic disorder caused by the lack of expression of paternal genes in a specific region on chromosome 15. Prader-Willi syndrome affects approximately 1 in 10,000–30,000 live births in the US, with no gender or race differentiation [1, 2]. The age of diagnosis continues to decrease with increased availability of genetic testing and, currently, generally ranges from 18 days old to 4.9 years old. Referrals for confirmatory genetic testing remain based on clinical suspicion, which can result in a delay in diagnosis and timely interventions [3].

The manifestation of PWS and expression of illness is caused by the absence of functional paternal alleles on chromosome 15q11.2–q13. There are several etiologies that can result in illness expression [2, 4–6]. The most common etiology is a de novo deletion of paternal alleles in the region 15q11.2–q13 (60-70%). Less common etiologies include maternal uniparental disomy (mUPD, 25-35%), in which two copies of the maternal allele are inherited and are, thus, inactive due to genomic imprinting. Less frequently (1–3%), other abnormalities in the 15q region, such as imprinting defects, can occur and, at times, result from microdeletions that account for some familial cases of inheritance [2, 4, 7].

The PWS neurobehavioral phenotype as well as the severity and frequency of other manifestations are associated with the genetic class of PWS [2, 4–6, 8–11]. The paternal deletion type is further classified into subtypes (Type 1 and Type 2) that are associated with the size of the deletion and impact illness severity [2, 4]. Type 1, which is the larger deletion and accounts for about 40% of patients,

J. Katz (✉)
Department of Child and Adolescent Psychiatry and Behavioral Sciences, Children's Hospital of Philadelphia, Philadelphia, PA, USA
e-mail: katzj10@chop.edu

R. P. Thom, C. J. McDougle (eds.), *Neuropsychiatric Care for Genetic Syndromes and Other Neurodevelopmental Disorders*,
https://doi.org/10.1007/978-3-031-76269-7_6

encompasses genes from breakpoint 1 to breakpoint 3. Type 2 encompasses a deletion from breakpoints 2 and 3. Individuals with Type 1 typically present with more severe neurobehavioral manifestations, such as intellectual disability (ID), compulsive behaviors, and self-injury, which are thought to be related to four genes located between breakpoint 1 and breakpoint 2 (*NIPA1, NIPA2, TUBGCP5*, and *CYFIP1*) [7]. In addition, the genes *SNORD116, MAGEL2,* and *IPW*, affected in Type 1 and Type 2 (located between breakpoints 2 and 3), were found to be prominent factors contributing to the PWS presentation [8, 12]. Work is ongoing to understand the interplay between the genes implicated in Type 1 versus Type 2 deletions and their respective contribution to the illness presentation. There are also neurobehavioral phenotypic differences between paternal deletion and mUPD, where individuals with mUPD have a higher risk for psychosis, anxiety, and autism spectrum disorder (ASD) compared to individuals with a paternal deletion subtype [6, 8, 10, 13].

PWS is characterized by several clinical phases that describe shifts in nutritional status. Phase 0 occurs in utero and is associated with growth restriction and decreased fetal movements. Phase 1a occurs during infancy (0–9 months) and includes hypotonia and feeding problems, resulting in failure to thrive. Infants will also present with craniofacial dysmorphism (narrow nasal bridge, almond-shaped palpebral features, downturned corners of the mouth, and narrow bifrontal diameter), small hands and feet, short stature, and hypogonadism [2, 4, 5, 11]. Phase 1b occurs between 9 and 25 months of age where improved nutritional status is observed. Following infancy, at around 2 years of age, PWS manifestations progress across several subsequent distinct phases that are associated with weight gain and feeding behavior. Toddlers initially present with weight gain independent of increased food intake (Phase 2a), followed by hyperphagia and increased appetite (phase 2b), resulting in further weight gain. At around 8 years of age (Phase 3), individuals with PWS rarely feel satiety, which results in hyperphagia. For some, hyperphagia attenuates in adulthood (Phase 4). The hyperphagia and lack of satiety associated with PWS are multifactorial, and studies are still ongoing to fully understand the neurobiological mechanisms contributing to this presentation. One factor is thought to be related to increased circulating ghrelin levels (an orexigenic hormone). A combination of decreased resting energy expenditure and high caloric intake are thought to contribute to weight gain [4, 14–16].

Other common clinical features of PWS include endocrine abnormalities associated with hypothalamic dysfunction such as central hypothyroidism, adrenal insufficiency, non-insulin-dependent diabetes, growth hormone deficiency, osteopenia, and osteoporosis [2, 4, 17, 18]. In addition, hypogonadism secondary to hypothalamic and primary gonadal deficiency are also often present. Precocious adrenarche is observed in about 15–20%, as well as primary amenorrhea or oligomenorrhoea and infertility in the majority of individuals with PWS [2, 4, 18]. Other physical manifestations include hip dysplasia (10–20%), scoliosis (40–80%), strabismus (60–70%), and sleep abnormalities such as obstructive sleep apnea, which is present in about 80% of children with PWS [2, 4, 19]. Furthermore, PWS individuals are at higher risk of comorbidities associated with hyperphagia and obesity including cardiac and respiratory issues, fatty liver, and gastrointestinal disorders [2, 4, 20].

Motor and language developmental delays are often observed, and by school age, most will be diagnosed with mild ID with an IQ ranging from 60 to 70 [4]. Patients with paternal deletion tend to have lower IQ scores compared to those with mUPD [6].

6.2 Signs and Symptoms of Common Psychiatric Comorbidities

Individuals with PWS often exhibit a range of challenging behaviors, both related and unrelated to food. Food-related behavior is often motivated by increased attention to obtaining food, which can manifest as talking about food excessively, planning or asking about future meals, and searching for or trying to obtain food and/or nonfood items that can be consumed. Anxiety and obsessive thoughts and actions about the availability of food and securing food can be present, as well as aggression in order to obtain food [10]. In addition to food-related challenging behaviors, many individuals with PWS also demonstrate challenging behaviors unrelated to food-seeking, such as impulsivity, compulsions and repetitive behaviors, skin picking, rigidity, and social impairment [2, 4, 10]. Another contributing factor to behavioral manifestations includes mild to moderate ID, as well as specific learning disorders, which together, are thought to contribute to the further development of mental health problems later in life [8, 10]. In addition, as individuals with PWS mature, they are more likely to develop depression, anxiety, and psychosis than other individuals with ID [9, 10, 21]. Furthermore, in a natural history study of individuals with PWS, Peleggi et al. found that the lifetime prevalence of suicidal ideation and suicide attempts was higher in adults with PWS than in the typically developing population [22].

6.2.1 Behavioral Dysregulation

Behavioral dysregulation occurs in about 80% of individuals with PWS and, generally, either remains stable throughout the lifetime or increases with age [9, 10, 21, 23]. Dysregulation often manifests with temper outbursts that appear to be disproportionate to a potential antecedent. Behaviors can consist of escalating distress that is initially expressed by crying and yelling that can escalate to include aggression and property destruction [10]. As noted above, this can be related to food-seeking behavior and denial of access to food; however, other potential contributing factors include poor frustration tolerance and emotion regulation in the setting of limited coping skills and executive function deficits [10, 24]. In addition, individuals with PWS also exhibit temper outbursts in response to deviations from their routine, which may stem from rigidity or social skill deficits. Schwartz et al. observed fewer behavioral outbursts following vagus nerve stimulation and hypothesized that autonomic nervous system dysregulation may play a role [10, 25].

6.2.2 Anxiety

Anxiety disorders were found to be highly comorbid with PWS, which is thought to be associated with both perceived food insecurity and hyperphagia, as well as other factors [10, 26, 27]. Some anxiety manifestations appear to be associated with insistence on sameness and distress when routine is disrupted. Other manifestations include checking behaviors, repetitive questioning, and repetitive movements. Other than behavioral dysregulation, caregivers noted that anxiety is the second most important behavioral symptom they would like to target in treatment [10, 28]. Some of the symptoms noted can resemble obsessive-compulsive disorder (OCD) symptoms, with rates of OCD diagnosis among this population ranging from 8% to 58% [10]. However, most of the compulsions observed by individuals with PWS appear to be ego-syntonic and associated with a desire for sameness and rigidity rather than fear or obsessive thoughts, suggesting a potentially different pathophysiology from typical OCD [9, 10, 21]. Of note, anxiety disorders were found to be generally higher in the mUPD genetic subtype of PWS compared to the deletion subtypes (73% vs 32%), while obsessive-compulsive-like symptoms appear to be higher in the PWS deletion subgroup [10].

6.2.3 Skin Picking

Skin picking behavior among individuals with PWS is common with a prevalence of >60%, compared to 1–4% in the general population [12, 29, 30]. This behavior appears to increase from early childhood to adolescence and has a potential association with the imprinting of the *NDN* gene [9, 12, 30]. A behavioral analysis study of skin picking showed that it occurs during moments of inattention by the individual and was maintained by automatic reinforcement via sensory stimulation rather than other behavioral motivations such as attention seeking [30]. However, in a study by Bull et al., they found that some individuals who engaged in skin picking were preoccupied with the activity, suggesting potential compulsive-like behavior as a mechanism in some patients. In addition, they found that the behavior was noted to be triggered or more associated with a preoccupation with an existing skin lesion or imperfection rather than intact skin [29]. Of note, individuals with PWS were found to have a higher pain threshold, which may also contribute to skin picking [12].

6.2.4 Social Impairment

Social difficulties are commonly observed in individuals with PWS, which in some cases is due to a comorbid diagnosis of ASD [13]. However, for most individuals with PWS, while the social difficulties can overlap with those observed in ASD, the severity either does not meet the threshold for an ASD diagnosis or appears to be different in quality. One factor that could account for this difference includes PWS patients having higher social motivation compared to individuals with ASD. The most frequently observed social challenges in PWS include reciprocal social communication, perspective-taking, and empathy [10]. Some estimates for the prevalence of ASD among individuals with PWS are about 25% [13, 31]; however, since most of the literature estimates are based on screening questionnaires rather than gold-standard clinical evaluations, this may be an overestimate [13]. A cross-sectional study that included 146 children and adolescents with PWS found that 12.3% met the criteria for ASD based on the Autism Diagnostic Observation Schedule (ADOS-2) [13]. Regarding repetitive behaviors observed both in PWS and ASD, Flores et al. found that individuals with PWS scored lower on the Repetitive Behavior Scale—Revised (RBS-R) compared to individuals with ASD, specifically in restricted, ritualistic, and self-injurious domains [13, 32]. Of note, individuals with mUPD or imprinting defects exhibited more severe symptoms and were more likely to be diagnosed with ASD compared to those with the deletion subtype [9, 10, 13]. Dykens et al. found that 78% of the individuals who met the criteria for ASD in their sample were found to have mUPD.

6.2.5 Psychosis

Individuals with mUPD experience elevated risk for psychosis, with an estimated 60–100% lifetime prevalence. The paternal deletion type does not appear to increase the risk for psychosis above that seen in the general population [8, 13, 33].

6.3 Assessment

When PWS is suspected based on the clinical symptoms noted above, genetic testing should be done to confirm the diagnosis. The initial recommended test is a DNA methylation analysis. Once DNA methylation confirms the diagnosis, either fluorescence in situ hybridization (FISH) or DNA chromosomal microarray analysis (CMA) is then utilized to further classify the molecular class of the disorder by evaluating the presence of a deletion [2, 4]. If a deletion is not found, a DNA polymorphism analysis is needed to assess the presence of mUPD or an imprinting defect [4]. While it is common for individuals with PWS to be diagnosed early in life due to failure to thrive, developmental delay, and/or hypotonia, it is important to consider this diagnosis in older individuals presenting to psychiatry, particularly if they are exhibiting ID, preoccupation with food, hyperphagia, obesity, and behavioral problems such as temper tantrums, skin picking, rigidity, and compulsive or repetitive behaviors.

6.4 Treatment

Treatment options for rare disorders are often limited by a paucity of rigorous, well-powered randomized controlled trials both for behavioral and pharmacological interventions. In part, this is due to the small number of available participants, which limits the ability to perform high-quality studies with adequate statistical power. Most of the interventions noted below are based on case reports, retrospective studies, and prospective open-label trials, highlighting the need for more rigorous studies. While the significant limitations of the literature to date preclude the author from providing definitive recommendations, the interventions noted below are ones to consider when providing care for individuals with PWS and have preliminary evidence to support their effectiveness.

6.4.1 Psychosocial Treatments

Initial behavioral problems most commonly arise in the setting of food-seeking and insecurity. One of the primary behavioral interventions focuses on limiting hyperphagia by restricting food and implementing supervision. However, since this approach alone can result in heightened anxiety due to food insecurity, this must be coupled with clear communication and expectations for when food will be available. Limiting access to food can be done by locking pantries and refrigerators and making food available only during meal and snack times. In addition, due to limited satiety during meals and the potential for obtaining food from others as well as nonfood items or scraps from the trash, constant supervision is recommended to limit this behavior [2, 34]. While constant supervision and food restriction are effective, their feasibility across the lifespan diminishes and warrants the incorporation of other interventions. Kennedy et al. suggested including elements of applied behavioral analysis (ABA), including using differential reinforcements and a token economy to reinforce desired behaviors as well as clear consequences and redirection of behaviors associated with food stealing and overeating [35]. While ABA research in individuals with PWS is limited, its efficacy in managing other problem behaviors among individuals with developmental disabilities suggests it can be applied to this population as well. In a case report of a 7-year-old girl with PWS, Lambert et al. used functional behavioral analysis to assess and inform the management of food-stealing behaviors. They then applied differential reinforcement using tokens to encourage behaviors other than stealing and provided redirection for undesired behaviors. The patient was motivated by earning tokens and was able to ask for food rather than steal it [34]. Other approaches can include mindfulness, which was studied by Singh et al. They found that teaching mindfulness strategies in association with food intake allowed for more sustained changes when working with a 17-year-old male with PWS on healthy eating and exercise [36]. In order to minimize anxiety associated with the uncertainty of receiving food, establishing a consistent and clear routine for mealtimes and snacks can be helpful. In addition, having a visual schedule that specifies mealtimes as well as preferred and non-preferred activities can assist with transitioning to and from meals and alleviate anxiety [2].

A range of psychosocial interventions has been described to address non-food-related behavioral challenges including emotion regulation, social challenges, skin picking, and cognitive deficits. Dimitropoulos et al. [37, 38] explored remotely delivered play therapy to address socio-emotional skill development among 15 school-aged children with PWS. This treatment was feasible and resulted in improvement in both flexibility of thoughts as well as affective and cognitive expression via play. The content was adapted from a curriculum designed for typically developing children and was delivered in 15–20 minutes sessions twice per week for six weeks. The program included three sections focusing on play skills, emotional expression, and coping skills [38]. Dykens et al. also explored a remote group-based intervention to address social skills impairment among 51 individuals with PWS with a mean age of 20 years (range: 14–33 years) [39]. The intervention was associated with increased prosocial behavior and reduced loneliness.

Lang et al. performed a systematic review examining behavioral interventions for chronic skin picking among individuals with developmental disabilities, with one of the studies exploring interventions for individuals with PWS specifically [40, 41]. The systematic review concluded that ABA-based principles such as interventions at the antecedent level and reinforcement-based interventions are effective in reducing skin picking [41]. Furthermore, similar interventions were also effective for individuals with other developmental disabilities suggesting treatment benefit, regardless of cognitive capacity.

Finally, as noted above, while there are no studies examining the use of other evidence-based behavioral treatments for this population, it is important to consider adapting interventions such as cognitive behavioral therapy (CBT), dialectical behavioral therapy (DBT), and acceptance and commitment therapy (ACT) to address emotion regulation, depression, anxiety, and other psychological comorbidities, in combination with functional behavioral analysis. A systematic review and meta-analysis by Vereenooghe and Langdon found that CBT can be an effective treatment modality for adults with ID for the management of anger and depression [42]. This work suggests CBT may also be effectively adapted for the PWS population. Furthermore, treatments like habit reversal therapy and exposure response prevention to target OCD symptoms and skin picking, respectively, are well-established treatments for the general population and warrant further exploration and/or adaptation for PWS.

6.4.2 Biological Treatments

There are no U.S. Food and Drug Administration (FDA)-approved pharmacological interventions to address psychiatric symptoms for individuals with PWS. However, in clinical practice, psychotropic medications are often prescribed to address the behavioral problems associated with PWS [43]. The most studied pharmacological interventions have been aimed at addressing some of the most frequent challenging behaviors associated with PWS including behavioral dysregulation, skin picking, and hyperphagia. While there are a limited number of randomized controlled trials (RCTs) examining these interventions, we summarize the most pertinent preliminary studies below.

While there are no RCTs to examine the efficacy of selective serotonin reuptake inhibitors (SSRIs) in PWS, there are two case reports on fluoxetine and a retrospective case series examining the use of sertraline to address behavioral dysregulation, which showed positive results [44]. Deest et al. examined 14 individuals with PWS with a mean age of 31 years who were treated with sertraline with dosages ranging from 25 mg to 100 mg for 6 months. They found an overall improvement in the frequency of temper outbursts in 13 of the patients, with no notable side effects, aside from severe sleep abnormalities in the 14th participant, resulting in discontinuation of treatment. Of note, half of the patients were on additional psychotropic medications. Two case reports, each with two patients, assessed the effect of fluoxetine on skin picking. The first report was on a 35-year-old woman and a 43-year-old man with PWS who both experienced benefits from fluoxetine for reducing skin picking [45]. The other case report included a 21-year-old man and an 18-year-old woman, neither of whom responded to fluoxetine for skin picking [46].

Among antipsychotic medications, the most frequently studied have been risperidone and aripiprazole. For risperidone, a case report on an 11-year-old boy and an open-label prospective trial including seven individuals ranging in age from 15 to 25 years showed improvement in anger outbursts, aggression, and impulsivity. Of note, both studies also reported an unexpected decrease in weight with the use of risperidone [47, 48]. The absence of weight gain, normally a prominent side effect of most antipsychotics, was also found by Elliott et al. who studied individuals with PWS who were either taking antipsychotics or started taking an antipsychotic during their inpatient stay [49]. For aripiprazole, one case report which included an 11-year-old girl showed improvement in aggression and OCD symptoms, and another case report involving a 16-year-old girl showed improvement in psychotic symptoms [50, 51]. Deest et al. examined the effectiveness of aripiprazole for addressing behavioral outbursts in a retrospective trial of ten individuals with PWS (mean age 35.8 years, range: 25–52 years) [52]. They found that seven of the ten patients showed an overall improvement (three of whom were on additional psychotropic medications); however, two required discontinuation of treatment due to severe daytime sleepiness. No significant weight change was noted at the six-month follow-up [52].

Topiramate was explored in several studies as a potential intervention to address behavioral difficulties as well as hyperphagia among individuals with PWS. Consoli et al. assessed the efficacy of topiramate in an 8-week, double-blind, randomized placebo-controlled trial among 62 individuals with PWS. While there was no significant impact on behavioral dysregulation, a significant improvement in hyperphagia was observed. This suggests topiramate might be a potential treatment option for obesity commonly experienced by individuals with PWS. The authors reported sedation and cognitive slowing as observed side effects, which should be considered, given the fatigue and cognitive difficulties already commonly experienced by individuals with PWS. In addition, changes in liver function tests and ammonia were also reported [53]. Two additional studies looking at topiramate use in open-label prospective trials found encouraging results as well; however, those are harder to interpret, given the study design and lack of use of standardized measures [54, 55]. Shapira et al. looked at three individuals with self-injurious behavior who were treated with topiramate and found improvement. Of note, two of the three patients were taking additional psychotropic medications [54]. Smathers et al. examined eight patients with PWS who were treated with topiramate and found improvement in mood, aggression, and eating behavior, resulting in weight stabilization (per parent report) for seven of the patients, as well as improvement in self-injurious behavior in two of the patients [55]. Thus, given the evidence provided above, topiramate should be considered for the management of hyperphagia and, potentially, aggression in individuals with PWS.

N-acetylcysteine (NAC) was also explored for its potential effectiveness in addressing skin picking in individuals with PWS. Miller and Angulo found an improvement in skin picking in all 35 patients enrolled in a 12-week open-label trial with minimal side effects [56]. Wieting et al. examined the effectiveness of NAC among 14 patients in a retrospective case series and found that 43% of individuals (six out of 14) had improved skin picking behavior but no effect on rectal picking which was also present in four patients [57].

Guanfacine extended release was evaluated by one retrospective cohort study with 20 patients with PWS between the ages of 6–26 years. It was found to improve symptoms of skin picking, aggression, and symptoms of attention-deficit/hyperactivity disorder (ADHD) for the majority of patients with no significant side effects [58].

The most studied medication in PWS is oxytocin, with five RCTs examining behavior and eating patterns [59–63]. Individuals with PWS have a reduction of oxytocin-producing neurons in the hypothalamic periventricular nucleus, which is also smaller in size [23]. Mouse models sharing some of the genes most implicated in PWS (*NDN* and *MAGEL2*) exhibited similar deficits in the oxytocin system [23, 64]. A review of clinical trials of intranasal oxytocin by Rice et al., in which four were RCTs [59–61, 63], showed some positive outcomes. However, the authors concluded that, given various study limitations associated with study design and measures, it would be challenging to draw conclusions regarding its efficacy [23]. Of note, studies exploring the potential efficacy of oxytocin are continuing, as evidenced by a recent Phase 3 RCT of carbetocin (oxytocin analog) by Roof et al. that showed improvement in hyperphagia and anxiety [65].

6.5 Common Medical Comorbidities

The most frequent medical comorbidities experienced by individuals with PWS are associated with hyperphagia and obesity and could lead to mortality associated with cardiorespiratory issues, complications secondary to diabetes, and gastric perforation or other gastrointestinal issues due to overeating [66]. Furthermore, mortality rates were found to be higher in PWS than in individuals with other developmental disabilities [4]. Currently, the only FDA-indicated medication to manage symptoms associated with PWS in childhood is growth hormone (GH) [17]. Growth hormone has repeatedly been found to alleviate hypotonia and change body composition, contributing to weight loss by reducing visceral fat and increasing lean body mass [2, 17, 67]. These changes were observed in children with PWS with and without GH deficiency, and treatment with GH is now the standard of care for children with PWS [68]. In addition, considering the favorable study outcomes observed in adult patients with PWS, the global community of PWS experts has recommended ongoing GH treatment in adults [68, 69]. Several studies found GH to be efficacious for improving the cognitive development of children with PWS [17, 70–72], as well as having a potential impact on behavior; however, this is still being explored based on mixed results and a negative finding in a recent meta-analysis [70, 73, 74].

Other relevant comorbidities that should be considered prior to prescribing psychotropic medications include sleep and endocrine disorders. Sleep apnea and other sleep disorders are common in PWS and might impact daytime energy levels as well as contribute to behavioral manifestations such as temper outbursts, anxiety, depression, and aggression [75]. Hypothyroidism should also be considered and TSH levels should be checked prior to psychiatric treatment, given the potential to mimic psychiatric comorbidities [2, 4, 76, 77]. In addition, patients' risk of further metabolic abnormalities should be considered and discussed prior to prescribing antipsychotics [2, 52, 78, 79]. Finally, Consoli et al. noted an increased risk of thermal dysregulation among individuals with PWS, and in light of reports of hyperthermia as a side effect of topiramate, prescribers should be mindful of this potential adverse effect [53]. In addition, two other potential side effects of topiramate that are important to consider in this population include the risk of renal tubular acidosis that can worsen osteoporosis, which is commonly present in individuals with PWS, as well as potential cognitive blunting that could further exacerbate executive function deficits that are often observed in this population [53].

Key Points to Remember

- Prader-Willi syndrome (PWS) is a neurodevelopmental genetic disorder caused by lack of expression of paternal genes on chromosome 15q11.2–q13, most commonly either due to the deletion of paternally inherited genes or inheritance of duplicated maternal genes (mUPD).
- PWS is characterized by hypotonia, developmental delay (motor and language), and failure to thrive in infancy, as well as dysmorphic features such as a narrow nasal bridge, almond-shaped palpebral features, downturned corners of the mouth and narrow bifrontal diameter, small hands and feet, short stature, hypogonadism, and hypopigmentation.

- The second phase of the disorder, most frequently presenting in early childhood, includes severe hyperphagia and obesity, which often result in medical comorbidities such as cardiorespiratory issues, gastrointestinal complications, and obstructive sleep apnea.
- Other common symptoms are associated with endocrine dysfunction secondary to hypothalamic impairment and include adrenal insufficiency, non-insulin-dependent diabetes, growth hormone deficiency, hypogonadism, osteopenia, and osteoporosis.
- Most individuals with PWS have mild intellectual disability (IQ range: 60–70) and present with behavioral concerns including temper tantrums, impulsivity, compulsions, repetitive behaviors, skin picking, rigidity, and social deficits.
- The neurobehavioral phenotype of PWS is associated with the genetic subtype of the disorder, with mUPD being associated with a higher likelihood for the development of psychosis, anxiety, and ASD.
- When PWS is suspected based on the clinical symptoms, DNA methylation analysis should be done, followed by a FISH test or CMA to classify the molecular class of the disorder.
- Growth hormone is often administered to children with PWS and has been found to assist with hypotonia and weight management. In addition, some studies have shown improvement in cognitive profile and behavior.
- Primary behavioral interventions associated with hyperphagia focus on limiting access to food such as supervision during mealtimes, locking pantries and refrigerators, and minimizing anxiety associated with food insecurity.
- Elements of applied behavioral analysis including using differential reinforcements or a token economy to reinforce desired behaviors other than food stealing and consequences as well as redirection for behaviors associated with food stealing appear to be helpful in managing behaviors associated with PWS.
- Selective serotonin reuptake inhibitors and atypical antipsychotics show promise in the management of behavioral dysregulation and aggression.
- Topiramate was found to be beneficial in the management of hyperphagia and, potentially, aggression.
- Effective medical care for PWS should involve a multidisciplinary team including primary care, endocrinologists, mental health providers, a nutritionist, and other specialties, as needed to address comorbidities.

Photographs of an individual with Prader-Willi Syndrome

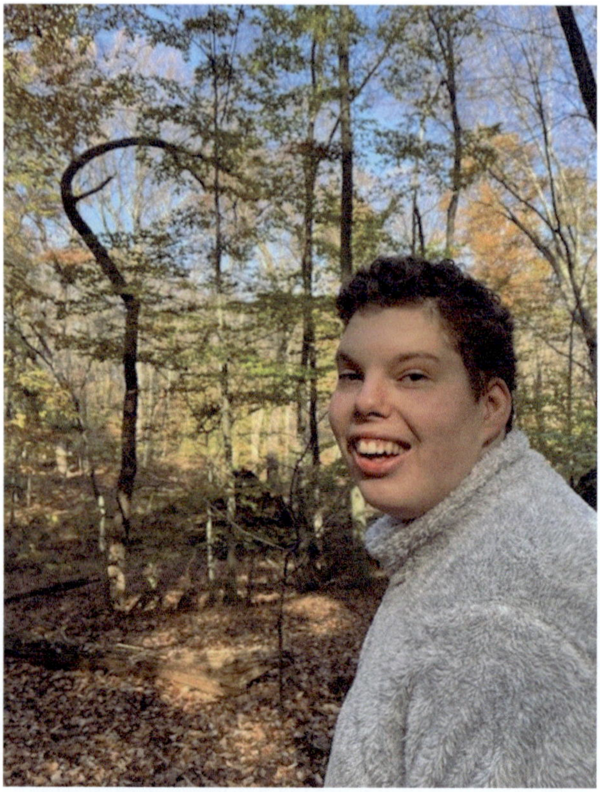

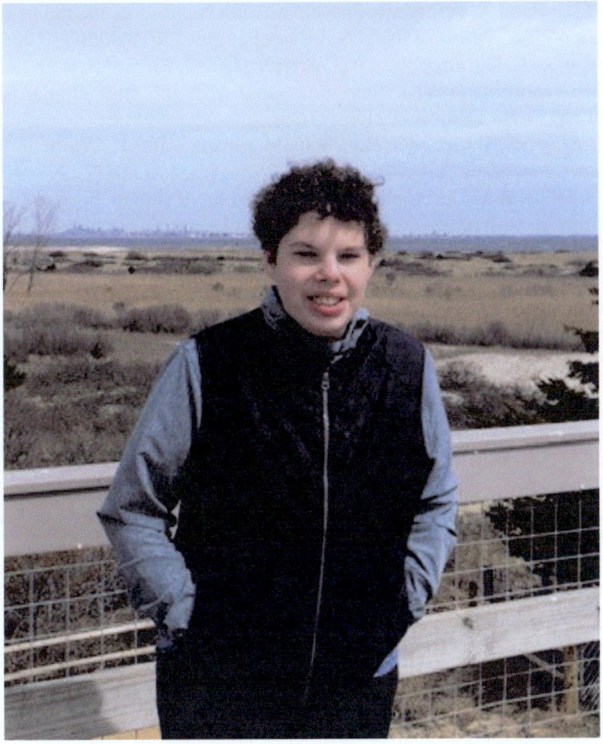

References

1. Bohonowych J, Miller J, McCandless SE, Strong TV. The global Prader–Willi syndrome registry: development, launch, and early demographics. Genes. 2019;10(9):713.
2. Butler MG, Miller JL, Forster JL. Prader-Willi syndrome—clinical genetics, giagnosis and treatment approaches: an update. Curr Pediatr Rev. 2019;15(4):207–44.
3. Mahmoud R, Singh P, Weiss L, Lakatos A, Oakes M, Hossain W, et al. Newborn screening for Prader–Willi syndrome is feasible: early diagnosis for better outcomes. Am J Med Genet A 2018;ajmg.a.60681.
4. Cassidy SB, Schwartz S, Miller JL, Driscoll DJ. Prader-Willi syndrome. Genet Med. 2012;14(1):10–26.
5. Butler MG, Thompson T. Prader-Willi syndrome: clinical and genetic findings. Endocrinologist. 2000;10(Suppl. 1):3S–16S.
6. Yang L, Zhan GD, Ding JJ, Wang HJ, Ma D, Huang GY, Zhou WH. Psychiatric illness and intellectual disability in the Prader-Willi syndrome with different molecular defects—a meta analysis. Veitia RA, editor. PLoS ONE. 2013;8(8):e72640.
7. Butler MG, Cowen N, Bhatnagar A. Prader-Willi syndrome, deletion subtypes, and magnesium: potential impact on clinical findings. Am J Med Genet A. 2022;188(11):3278–86.
8. Holland AJ, Aman LCS, Whittington JE. Defining mental and behavioural disorders in genetically determined neurodevelopmental syndromes with particular reference to Prader-Willi syndrome. Genes. 2019;10(12):1025.

9. Whittington J, Holland A. A review of psychiatric conceptions of mental and behavioural disorders in Prader-Willi syndrome. Neurosci Biobehav Rev. 2018;95:396–405.
10. Schwartz L, Caixàs A, Dimitropoulos A, Dykens E, Duis J, Einfeld S, et al. Behavioral features in Prader-Willi syndrome (PWS): consensus paper from the international PWS clinical trial consortium. J Neurodev Disord. 2021;13(1):25.
11. Holm VA, Cassidy SB, Butler MG, Hanchett JM, Greenswag LR, Whitman BY, et al. Prader-Willi syndrome: consensus diagnostic criteria. Pediatrics. 1993;91(2):398–402.
12. Whittington J, Holland A. Developing an understanding of skin picking in people with Prader-Willi syndrome: a structured literature review and re-analysis of existing data. Neurosci Biobehav Rev. 2020;112:48–61.
13. Dykens EM, Roof E, Hunt-Hawkins H, Dankner N, Lee EB, Shivers CM, et al. Diagnoses and characteristics of autism spectrum disorders in children with Prader-Willi syndrome. J Neurodev Disord. 2017;9(1):18.
14. DelParigi A, Tschöp M, Heiman ML, Salbe AD, Vozarova B, Sell SM, et al. High circulating ghrelin: a potential cause for hyperphagia and obesity in Prader-Willi Syndrome. J Clin Endocrinol Metab. 2002;87(12):5461–4.
15. Erdie-Lalena CR, Holm VA, Kelly PC, Frayo RS, Cummings DE. Ghrelin levels in young children with Prader-Willi syndrome. J Pediatr. 2006;149(2):199–204.
16. Butler MG, Theodoro MF, Bittel DC, Donnelly JE. Energy expenditure and physical activity in Prader-Willi syndrome: comparison with obese subjects. Am J Med Genet A. 2007;143A(5):449–59.
17. Di Lorenzo R, Sberveglieri S, Marrama D, Landi G, Ferri P. Weight control and behavior rehabilitation in a patient suffering from prader willi syndrome. BMC Res Notes. 2016;9(1):199.
18. Alves C, Franco RR. Prader-Willi syndrome: endocrine manifestations and management. Arch Endocrinol Metab. 2020;64(3):223–34.
19. Sedky K, Bennett DS, Pumariega A. Prader willi syndrome and obstructive sleep apnea: co-occurrence in the pediatric population. J Clin Sleep Med. 2014;10(04):403–9.
20. Tauber M, Diene G, Molinas C, Hébert M. Review of 64 cases of death in children with Prader–Willi syndrome (PWS). Am J Med Genet A. 2008;146A(7):881–7.
21. Ho A, Dimitropoulos A. Clinical management of behavioral characteristics of Prader–Willi syndrome. Neuropsychiatr Dis Treat. 2010;107
22. Peleggi A, Bohonowych J, Strong TV, Schwartz L, Kim SJ. Suicidality in individuals with Prader-Willi syndrome: a review of registry survey data. BMC Psychiatry. 2021;21(1):438.
23. Rice LJ, Einfeld SL, Hu N, Carter CS. A review of clinical trials of oxytocin in Prader-Willi syndrome. Curr Opin Psychiatry. 2018;31(2):123–7.
24. Tunnicliffe P, Woodcock K, Bull L, Oliver C, Penhallow J. Temper outbursts in Prader-Willi syndrome: causes, behavioural and emotional sequence and responses by carers: temper outbursts in Prader-Willi syndrome. J Intellect Disabil Res. 2014;58(2):134–50.
25. Manning KE, Beresford-Webb JA, Aman LCS, Ring HA, Watson PC, Porges SW, et al. Transcutaneous vagus nerve stimulation (t-VNS): A novel effective treatment for temper outbursts in adults with Prader-Willi syndrome indicated by results from a non-blind study. Phan TG, editor. PLoS ONE. 2019;14(12):e0223750.
26. Manzardo AM, Weisensel N, Ayala S, Hossain W, Butler MG. Prader-Willi syndrome genetic subtypes and clinical neuropsychiatric diagnoses in residential care adults. Clin Genet. 2018;93(3):622–31.
27. Feighan S-M, Hughes M, Maunder K, Roche E, Gallagher L. A profile of mental health and behaviour in Prader-Willi syndrome. J Intellect Disabil Res. 2020;64(2):158–69.
28. Tsai JH, Scheimann AO, McCandless SE, Strong TV, Bridges JFP. Caregiver priorities for endpoints to evaluate treatments for Prader-Willi syndrome: a best–worst scaling. J Med Econ. 2018;21(12):1230–7.
29. Bull LE, Oliver C, Woodcock KA. Skin picking in people with Prader-Willi Syndrome: phenomenology and management. J Autism Dev Disord. 2021;51(1):286–97.
30. Hall SS, Hustyi KM, Chui C, Hammond JL. Experimental functional analysis of severe skin-picking behavior in Prader-Willi syndrome. Res Dev Disabil. 2014;35(10):2284–92.

31. Bennett JA, Germani T, Haqq AM, Zwaigenbaum L. Autism spectrum disorder in Prader-Willi syndrome: a systematic review. Am J Med Genet A. 2015;167(12):2936–44.
32. Flores CG, Valcante G, Guter S, Zaytoun A, Wray E, Bell L, et al. Repetitive behavior profiles: consistency across autism spectrum disorder cohorts and divergence from Prader-Willi syndrome. J Neurodev Disord. 2011;3(4):316–24.
33. Vogels A, Hert MD, Descheemaeker MJ, Govers V, Devriendt K, Legius E, et al. Psychotic disorders in Prader-Willi syndrome. Am J Med Genet. 2004;127A(3):238–43.
34. Lambert JM, Parikh N, Stankiewicz KC, Houchins-Juarez NJ, Morales VA, Sweeney EM, et al. Decreasing food stealing of child with Prader-Willi syndrome through function-based differential reinforcement. J Autism Dev Disord. 2019;49(2):721–8.
35. Kennedy D, Marten H, O'Sullivan C, Catrone R. Biological, behavioral, and ethical considerations of Prader-Willi syndrome: a primer for behavior analysts. Behav Anal Pract. 2022;15(2):562–70.
36. Singh NN, Hwang YS. Mindfulness-based programs and practices for people with intellectual and developmental disability. Curr Opin Psychiatry. 2020;33(2):86–91.
37. Dimitropoulos A, Zyga O, Russ S. Evaluating the feasibility of a play-based telehealth intervention program for children with Prader-Willi syndrome. J Autism Dev Disord. 2017;47(9):2814–25.
38. Dimitropoulos A, Zyga O, Doernberg E, Russ SW. Show me what happens next: preliminary efficacy of a remote play-based intervention for children with Prader-Willi syndrome. Res Dev Disabil. 2021;108:103820.
39. Dykens EM, Roof E, Hunt-Hawkins H, McDonald C. The feasibility and effectiveness of a novel, on-line social skills intervention for individuals with Prader-Willi syndrome. Front Psych. 2022;13:863999.
40. Stokes JV, Luiselli JK. Applied behavior analysis assessment and intervention for health threatening self-injury in an adult with Prader–Willi syndrome. Clin Case Studies. 2009;8:38–47.
41. Lang R, Didden R, Machalicek W, Rispoli M, Sigafoos J, Lancioni G, et al. Behavioral treatment of chronic skin-picking in individuals with developmental disabilities: a systematic review. Res Dev Disabil. 2010;31(2):304–15.
42. Vereenooghe L, Langdon PE. Psychological therapies for people with intellectual disabilities: a systematic review and meta-analysis. Res Dev Disabil. 2013;34(11):4085–102.
43. Soni S, Whittington J, Holland AJ, Webb T, Maina E, Boer H, et al. The course and outcome of psychiatric illness in people with Prader-Willi syndrome: implications for management and treatment. J Intellect Disabil Res. 2007;51(1):32–42.
44. Deest M, Jakob MM, Seifert J, Bleich S, Frieling H, Eberlein C. Sertraline as a treatment option for temper outbursts in Prader-Willi syndrome. Am J Med Genet A. 2021;185(3):790–7.
45. Warnock JK. Pharmacologic treatment of severe skin-picking behaviors in Prader-Willi syndrome: two case reports. Arch Dermatol. 1992;128(12):1623.
46. Schepis C, Failla P, Siragusa M, Palazzo R, Romano C. Failure of fluoxetine to modify the skin-picking behaviour of Prader-Willi syndrome. Australas J Dermatol. 1998;39(1):57–60.
47. Araki S, Ohji T, Shiota N, Dobashi K, Shimono M, Shirahata A. Successful risperidone treatment for behavioral disturbances in Prader-Willi syndrome. Pediatr Int. 2010;52(1):e1–3.
48. Durst R, Rubin-Jabotinsky K, Raskin S, Katz G, Zislin J. Risperidone in treating behavioural disturbances of Prader-Willi syndrome: risperidone in Prader-Willi syndrome. Acta Psychiatr Scand. 2000;102(6):461–5.
49. Elliott JP, Cherpes G, Kamal K, Chopra I, Harrison C, Riedy M, et al. Relationship between antipsychotics and weight in patients with Prader-Willi Syndrome. Pharmacother J Hum Pharmacol Drug Ther. 2015;35(3):260–8.
50. Briegel W. Clinical usefulness of aripiprazole treatment in a girl with Prader-Willi syndrome and psychosis. Clin Psychopharmacol Neurosci. 2018;16(4):497.
51. Akça ÖF, Yilmaz S. Aripiprazole in the treatment of obsessive compulsive disorder and aggressive behaviors in a child with Prader-Willi syndrome: a case report. J Clin Psychopharmacol. 2016;36(5):526–8.

52. Deest M, Wieting J, Jakob MM, Deest-Gaubatz S, Groh A, Seifert J, et al. Aripiprazole treatment for temper outbursts in Prader-Willi syndrome. Orphanet J Rare Dis. 2022;17(1):324.
53. Consoli A, Çabal Berthoumieu S, Raffin M, Thuilleaux D, Poitou C, Coupaye M, et al. Effect of topiramate on eating behaviours in Prader-Willi syndrome: TOPRADER double-blind randomised placebo-controlled study. Transl Psychiatry. 2019;9(1):274.
54. Shapira NA, Lessig MC, Murphy TK, Driscoll DJ, Goodman WK. Topiramate attenuates self-injurious behaviour in Prader–Willi syndrome. Int J Neuropsychopharmacol. 2002;5(2):141–5. https://doi.org/10.1017/S1461145702002833.
55. Smathers SA, Wilson JG, Nigro MA. Topiramate effectiveness in Prader-Willi syndrome. Pediatr Neurol. 2003;28(2):130–3.
56. Miller JL, Angulo M. An open-label pilot study of N -acetylcysteine for skin-picking in Prader-Willi syndrome. Am J Med Genet A. 2014;164(2):421–4.
57. Wieting J, Deest M, Bleich S, Frieling H, Eberlein C. N -Acetylcysteine provides limited efficacy as treatment option for skin picking in Prader-Willi syndrome. Am J Med Genet A. 2022;188(3):828–35.
58. Singh D, Wakimoto Y, Filangieri C, Pinkhasov A, Angulo M. Guanfacine extended release for the reduction of aggression, attention-deficit/hyperactivity disorder symptoms, and self-injurious behavior in Prader-Willi syndrome—a retrospective cohort study. J Child Adolesc Psychopharmacol. 2019;29(4):313–7.
59. Einfeld SL, Smith E, McGregor IS, Steinbeck K, Taffe J, Rice LJ, et al. A double-blind randomized controlled trial of oxytocin nasal spray in prader willi syndrome. Am J Med Genet A. 2014;164(9):2232–9.
60. Miller JL, Tamura R, Butler MG, Kimonis V, Sulsona C, Gold JA, et al. Oxytocin treatment in children with Prader-Willi syndrome: a double-blind, placebo-controlled, crossover study. Am J Med Genet A. 2017;173(5):1243–50.
61. Kuppens RJ, Donze SH, Hokken-Koelega ACS. Promising effects of oxytocin on social and food-related behaviour in young children with Prader-Willi syndrome: a randomized, double-blind, controlled crossover trial. Clin Endocrinol (Oxf). 2016;85(6):979–87.
62. Hollander E, Levine KG, Ferretti CJ, Freeman K, Doernberg E, Desilva N, et al. Intranasal oxytocin versus placebo for hyperphagia and repetitive behaviors in children with Prader-Willi syndrome: a randomized controlled pilot trial. J Psychiatr Res. 2021;137:643–51.
63. Tauber M, Mantoulan C, Copet P, Jauregui J, Demeer G, Diene G, et al. Oxytocin may be useful to increase trust in others and decrease disruptive behaviours in patients with Prader-Willi syndrome: a randomised placebo-controlled trial in 24 patients. Orphanet J Rare Dis. 2011;6:47.
64. Althammer F, Muscatelli F, Grinevich V, Schaaf CP. Oxytocin-based therapies for treatment of Prader-Willi and Schaaf-Yang syndromes: evidence, disappointments, and future research strategies. Transl Psychiatry. 2022;12(1):318.
65. Roof E, Deal CL, McCandless SE, Cowan RL, Miller JL, Hamilton JK, et al. Intranasal carbetocin reduces hyperphagia, anxiousness, and distress in Prader-Willi syndrome: CARE-PWS Phase 3 trial. J Clin Endocrinol Metab. 2023:dgad015.
66. Manzardo AM, Loker J, Heinemann J, Loker C, Butler MG. Survival trends from the Prader-Willi syndrome Association (USA) 40-year mortality survey. Genet Med. 2018;20(1):24–30.
67. CDGB P, Franco RR, Ito SS, Trindade E, Polak M, Damiani D, et al. Growth hormone treatment in Prader-Willi syndrome patients: systematic review and meta-analysis. BMJ Paediatr Open. 2020;4(1):e000630.
68. Rosenberg AGW, Passone CGB, Pellikaan K, Damiani D, van der Lely AJ, Polak M, et al. Growth Hormone treatment for adults with Prader-Willi syndrome: a meta-analysis. J Clin Endocrinol Metab. 2021;106(10):3068–91.
69. The Clinical and Scientific Advisory Board of The International Prader-Willi Syndrome Organisation, Höybye C, Holland AJ, Driscoll DJ. Time for a general approval of growth hormone treatment in adults with Prader–Willi syndrome. Orphanet J Rare Dis. 2021;16(1):69.

70. Mahmoud R, Swanson HD, Butler MG, Flodman P, Gold JA, Miller JL, et al. Molecular classes and growth hormone treatment effects on behavior and emotion in patients with Prader-Willi syndrome. J Clin Med. 2022;11(9):2572.
71. Dykens EM, Roof E, Hunt-Hawkins H. Cognitive and adaptive advantages of growth hormone treatment in children with Prader-Willi syndrome. J Child Psychol Psychiatry. 2017;58(1):64–74.
72. Butler MG, Matthews NA, Patel N, Surampalli A, Gold J, Khare M, et al. Impact of genetic subtypes of Prader-Willi syndrome with growth hormone therapy on intelligence and body mass index. Am J Med Genet A. 2019:ajmg.a.61293.
73. Luo Y, Zheng Z, Yang Y, Bai X, Yang H, Zhu H, et al. Effects of growth hormone on cognitive, motor, and behavioral development in Prader-Willi syndrome children: a meta-analysis of randomized controlled trials. Endocrine. 2021;71(2):321–30.
74. Ji NY, Findling RL. Pharmacotherapy for mental health problems in people with intellectual disability. Curr Opin Psychiatry. 2016;29(2):103–25.
75. Duis J, Pullen LC, Picone M, Friedman N, Hawkins S, Sannar E, et al. Diagnosis and management of sleep disorders in Prader-Willi syndrome. J Clin Sleep Med. 2022;18(6):1687–96.
76. Yang-Li D, Fei-Hong L, Hui-Wen Z, Ming-Sheng M, Xiao-Ping L, Li L, et al. Recommendations for the diagnosis and management of childhood Prader-Willi syndrome in China. Orphanet J Rare Dis. 2022;17(1):221.
77. Bauer M, Whybrow PC. Thyroid hormone, neural tissue and mood modulation. World J Biol Psychiatry. 2001;2(2):59–69.
78. Bonnot O, Cohen D, Thuilleaux D, Consoli A, Cabal S, Tauber M. Psychotropic treatments in Prader-Willi syndrome: a critical review of published literature. Eur J Pediatr. 2016;175(1):9–18.
79. McIntyre RS, McCann SM, Kennedy SH. Antipsychotic metabolic effects: weight gain, diabetes mellitus, and lipid abnormalities. Can J Psychiatry. 2001;46(3):273–81.

Further Reading

Bonnot O, Cohen D, Thuilleaux D, Consoli A, Cabal S, Tauber M. Psychotropic treatments in Prader-Willi syndrome: a critical review of published literature. Eur J Pediatr. 2016;175(1):9–18.
Butler MG, Miller JL, Forster JL. Prader-Willi syndrome—clinical genetics, diagnosis and treatment approaches: an update. Curr Pediatr Rev. 2019;15(4):207–44.
Cassidy SB, Schwartz S, Miller JL, Driscoll DJ. Prader-Willi syndrome. Genet Med. 2012;14(1):10–26.
Duis J, Pullen LC, Picone M, Friedman N, Hawkins S, Sannar E, et al. Diagnosis and management of sleep disorders in Prader-Willi syndrome. J Clin Sleep Med. 2022;18(6):1687–96.
Rice LJ, Einfeld SL, Hu N, Carter CS. A review of clinical trials of oxytocin in Prader–Willi syndrome. Curr Opin Psychiatry. 2018;31(2):123–7.
Schwartz L, Caixàs A, Dimitropoulos A, Dykens E, Duis J, Einfeld S, et al. Behavioral features in Prader-Willi syndrome (PWS): consensus paper from the International PWS clinical trial consortium. J Neurodev Disord. 2021;13(1):25.
Tan Q, Orsso CE, Deehan EC, Triador L, Field CJ, Tun HM, et al. Current and emerging therapies for managing hyperphagia and obesity in Prader-Willi syndrome: a narrative review. Obes Rev. 2020;21(5)

Fragile X Syndrome

7

Elizabeth Berry-Kravis and Craig Erickson

7.1 Overview of Fragile X Syndrome

Fragile X syndrome (FXS) occurs in about 1:4000 males and females and is the most common known genetic cause of autism spectrum disorder (ASD) and inherited cause of intellectual disability (ID). Fragile X syndrome results from a trinucleotide repeat (CGG) expansion mutation of greater than 200 repeats (full mutation) in the promoter of the *FMR1* (*Fragile X Messenger Ribonucleoprotein 1*) gene, which leads to the transcriptional silencing of *FMR1* and either the loss or significant reduction of expression of the gene product, fragile X messenger ribonucleoprotein (FRMP) [1–3]. Fragile X messenger ribonucleoprotein is an RNA-binding protein that associates with ribosomes in a protein complex and regulates activation-dependent dendritic translation through multiple signaling pathways. Loss of FMRP in the FXS mouse model results in morphologically immature dendritic spines and impaired synaptic plasticity [1–3].

Fragile X syndrome is associated with characteristic but variably present physical features like large ears, long face, hyperflexible joints, and large testes. However, based on the synaptic and neural deficits, the major functional challenge in FXS is related to ID and associated impaired adaptive, social, and language functioning, combined at times, with behavioral difficulties including distractibility, hyperactivity, anxiety, perseveration, irritability, and aggression [2, 3]. This complex mix of manifestations of neural miswiring results in long-term limitations to independent

E. Berry-Kravis (✉)
Departments of Pediatrics, Neurological Sciences, Anatomy and Cell Biology, Rush University Medical Center, Chicago, IL, USA
e-mail: elizabeth_berry-kravis@rush.edu

C. Erickson
Division of Child and Adolescent Psychiatry, Cincinnati Children's Hospital Medical Center, Cincinnati, OH, USA

R. P. Thom, C. J. McDougle (eds.), *Neuropsychiatric Care for Genetic Syndromes and Other Neurodevelopmental Disorders*,
https://doi.org/10.1007/978-3-031-76269-7_7

functioning, self-support, community access, and vocational and social options. Females with FXS are typically less affected due to the expression of FMRP from the normal gene in cells in which the normal X is the active chromosome. The manifestations of FXS are currently addressed with supportive management, including addressing medical issues, implementing therapy, optimizing educational support, and managing behavior with behavioral therapy and medications.

The Fragile X Clinical and Research Consortium (FXCRC) was created in 2006 to help ensure patient and family access to expert supportive management of FXS, standardize care delivery, and provide a clinic network that could increase research cohort size, collect data on the natural history of FXS, and form a clinical trial network for upcoming trials of disease-targeted treatments [4]. This network now includes 34 FXS clinics across the United States. Treatment and Intervention Recommendations documents were created to provide families, educators, and clinicians information on best practice management of many issues that are relevant to persons with FXS. These are posted on the National Fragile X Foundation (NFXF) website (see Further Reading) and can be downloaded in PDF format. The documents are updated periodically based on new information continuously becoming available from the Fragile X Online Registry With Accessible Research Database (FORWARD), the natural history study of FXS being carried out at FXCRC clinics from 2009 to 2020 [5]. and FORWARD Multiple Assessments for Research Characterization (FORWARD-MARCH), the current natural history study. The FORWARD project has also generated multiple publications in the literature providing information on problems seen in FXS to facilitate anticipatory guidance and management recommendations [6].

7.1.1 Developmental and Cognitive Characteristics of FXS

The majority of males with FXS will meet the criteria for mild-to-severe ID [7]. The average IQ in adult males with FXS is 40–50, with a mental age equivalent of about 5 or 6 years. About 25% of females with FXS have ID, with others frequently being diagnosed with learning disabilities [8]. The average IQ in females is around 80, ranging from severe impairment to normal or even superior cognitive ability. There is a relatively consistent pattern of intellectual weaknesses and strengths distinct to FXS. Most research indicates that FXS is associated with deficiencies in visuospatial skills, processing of sequential information, and executive functioning skills such as working memory and attention [9]. Areas of relative strength include vocabulary, receptive language, visual memory, simultaneous processing, and long-term memory. Standard scores on intelligence and adaptive tests drop with age during childhood; however, this does not represent a true decline but rather a failure to keep pace with the rate of development in typical peers [10–12].

7.1.2 Language in FXS

Language development is delayed starting early in life for most males and some females with FXS [13, 14]. It is not uncommon for individuals with FXS to remain as prelinguistic communicators, i.e., using gestures, vocalizations, and maybe a few single words, much later in life than is seen in typical development. The majority of males and females with FXS obtain spoken language at some point, and they will continue to gain language skills throughout their lifespan [13–17]. The gap in language ability between individuals with FXS and their typically developing peers, however, widens with time, resulting in lower standard scores on language tests with advancing age, again reflecting slower development rather than individual decline [18]. In general, individuals with FXS have stronger receptive than expressive language skills [16, 17].

Individuals with FXS show delays in pragmatic language very early in development. Young children with FXS have difficulty reciprocating positive facial expressions, for example [13]. Joint attention in infants and toddlers with FXS is reduced, and this may cause delays or abnormal development of behaviors such as pointing or following eye gaze, as well as decreased turn-taking [19]. Deficits in pragmatic skills continue to surface as individuals develop. Studies indicate that males with FXS demonstrate high rates of tangential (off-topic) language, overly literal interpretation of language, and decreased topic initiation and maintenance [20]. Repetitive language is a hallmark of FXS and one that causes significant social difficulty and may reduce the intelligibility of speech, particularly when perseverative speech is rapid. This repetition can occur at the sound, word, and phrase level, such as repeating a certain phrase over and over, or it may be a refusal to allow a conversation to transition away from a preferred topic.

7.2 Signs and Symptoms of Common Psychiatric Comorbidities

7.2.1 Autism Spectrum Disorder (ASD)

Fragile X syndrome accounts for about 2 or 3% of all cases of ASD [21]. A variety of studies of FXS cohorts have suggested that about 18–67% of males and 20% of females with FXS meet the diagnostic criteria for ASD [22]. In the FORWARD study, 51% of males and 18% of females had ASD based on the Diagnostic and Statistical Manual of Mental Disorders, Fifth Edition (DSM-5) criteria [23]. Behavioral and neurological phenotypes common to FXS and ASD include social-interactional and communication/language deficits, poor eye contact, repetitive motor movements such as stereotypies, unusual reactions to sensory input, including hypersensitivity (e.g., tactile defensiveness) and hyposensitivity (e.g., high tolerance for pain), cognitive strength in visual memory, increased prevalence of seizures relative to the general population (although peak incidence is in childhood in FXS, compared to adolescence in ASD), macrocephaly, difficulties with the regulation of attention, activity level, emotional behavior, and mood, often leading to additional diagnoses (e.g., ADHD, anxiety, and mood disorder), other problematic behaviors (e.g., aggression, noncompliance, and self-injury), and sleep problems. Some behavioral characteristics or symptoms are seen in both ASD and FXS but for different underlying reasons. Individuals with FXS, for example, typically avoid eye contact directly [24]. looking away from people so as to help with coping with emotional discomfort that is driven by social anxiety [25, 26]. Thus, lack of social initiation and poor eye contact are thought to be mostly due to anxiety [27]. in FXS, rather than a lack of social awareness or failure to process social cues, which are commonly seen in ASD.

Characteristics that tend to differ between the FXS and ASD phenotypes include a higher rate of ID in FXS than idiopathic ASD, significantly more severe motor coordination deficits in FXS than ASD, generally higher interest in socialization in FXS (although limited by anxiety), and better imitation skills in FXS than ASD. Based on FORWARD data, individuals with FXS and ASD, relative to those with FXS alone, have less developed language skills, lower IQ, and adaptive skills, are less likely to toilet train, are more likely to have seizures and sleep problems, are more likely to demonstrate irritability, and are more likely to be on antipsychotic medication. Although individuals with FXS and comorbid ASD have a behavioral phenotype more similar to idiopathic ASD than those with FXS alone, these individuals still have a characteristic pattern of ASD with higher levels of hyperarousal, social and generalized anxiety, and repetitive behaviors [24, 27, 28].

7.2.2 Behavior and Comorbid Psychiatric Diagnoses Related to Behavior in FXS

The behavioral phenotype in males with FXS covers a wide spectrum although there are certain key behaviors that are considered hallmarks of the disorder. These behaviors fall into the broad categories of inattention/hyperactivity, hyperarousal, anxiety, perseveration, and aggression. Females can have problems in any of these behavioral categories but tend to be less frequently aggressive and typically struggle the most with anxiety and inattention.

In attention, hyperactivity, and impulsivity are very common in FXS, and an attention-deficit/hyperactivity disorder (ADHD) diagnosis has been reported in as many as 73% of males with FXS [29]. For females, there is an increased risk of ADHD symptoms, although the rate of actual diagnosis of ADHD is lower, between 30–63% [30]. For both sexes, these rates are higher than what is found in populations with individuals with learning disabilities not related to FXS, and the symptoms do not seem to be attributable solely to cognitive or developmental level [31].

Another key area of difficulty for individuals with FXS is anxiety. One study found that 86.2% of males with FXS and 76.9% of females with FXS met the criteria for an anxiety disorder [32]. Although individuals with FXS manifest high rates of generalized anxiety disorder, and of virtually all of the anxiety disorders, the anxiety disorders most frequently found in the literature are specific phobias and social anxiety disorder [32]. Social anxiety and consequent social avoidance appear to begin as early as during the preschool years and continue through adulthood. The severity of social anxiety may increase in adulthood, leading to significant avoidance and reclusiveness. At its most severe, social avoidance can manifest itself as selective mutism, a condition in which an individual is unable to speak in certain environments. This condition was found in 28% of the individuals with FXS and is dramatically higher than the prevalence rate of <0.1% found in the general population [32]. A recent family survey yielded four main categories of behaviors associated with anxiety: (1) increased irritability, aggression, and self-injury, (2) increased physical movement, nervous activity, and restlessness, (3) avoidance, freezing, and physical/physiological features of anxiety such as flushing and palpitations, and (4) gastrointestinal symptoms [33].

Hyperarousal and sympathetic overactivity are commonly seen in FXS. These hypersensitivities are triggered by a wide range of situations, including but not limited to noises, new environments, crowds, interpersonal distance, eye contact, and new people. The effects of hyperarousal are widespread including potentially physical hyperactivity (e.g., running and jumping), stereotypic motor movements (e.g., hand-flapping), gaze aversion, and an increase in perseverative behaviors [34].

Perseverative behavior can take many forms, including perseverative speech. Perseveration on a certain movie, or part of a movie, as well as fixating on a particular theme (e.g., only being interested in movies that show one preferred character) is also very common [34]. These extremely restricted interests are difficult to expand and cause difficulties in social interactions as the individual may be unwilling to deviate from their preferred activities.

Irritability, agitation, aggression, and self-injurious (IAAS) behaviors are especially detrimental to family functioning in FXS as they can significantly impede an individual's ability to participate in daily activities. In a large parental report study, 41% of males and 17% of females with FXS were described as having self-injured at some point in their lifetime [35]. Based on this report, self-injurious behaviors (SIB) typically appear fairly early in development, with an onset between 1 and 3 years of age for most individuals. There are a wide variety of types of SIB, including self-hitting, biting, pulling, picking, and scratching. Aggression can occur early in life but often becomes worse during the pubescent and postpubescent periods. In the FORWARD dataset, IAAS behaviors occurred in 50.1% of individuals with FXS, and 43.5% were treated with medication targeting IAAS [36]. Another report noted that 31% of caregivers of males with FXS and 17% of females reported being injured by that individual with FXS during the previous year. Of those caregivers of males, there was a mean number of 16 injuries per year, with 2.7 being serious enough to require medical care [37]. Research from FORWARD indicates that a comorbid diagnosis of FXS and ASD is associated with a significantly higher rate of aggressive behaviors and that overall IAAS behaviors in FXS are associated with male sex, lower IQ, anxiety, and increased need for antipsychotic use [36].

Among the 1,626 individuals with FXS in FORWARD, behavior problems have been described as a limiting issue in 87% of patients. The behavioral picture described in the FORWARD cohort is complex with life-limiting problems in multiple behavioral domains. Sixty-five percent of patients have multiple comorbid diagnoses, and half of the individuals with FXS are treated with psychiatric medications [6]. In this patient population, increasing severity of ID has been associated with increased psychiatric medication use overall, specifically of antipsychotic medications [38].

7.3 Assessment/Diagnosis of FXS

A simple DNA test based on polymerase chain reaction (PCR) can be used to detect the CGG repeat mutation of >200 repeats and diagnose FXS. The PCR test will also show alleles less than 200 repeats if the individual is mosaic for a premutation or normal allele. The methylation status of *FMR1* can be determined by Southern blot or by methylation PCR. Other medical and psychological assessments are based on the specific needs of the individual being assessed.

7.4 Psychosocial Treatment of FXS

7.4.1 Supportive Therapies

Given the global developmental delay most individuals with FXS display, it is likely that they will qualify for multiple therapy services at a young age. Occupational therapy, physical therapy, and speech therapy should all be accessed as much as possible to maximize early developmental progress. If verbal language is extremely delayed, families may find it beneficial to pursue another form of communication such as sign language or a picture exchange system in order to minimize frustration. Individuals with FXS who are minimally verbal may find an alternative augmented communication (AAC) device helpful for communication.

Occupational therapy (OT) will often target both the fine motor and sensory difficulties found in FXS. Fine motor skills are often significantly delayed and OT services may continue throughout the school years. If writing skills are delayed enough to inhibit performance at school, it is recommended the child with FXS have access to a keyboard for typing or an option to dictate responses. Physical therapy (PT) is usually implemented for younger children with FXS due to hypotonia and to work on gait skills. Most children with FXS need PT less as they are older, but some can benefit from an adaptive physical education program at school.

Therapy techniques that have been validated for ASD are often helpful in FXS. However, it is important to modify them based on what is known about the FXS phenotype. For example, Applied Behavioral Analysis (ABA) approaches are systematic methods of behavioral modification that have been shown to be effective for individuals with ASD. This approach is often suggested as an intervention for individuals with FXS, but a common early goal in many ABA-based interventions is to increase eye contact. This may not be appropriate for some individuals with FXS, as eye contact increases hyperarousal in FXS and decreases the ability to interact appropriately. Approaches used in ASD also do not take advantage of the natural desire for social engagement found in FXS, a significant strength that should be utilized. Therefore, modified ABA or therapy following the Early Start Denver Model may be recommended for children with FXS.

7.4.2 Supportive Educational Management

Educational interventions that match the cognitive and behavioral profile in FXS are important to optimize learning and minimize frustration, which can lead to behavioral problems. Most males and a high percentage of females with FXS will need an Individualized Education Program (IEP) for special education services and support in school. Inclusion is typically recommended to the extent possible for children with FXS, as this will provide better opportunities to benefit from peer modeling. Given the strength in imitation found in FXS, indirect teaching using peers can be an excellent tool for teaching. In order for inclusion to be successful, it is vital to provide the support needed by the individual, such as a one-on-one aide to adapt the curriculum and help with redirection and classroom integration for the child with FXS. These supports should be provided systematically and consistently throughout the child's academic environment.

In general, individuals with FXS benefit from a structured approach to academics that relates to their areas of interest. This could mean counting activities during which the individual counts a high-interest item or targeting sight words from a preferred television program. As individuals with FXS frequently display limited but intense interests, this is a simple way to increase engagement in an activity. Mathematics is often an area of academic weakness with severely impaired quantity sense. Visual and/or manipulative-based strategies may be useful for this area.

The visual memory strengths in FXS make reading approaches focused on sight words usually more successful. The weaknesses in working memory and sequencing common to FXS may make phonics-based approaches more frustrating, and many individuals with FXS may struggle with them. Many individuals with FXS are able to acquire some reading skills, and it is important for them to have consistent exposure to written content at the appropriate level to ensure that those skills are retained.

As individuals with FXS transition to higher levels of education, there is at times, a need to transition to vocational training as opposed to a strictly academic curriculum. The degree to which academics are continued depends on the needs of the individual. Some may plan to attend a postgraduation academic program that would require additional academic preparation.

Throughout the school-age years, it is necessary to provide intentional and planned opportunities for socialization, including, for example, peer buddy programs and socialization therapy to ensure that interaction skills continue to develop. Social goals should be included in the IEP so that they can be targeted directly during the school day.

Treatment recommendation documents outlining the above strategies and additional more detailed recommendations for general educational programming for children with FXS, as well as specific documents for preschool, elementary school, middle-high school, and transition programming are available on the NFXF website (see Further Reading). These documents are quite helpful for families to provide to educators when planning the IEP for a child with FXS.

7.4.3 Supportive Behavioral Approaches

While the behavioral phenotype of FXS is often challenging, there are some relatively simple strategies that can be implemented to lessen their impact on daily functioning.

In order to manage anxiety, it is helpful to use visual schedules that provide a clear picture of when an activity will end and what will happen next. Changes to routine and transitions are frequently problematic; so extra support at these times can be extremely helpful. Social stories are often useful for explaining appropriate behavior for a given situation. Counseling can be helpful for some higher and even lower functioning individuals with FXS to help them manage anxiety and learn to take themselves out of situations when upset or develop coping skills such as relaxation breathing or counting.

Hyperarousal is an ongoing issue in FXS, and there are several strategies that may be used to lessen its effect. Maintaining a calm environment will minimize the excessive stimuli that often result in hyperarousal. This can involve minimizing the extraneous noise from heating/cooling systems, dimming lights, and limiting excessive visual stimulation. Sensory diets, which are a schedule of sensory breaks and activities designed to keep the individual regulated, can be developed with an OT. Sensory diets are most effective when used to prevent hyperarousal from occurring, instead of being used reactively when the individual is already in a state of hyperarousal.

Many more helpful suggestions for managing behavior in FXS can be found in the Treatment Recommendations document on Behavioral Challenges in FXS on the NFXF website (see Further Reading).

For supportive management strategies in general, it is important to bear in mind that there is a wide spectrum of abilities in FXS, and the approach will need to be individualized to fit the strengths, weaknesses, and preferences of the individual. Individuals with FXS have been shown to display better behavioral and adaptive functioning when their environment and supportive programming are well-matched to their needs [43], and therefore, a highly individualized behavioral, therapeutic, and educational intervention plan is needed both for home and school or work environments.

7.5 Biological Treatments

7.5.1 Psychopharmacology for Behavior—General

Given the severity of behavior frequently seen in FXS that may prevent an individual from working or engaging in typical life activities and frequently causes a substantial burden for caregivers [37], psychopharmacological treatment is often used to ameliorate behavioral symptoms. Medication for behavior may be prescribed because an individual with FXS is causing injury or property destruction, because an individual is cognitively and/or behaviorally incapable of participating in normal life, or it is perceived that an individual could perform better or be in more inclusive settings if behavior (e.g., attention) was better managed. Thus, although little to no formal clinical trial data regarding efficacy for symptomatic drug treatment in FXS is available, psychopharmacologic treatment of ADHD symptoms, anxiety, hyperarousal, and IAAS behaviors with medications, such as stimulants, SSRIs, alpha-agonists, mood stabilizers, and antipsychotics, is often employed for individuals with FXS in clinical settings [44–46]. Indeed, in the FORWARD project, at a time when 975 individuals with FXS were enrolled, 66% of males (76% of those over age 4 years) and 54% of females were treated with medication for behavior [38]. The type of treatment needed varies with age as the behavioral phenotype tends to evolve, such that ADHD-like symptoms are more common in young children, while anxiety and irritability/aggression increase during the adolescent years into young adulthood [45, 47]. Thus, although there is overlap in behavioral symptoms, and all classes of medication are used at all ages, males with FXS under the age of 18 years are most commonly treated with stimulants and/or alpha-agonists, and males over the age of 18 years and females with FXS are most commonly treated with antidepressants. There is an increasing use of antipsychotics as males become older [44–46]. Successful treatment of targeted behaviors in FXS in a clinic setting, as defined by stringent clinical criteria for behavioral improvement based on reports from two sources over 6 months of treatment, ranges from 53% to 62% for trials of different classes of psychoactive medications [45, 47]. In several studies, the rate of success improved with sequential trials of medications within a class to find the most effective and best-tolerated medication, such that ultimately targeted behaviors were perceived as improved for about 73–77% of individuals with FXS on psychopharmacological treatment [45, 46]. Since only data from clinic surveys is available, these response data are likely somewhat inflated due to placebo responses.

Available data does, however, suggest that psychopharmacology targeted to ADHD-like, anxiety, and irritability symptoms in FXS can be quite helpful and appears to have fairly high effectiveness in a clinical setting. Several trials of medicines from a particular class, however, may be needed to achieve successful treatment without problematic side effects. The majority of individual treatment failures occur because the medication is not helpful for the targeted symptom although over a third of stimulant and antipsychotic trials fail because of side effects [46]. Although behavior in FXS is often difficult to analyze, and many patients have behaviors that fall into multiple categories and sometimes need treatment with a combination of medications to fully address their symptoms, it is important to identify the most problematic symptom and start one medication at a time targeted to this problem. Doses should start low and be titrated systematically to clinical effectiveness or side effects. Once an effective dose of medication treating the most significant problem has been achieved, then a second and additional problems can be targeted in sequence, if needed. The following subsections will address treatment based on common symptom complexes seen in FXS.

7.5.2 Treatment for ADHD Symptoms: Inattention, Hyperactivity, and Impulsivity

Stimulants are the most commonly used and, most often, effective class of medications in treating ADHD symptoms in youth with FXS. A 67% response rate was seen with methylphenidate in 15 patients in the one placebo-controlled study evaluating stimulants in FXS [48]. This is consistent with the report that 73% of individuals with FXS responded without major side effects to some preparation of stimulants in a large FXS cohort in a clinical setting [46]. Electrodermal studies, measuring an enhanced sweat response to stimuli in children with FXS, showed a decrease in electrodermal response after stimulant treatment, suggesting that FXS patients are responsive to the enhancement of inhibitory systems that occur with stimulant use for ADHD [49]. Although adult males with FXS tend to be less hyperactive and more anxious, leading to a medication shift toward the use of antidepressants and antipsychotics, some individuals still benefit substantially from the use of stimulants through adulthood.

In some individuals with FXS, stimulants exacerbate anxiety, irritability, or aggressive tendencies and must be abandoned. Indeed 40% of stimulant trials in a clinical setting were reported to fail because of side effects, which mostly consisted of aggravation of anxiety/irritability/aggressiveness but could occasionally include appetite suppression with occasional weight loss, stomach discomfort, lethargy, suppression of exuberance, and reduced speech output [46]. Stimulants now come in many different long-acting forms that may be quite useful in eliminating swings in mood and behavior during the day seen on multiple-dose regimens of fast-acting preparations. Stimulants may induce excessive side effects or may not be effective in children with FXS less than five or six years old, although they may be effective if reintroduced at an older age. One study suggested that stimulant preparations of the two major classes, methylphenidate and amphetamine salts, have similar overall response rates and the same profile of reasons for failure in FXS [46]. Distinct groups of patients with FXS, however, may respond to or have side effects on only one class of stimulant, suggesting that both classes should be tried before making a determination about whether stimulants are helpful for a given patient with FXS.

The alpha-2 agonists, clonidine and guanfacine, showed a response rate of about 62% on a clinic chart review in treating hyperactive, hyper-aroused, hypersensitive, impulsive, and aggressive behaviors in boys with FXS [46], consistent with a survey study showing an 80% response rate for the management of hyperarousal and hyperactivity [50]. Alpha-2 agonists may be particularly effective in young children who do not tolerate or respond to stimulants and can also be quite helpful for sleep problems, although sedation can also be a problematic side effect. Sedation is often most prominent in the first few weeks after medication initiation and dose increases and often abates after that. Extended-release preparations of both clonidine and guanfacine now exist that can minimize sedation and eliminate the need for multiple daily doses of these agents.

7.5.3 Treatment for Anxiety/Mood Symptoms

Antidepressants are helpful in the clinical setting to target anxiety and mood symptoms and, to some extent, perseverative behaviors. In a large clinic cohort report, 77% of individuals with FXS responded to at least one antidepressant without major side effects limiting treatment [46]. This is consistent with data from a self-report survey of the effects of fluoxetine in adults with FXS, which revealed improvements in anxiety and mood in about 70% of treated individuals [51]. A placebo-controlled trial of sertraline in children with FXS aged 3–6 years showed no safety concerns and no improvement in primary outcomes, but analysis of secondary outcome measures showed significant improvements in motor and visual perceptual abilities and social participation in the sertraline-treated group relative to placebo [52]. Selective serotonin reuptake inhibitors are used across all ages in FXS but are the most commonly utilized form of treatment for females and adults with FXS [38] and appear to be particularly helpful for social anxiety and withdrawal in females with FXS. Fluoxetine has been previously reported to be effective for selective mutism in females with FXS and extreme shyness [53]. Taken together, the available studies suggest that SSRIs can be useful for the management of anxiety and behavioral/emotional symptoms in individuals with FXS.

The predominant side effect of SSRIs in FXS is behavioral activation with an increase in hyperactivity and disinhibited behaviors although nausea, diarrhea, and sedation are also seen sometimes. Insomnia is uncommon as an SSRI side effect in FXS [46]. Less activating SSRIs, such as sertraline or escitalopram, may be better tolerated in individuals with FXS who have higher levels of hyperactivity and impulsive behavior. The tricyclic antidepressants can also work well for bedwetting and sleep dysregulation [54], although electrocardiograms must be monitored, as sudden death, presumed due to cardiac dysrhythmias, has been described in rare individuals with FXS. Bupropion, which increases dopamine levels more than other antidepressants, can help with both attention and mood/anxiety issues. Bupropion can precipitate seizures in at-risk individuals and, therefore, should not be used in individuals with FXS and active seizures. Finally, trazodone can help with sleep dysregulation as well as anxiety.

7.5.4 Treatment for IAAS Behaviors

Antipsychotics are generally reserved for individuals with FXS who exhibit more extreme behaviors, and use rates are, thus, lower than for stimulants and antidepressants. They were helpful in a clinical setting to target irritability and aggression in 76% of individuals with FXS who had treatment trials with one or multiple antipsychotics [46]. The most problematic side effect of antipsychotics is weight gain, although nausea, vomiting, lethargy, and extrapyramidal symptoms can also occur [46]. Risperidone was effective clinically in FXS with high response rates for aggressive behavior in older males with FXS and other aberrant and undesired behaviors in young boys with FXS and autistic traits. This is consistent with the finding that risperidone is safe and effective for aggressive and aberrant behaviors in double-blind placebo-controlled trials in individuals with ASD [55]. Other atypical antipsychotics (quetiapine and ziprasidone) have less effect on weight and have been helpful for aggressive behavior in some patients with excessive weight gain on risperidone or olanzapine. Aripiprazole also has less effect on weight and appears to have high response rates in individuals with FXS in clinic cohorts [46] and resulted in a significant reduction in irritability in an open-label trial [56]. The pharmacological profile of aripiprazole may allow it to target multiple problematic areas including distractibility, aggressive and agitated behavior, and aberrant social behaviors. Some individuals with FXS, however, simply cannot tolerate aripiprazole because of side effects similar to those seen with stimulants including aggravation of irritable and perseverative behaviors, likely resulting from partial dopamine agonist activity. Although the newer atypical antipsychotics are less sedating and have a more favorable motor side effect profile than older antipsychotics like haloperidol and thioridazine, side effects, particularly weight gain, more so in children than adults, are still more frequent with atypical antipsychotics than for other classes of medications [46]. Metformin has been used to help with weight gain on antipsychotics in FXS, particularly as the FXS mouse and fly models have shown reversal of some phenotypes with metformin due to stabilization of insulin over-signaling [6]. In some cases, anticonvulsant mood stabilizers or lithium may be used for severe mood lability and behavioral outbursts in FXS, even in the absence of seizures.

In summary, the psychopharmacologic treatment of ADHD symptoms, anxiety, hyperarousal, and irritable/aggressive behaviors with medications such as stimulants, SSRIs, alpha-2 agonists, and antipsychotics, appears to be helpful in clinical settings, but response is typically incomplete. For example, data from a National Survey on FXS showed that about 10–20% of survey respondents felt that medication was not helpful for the behavior problems being treated in their child with FXS, while only about 40% felt the medication was helping a lot [47]. There is clearly an unmet need in FXS for better medications to treat behavior and for the development of treatments that target cognitive deficits. Treatments in development that appear to modify the underlying disorder in animal models would be a tremendously important advancement.

7.6 Common Medical Comorbidities and Management

The following conditions have been reported to be more common and clinically important in the FXS population relative to typical populations, based on data from the FORWARD project: strabismus, recurrent otitis media, obstructive sleep apnea (OSA), gastrointestinal problems such as loose stools and gastroesophageal reflux disease (GERD), seizures, and excessive weight gain [39]. Treatment of medical problems is important as, if these problems go untreated, they can impact development or behavior. The pediatrician should look for and ask about symptoms that might be related to these problems at routine yearly well-child visits and should refer to specialists for further evaluation and management if needed [39].

Since children with FXS have expressive language delays and recurrent otitis media (affecting 53% of children with FXS) [39], this may lead to conductive hearing loss and further language and articulation issues. It is important that all otitis media and/or any otologic issues be treated promptly and appropriately, with hearing monitoring and a relatively low threshold for early myringotomy tube placement in children with FXS and recurrent otitis media. It is important to recognize that children with FXS may not communicate pain well, and behavioral issues like head banging may be a sign of pain from acute otitis media. If chronically infected adenoids and tonsils become a problem, adenoidectomy and/or tonsillectomy may be performed at the same time as the myringotomy tubes are inserted.

Although vision monitoring is important for children with FXS, it can be difficult to obtain good vision screening for children with FXS due to communication and behavioral issues. Children with FXS who cannot cooperate with standard vision screening should be referred to a professional who can obtain a good vision assessment every few years during childhood to ensure that any acuity issues are being addressed. This is important so that these issues with vision do not compound problems with reading and academics. When present, strabismus, occurring in 16% of children with FXS [39], should be managed with eye patching, vision therapy, or surgery to avoid amblyopia and compounding of visual processing problems.

For concerns about episodes that might be seizures, which occurred in 13% of the 1,626 children with FXS in the FORWARD project [40], an electroencephalogram (EEG) should be obtained, along with a neurology referral. Ambulatory EEG can be used to distinguish behavioral spells from seizures. Typically, anticonvulsants that are least likely to cause sedation or behavioral aggravation are started after two documented seizures, with a plan to discontinue treatment after an individual with FXS is seizure-free for two years. The anticonvulsants most commonly used in FXS are levetiracetam, oxcarbazepine, lamotrigine, and valproic acid [40]. About 15% of individuals treated with levetiracetam develop behavioral deterioration. This may be ameliorated by co-treatment with pyridoxine, but in some cases, the levetiracetam must be discontinued. Oxcarbazepine, lamotrigine, and valproic acid can help with behavior and mood stabilization in some cases, allowing the management of both mood and seizures.

Children, especially those with ID, require adequate sleep for optimal development, learning, and functioning. Monitoring and managing OSA and other sleep problems [41] are of particular importance in FXS due to their relationship to decrements in daytime performance and behavior. The primary care physician should inquire about potential sleep problems in children with FXS at every well-child visit. Depending on the severity of the sleep problems, these may require behavioral and/or medical treatment or a referral to a sleep specialist. When symptoms of OSA are clearly present, management with tonsillectomy/adenoidectomy is indicated to prevent cognitive and behavioral aggravation.

Growth patterns identified in children with FXS suggest an increased risk for being overweight and having somewhat diminished height in adulthood [42]. It is important to encourage a healthy diet, food restriction when necessary, and exercise for 30–40 min, four or five times a week to minimize problems associated with increased weight.

When GERD is present, occurring in about 11% of those with FXS [39], medication should be used, when needed, to prevent pain, esophagitis, and resulting behavioral decompensation. As individuals with FXS are not always able to describe heartburn, the only signs of GERD may be behavioral outbursts occurring in patterns during the day in relation to meals or sleep dysfunction with frequent nighttime awakenings.

Finally, some individuals with FXS benefit from orthotics or shoe inserts for foot pronation and flat feet to help with motor development when young and avoid leg pain and reduce gait problems when older.

Key Points to Remember

- Fragile X syndrome is associated with a complex mix of behavioral and psychiatric comorbidities, often requiring multimodal interventions including tailored educational services, behavioral, speech, and occupational therapies, and at times, psychopharmacologic treatments.
- Characteristic behavioral problems in FXS evolve from hyperactivity, hyperarousal, and predominant ADHD symptoms in early childhood to anxiety, avoidance, reclusiveness, and sometimes, IAAS behaviors in adolescence and adulthood although the full range of associated behaviors can be seen at any age.
- While overall developmental and behavioral challenges on average are increased in males with FXS, females with FXS exhibit significant phenotypic heterogeneity with presentations on an individual patient level that may significantly overlap with common behaviors and concerns present in males with FXS.

Photographs of Individuals with the Syndrome

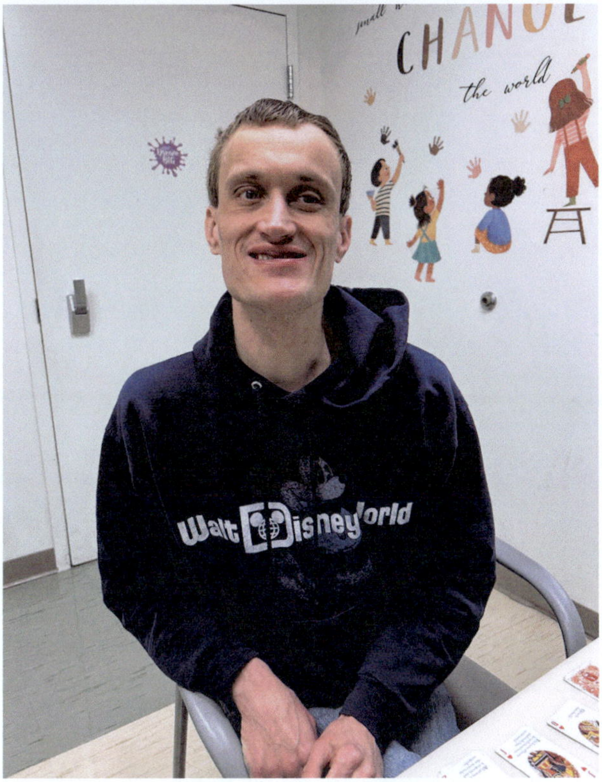

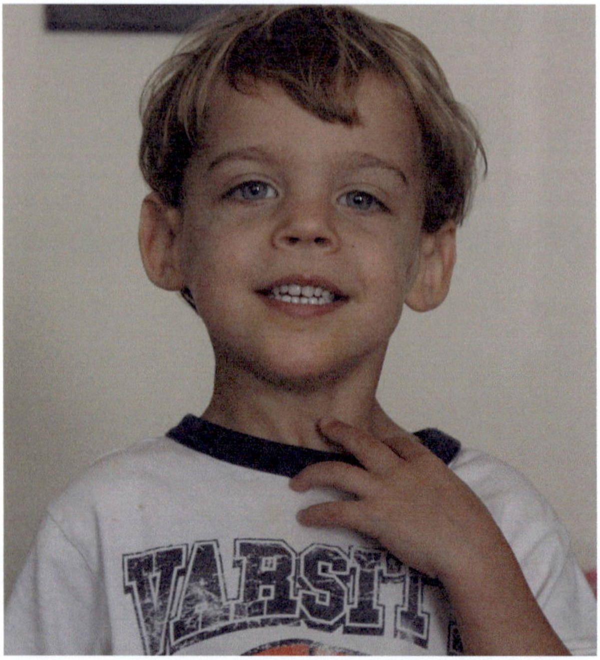

References

1. Berry-Kravis E, Lindemann L, Jønch AE, Apostol G, Bear MF, Carpenter RL, Crawley JN, Curie A, Des Portes V, Hossain F, Gasparini F, Gomez-Mancilla B, Hessl D, Loth E, Scharf SH, Wang PP, Von Raison F, Hagerman R, Spooren W, Jacquemont S. Drug development for neurodevelopmental disorders: lessons learned from fragile X syndrome. Nat Rev Drug Discov. 2018;17(4):280–99. https://doi.org/10.1038/nrd.2017.221.
2. Gross C, Hoffmann A, Bassell GJ, Berry-Kravis EM. Therapeutic strategies in fragile X syndrome: from bench to bedside and back. Neurotherapeutics. 2015;12(3):584–608. https://doi.org/10.1007/s13311-015-0355-9.
3. Hagerman RJ, Berry-Kravis E, Hazlett HC, Bailey DB, Moine H, Kooy RF, Tassone F, Gantois I, Sonenberg N, Mandel JL, Hagerman PJ. Fragile X syndrome. Nat Rev Dis Primers. 2017;3(1):1–19. https://doi.org/10.1038/nrdp.2017.65.
4. Liu JA, Hagerman RJ, Miller RM, Craft LT, Finucane B, Tartaglia N, Berry-Kravis EM, Sherman SL, Kidd SA, Cohen J. Clinicians' experiences with the fragile X clinical and research consortium. Am J Med Genet A. 2016;170(12):3138–43. https://doi.org/10.1002/ajmg.a.37948.
5. Sherman SL, Kidd SA, Riley C, Berry-Kravis E, Andrews HF, Miller RM, Lincoln S, Swanson M, Kaufmann WE, Brown WT. Forward: a registry and longitudinal clinical database to study fragile X syndrome. Pediatrics. 2017;139(Suppl. 3):S183–93. https://doi.org/10.1542/peds.2016-1159E.
6. Berry-Kravis E. Disease-targeted treatment translation in Fragile X syndrome as a model for neurodevelopmental disorders. J Child Neurol. 2022;37(10-11):797–812.
7. Kaufmann WE, Abrams MT, Chen W, Reiss AL. Genotype, molecular phenotype, and cognitive phenotype: Correlations in fragile X syndrome. Am J Med Genet. 1999;83(4):286.

8. de Vries BB, Wiegers AM, Smits AP, et al. Mental status of females with an FMR1 gene full mutation. Am J Hum Genet. 1996;58(5):1025.
9. Dykens EM, Hodapp RM, Leckman JF. Strengths and weaknesses in the intellectual functioning of males with fragile X syndrome. Am J Ment Def. 1987;92(2):234.
10. Fisch GS, Carpenter N, Holden JJA, et al. Longitudinal changes in cognitive and adaptive behavior in fragile X females: a prospective multicenter analysis. Am J Med Genet. 1999;83(4):308.
11. Fisch GS, Simensen R, Tarleton J, et al. Longitudinal study of cognitive abilities and adaptive behavior levels in fragile X males: a prospective multicenter analysis. Am J Med Genet. 1996;64(2):356.
12. Klaiman C, Quintin E-M, Jo B, et al. Longitudinal profiles of adaptive behavior in fragile X syndrome. Pediatrics. 2014;134(2):315–24.
13. Roberts JE, Mirrett P, Anderson K, Burchinal M, Neebe E. Early communication, symbolic behavior, and social profiles of young males with fragile X syndrome. Am J Speech Lan Pathol. 2002;11(3):295–304.
14. Roberts JE, Mirrett P, Burchinal M. Receptive and expressive communication development of young males with fragile X syndrome. Am J Ment Retard. 2001;106(3)
15. Abbeduto L, Hagerman RJ. Language and communication in fragile X syndrome. Ment Retard Dev Disabil Res Rev. 1997;3(4):313.
16. Lewis P, Abbeduto L, Murphy M, et al. Cognitive, language and social-cognitive skills of individuals with fragile X syndrome with and without autism. J Intellect Develop Disabil. 2006;50(7):532–45.
17. McDuffie A, Kover S, Abbeduto L, Lewis P, Brown T. Profiles of receptive and expressive language abilities in boys with comorbid Fragile X syndrome and autism. Am J Intellect Dev Disabil. 2012;117(1):18.
18. Hoffmann A, Wang A, Berger N, Cordeiro L, Shaffer R, Tartaglia N, Erickson C, Berry-Kravis E. Language across the lifespan in Fragile X syndrome: characteristics and considerations for assessment. Brain Sci. 2020;10:212.
19. Murphy MM, Abbeduto L. Indirect genetic effects and the early language development of children with genetic mental retardation syndromes: the role of joint attention. Infant Young Child. 2005;18(1):47–59.
20. Belser RC, Sudhalter V. Conversational characteristics of children with Fragile X syndrome: repetitive speech. J Info. 2001;106(1)
21. Schaefer GB, Mendelsohn NJ. Genetics evaluation for the etiologic diagnosis of autism spectrum disorders. Genet Med. 2008;10(1):4–12.
22. Wang LW, Berry-Kravis E, Hagerman RJ. Fragile X: Leading the way for targeted treatments in autism. Neurotherapeutics. 2010;7(3):264–74.
23. Kaufmann WE, Kidd SA, Andrews HF, Budimirovic DB, Esler A, Haas-Givler B, Stackhouse T, Peacock G, Riley C, Sherman SL, Brown WT, Berry-Kravis E. Autism spectrum disorder in Fragile X syndrome: Characterization using FORWARD. Pediatrics. 2017;139(Suppl. 3):S194–206.
24. Hall SS, Lightbody AA, Hirt M, Rezvani A, Reiss AL. Autism in fragile X syndrome: a category mistake? J Am Acad Child Adolesc Psychiatry. 2010;49(9):921–33.
25. Budimirovic DB, Kaufmann WE. What can we learn about autism from studying Fragile X syndrome? Dev Neurosci. 2011;33(5):379–94.
26. Watson C, Hoeft F, Garrett AS, Hall SS, Reiss AL. Aberrant brain activation during gaze processing in boys with Fragile X syndrome. Arch Gen Psychiatry. 2008;65(11):1315–23.
27. Talisa VB, Boyle L, Crafa D, Kaufmann WE. Autism and anxiety in males with fragile X syndrome: an exploratory analysis of neurobehavioral profiles from a parent survey. Am J Med Genet B. 2014;164A(5):1198–203.
28. Abbeduto L, McDuffie A, Thurman AJ. The Fragile X syndrome–autism comorbidity: what do we really know? Front. Genetics. 2014:5.
29. Baumgardner TL, Reiss AL, et al. Specification of the neurobehavioral phenotype in males with fragile X syndrome. Pediatrics. 1995;95(5):744.

30. Mazzocco MM, Pennington BF, Hagerman RJ. The neurocognitive phenotype of female carriers of fragile X: additional evidence for specificity. J Dev Behav Pediatr. 1993;14(5):328–35.
31. Turk J. Fragile X syndrome and attentional deficits. J Appl Res Intell Disab. 1998;11(3):175.
32. Cordeiro L, Ballinger E, Hagerman R, Hessl D. Clinical assessment of DSM-IV anxiety disorders in Fragile X syndrome: prevalence and characterization. J Neurodev Disord. 2011;3(1):57–67.
33. Lozano R, Thompson T, Dixon-Weber J, Erickson CA, Berry-Kravis E, Williams S, Smith E, Frazier JA, Rosselot H, Farmer C, Hessl D. Observable symptoms of anxiety in individuals with Fragile X syndrome: parent and caregiver perspectives. Genes (Basel). 2022;13(9):1660.
34. Reisinger DL, Shaffer RC, Tartaglia N, Berry-Kravis E, Erickson CA. Delineating repetitive behavior profiles across the lifespan in Fragile X syndrome. Brain Sci. 2020;10:239.
35. Symons FJ, Byiers BJ, Raspa M, Bishop E, Bailey DB Jr. Self-injurious behavior and Fragile X syndrome: findings from the national fragile X survey. Am J Intellect Dev Disabil. 2010;115(6):473–81.
36. Eckert EM, Dominick KC, Pedapati EV, Wink LK, Shaffer RC, Andrews H, Choo TH, Chen C, Kaufmann WE, Tartaglia N, Berry-Kravis EM, Erickson CA. Pharmacologic interventions for irritability, aggression, agitation and self-injurious behavior in fragile X syndrome: an initial cross-sectional analysis. J Autism Dev Disord. 2019;49:4595–602.
37. Bailey DB Jr, Raspa M, Bishop E, Mitra D, Martin S, Wheeler A, Sacco P. Health and economic consequences of Fragile X syndrome for caregivers. J Dev Behav Pediatr. 2012;33:705–12.
38. Dominick KC, Andrews HF, Kaufmann WE, Berry-Kravis E, Erickson CA. Psychotropic drug treatment patterns in persons with fragile X syndrome. J Child Adolesc Psychopharmacol. 2021;31:659–69.
39. Kidd S, Lachiewicz A, Barbouth D, Blitz RK, Delahunty C, McBrien D, Visootsak J, Berry-Kravis E. Fragile X syndrome: a review of associated medical problems. J Pediatr. 2014;134:995–1005.
40. Berry-Kravis E, Filipink RA, Frye RE, Golla S, Morris SM, Andrews H, Choo TH, Kaufmann WE, FORWARD Consortium. Seizures in Fragile X syndrome: associations and longitudinal analysis of a large clinic-based cohort. Front Pediatr. 2021;9:736255. https://doi.org/10.3389/fped.2021.736255.
41. Budimirovic DB, Protic DD, Delahunty CM, Andrews HF, Choo TH, Xu Q, Berry-Kravis E, Kaufmann WE, FORWARD Consortium. Sleep problems in Fragile X syndrome: cross-sectional analysis of a large clinic-based cohort. Am J Med Genet A. 2021; Epub ahead of print
42. Choo TH, Xu Q, Budimirovic D, Lozano R, Esler AN, Frye RE, Andrews H, Velinov M. Height and BMI in Fragile X syndrome: a longitudinal assessment. Obesity (Silver Spring). 2022;30:743–50.
43. Hessl D, Dyer-Friedman J, Glaser B, et al. The influence of environmental and genetic factors on behavior problems and autistic symptoms in boys and girls with fragile X syndrome. Pediatrics. 2001;108(5):e88.
44. Amaria R, Billeisen L, Hagerman R. Medication use in Fragile X syndrome. Mental Health Aspects Dev Disabil. 2001;4:143–7.
45. Berry-Kravis E, Potanos K. Psychopharmacology in fragile X syndrome—present and future. Ment Retard Dev Disabil Res Rev. 2004;10(1):42–8.
46. Berry-Kravis E, Sumis A, Hervey C, Mathur S. Clinic-based retrospective analysis of psychopharmacology for behavior in fragile x syndrome. Int J Pediatr. 2012;2012(5):843016–1.
47. Bailey DB, Raspa M, Bishop E, Olmsted M, Mallya UG, Berry-Kravis E. Medication utilization for targeted symptoms in children and adults with Fragile X syndrome: US survey. J Dev Behav Ped. 2012;33(1):62–9.
48. Hagerman RJ, Murphy MA, Wittenberger MD. A controlled trial of stimulant medication in children with the fragile X syndrome. Am J Med Genet. 1988;30(1-2):377–92.
49. Hagerman RJ, Miller LJ, McGrath-Clarke J, et al. Influence of stimulants on electrodermal studies in Fragile X syndrome. Microsc Res Techniq. 2002;57(3):168–73.
50. Hagerman R, Riddle J, Roberts L, Breese K, Fulton M. Survey of the efficacy of clonidine in Fragile X syndrome. Dev Brain Dysfunct. 1995;8(4–6):336–44.

51. Hagerman RJ, Fulton MJ, Leaman A, Riddle J. A survey of fluoxetine therapy in fragile X syndrome. Dev Brain Dysfunct. 1994;
52. Greiss Hess L, Fitzpatrick SE, Nguyen DV, Chen Y, Gaul KN, Schneider A, Lemons Chitwood K, Eldeeb MA, Polussa J, Hessl D, Rivera S, Hagerman RJ. A randomized, double-blind, placebo-controlled trial of low-dose sertraline in young children with Fragile X syndrome. J Dev Behav Pediatr. 2016;37(8):619–28. https://doi.org/10.1097/DBP.0000000000000334.
53. Hagerman R, Hills J, Scharfenaker S, Lewis H. Fragile X syndrome and selective mutism. Am J Med Genet. 1999;83(4):313–7.
54. Hilton DK, Martin CA, Heffron WM, Hall BD, Johnson GL. Imipramine treatment of ADHD in a Fragile X child. J Am Acad Child Adolesc Psychiatry. 1991;30(5):831–4.
55. McCracken JT, McGough J, Shah B, et al. Risperidone in children with autism and serious behavioral problems. N Engl J Med. 2002;347(5):314–21.
56. Erickson CA, Stigler KA, Wink LK, et al. A prospective open-label study of aripiprazole in fragile X syndrome. Psychopharmacology. 2011;216(1):85–90.

Further Reading

Berry-Kravis E. Disease-targeted treatment translation in Fragile X Syndrome as a model for neurodevelopmental disorders. J Child Neurol. 2022;37(10-11):797–812.

NFXF Treatment and Recommendation Documents. n.d.. https://fragilex.org/our-research/treatment-recommendations/.

Duplication 15q Syndrome

8

Dana Q. Tran

8.1 Overview

8.1.1 Epidemiology

The prevalence of maternal 15q duplication syndrome (Dup15q) in the general population remains unknown. Maternal 15q duplication syndrome is one of the most frequent genetic mutations in individuals with autism spectrum disorder (ASD). Prevalence rates of Dup15q have been estimated to vary between 0.2% and 3% in patients with ASD [1–4].

8.1.2 Genetic/Neurobiological Mechanisms

Maternal 15q duplication syndrome originates from maternally derived repeats of segments on the long arm of chromosome 15 (15q). There are five segments of chromosome 15q that are susceptible to genetic rearrangement. These segments are called B1, B2, B3, B4, and B5, and they make up the 15q11.2–q13.1 region [5–7]. Genes in the 15q11.2–q13.1 region, known as the Prader-Willi/Angelman Critical Region (PWACR), are subject to imprinting, an epigenetic phenomenon that determines gene expression depending on the parent of origin [8]. Deletions in this region can result in either Angelman syndrome if derived from the mother or Prader-Willi syndrome if derived from the father. The duplication phenotype appears almost exclusively in cases of maternal origin, although paternal duplications with

D. Q. Tran (✉)
Massachusetts General Hospital Lurie Center for Autism, Lexington, MA, USA

Harvard Medical School, Boston, MA, USA
e-mail: dtran11@mgh.harvard.edu

R. P. Thom, C. J. McDougle (eds.), *Neuropsychiatric Care for Genetic Syndromes and Other Neurodevelopmental Disorders*,
https://doi.org/10.1007/978-3-031-76269-7_8

variable phenotypes have also been reported [9]. Usually, however, paternally derived 15q11.2–q13.1 duplications result in a normal phenotype [1, 10].

There are two common forms of maternally derived 15q duplications, each associated with a relatively distinct clinical profile. The maternal interstitial subtype (int[15]) is caused by an extra copy of 15q11.2–q13.1 within the 15q chromosome (~20–40%), resulting in trisomy for 15q11.2–q13.1. The maternal isodicentric subtype (idic(15)) is caused by a supernumerary chromosome, which typically contains two extra copies of 15q11.2–q13.1 (~60–80%), resulting in tetrasomy of this genetic region [11–13, 15]. More severe presentations are typically seen in patients with idic(15) [14]. The penetrance is generally complete for both subtypes and equivalent in males and females [15].

The duplication of 15q11.2–q13.1 involves various genes that give rise to some of the common issues seen clinically. However, no single gene has been identified as causing Dup15q on its own. *UBE3A*, the gene involved in Angelman syndrome, is also thought to be the primary gene responsible for intellectual impairment, anxiety, and the reduced seizure threshold seen in Dup15q [16]. Maternal duplication of *UBE3A* also underlies the ASD phenotype seen in this syndrome [2, 17, 18]. *GABRB3*, *GABRA5,* and *GABRG3* are genes that encode $GABA_A$ receptor subunits and are involved in the seizures commonly seen in Dup15q [8, 19–21].

8.1.3 Common Clinical Features

Dysmorphic features tend to be mild and include a flat occiput, down-slanting palpebral fissures, a depressed nasal bridge, a short nose with an upturned nasal tip, low-set ears, a long philtrum, a high-arched palate, a thick vermilion of the upper and lower lips, and micrognathia. As features tend to be subtle, they can be missed in infancy [8, 9, 22, 23].

Maternal 15q duplication syndrome is often accompanied by developmental delay and associated features, with common traits and differences between the interstitial and isodicentric subtypes. Individuals with Dup15q usually meet the criteria for ASD [1, 2]. Other common characteristics of Dup15q include intellectual disability (ID), central hypotonia resulting in motor delays, moderate-to-profound language impairment, and early-onset epilepsy that is often treatment-resistant [12, 13, 24–26]. Overall, the phenotype of int(15) is milder than that seen in idic(15). Although ID is part of both profiles, the severity of ID in int(15) is typically mild-to-moderate, whereas individuals with idic(15) typically have moderate-to-profound ID [9, 12, 13]. Higher rates of ASD are also found in idic(15) compared to int(15), with approximately ≥80% and ≥50% meeting the criteria for ASD, respectively [8, 9, 24, 25]. Individuals with the idic(15) subtype also have greater impairment across cognitive, language, motor, and adaptive domains, especially if the presentation is accompanied by epilepsy [27].

More recent studies in the past decade have sought to further specify neurodevelopmental and functional characteristics of Dup15q, as well as to distinguish the profile from non-syndromic ASD. With regard to daily functioning, adaptive skills in Dup15q are relatively impaired across domains. Compared to children with nonsyndromic ASD, daily living and motor skills in youth with Dup15q are more severely affected [26]. Adaptive behaviors are highly correlated with the level of both verbal and nonverbal cognitive abilities [27]. Socially, eye contact in Dup15q is poorly modulated and very similar to classical ASD. However, in comparison to idiopathic ASD, children with Dup15q show significantly better performance on the Autism Diagnostic Observation Schedule (ADOS)-specific observations of "responsive social smile" and "facial expressions directed to others" [26]. Due to the relative strength in specific socialization skills, research suggests that the social pragmatic profile of Dup15q is more similar to other neurogenic syndromes than to idiopathic ASD. As for cognitive functioning, there is a high correlation between verbal and nonverbal cognitive abilities with consistency across subdomains [27].

8.2 Psychiatric Comorbidities

8.2.1 Anxiety

Although there is still a dearth of literature on the presence and nature of comorbid psychiatric illnesses, anxiety has been reported in Dup15q. Anxiety may stem from simple demands [22]. Generalized anxiety disorder (GAD), social anxiety disorder, and separation anxiety disorder have all been reported [4].

8.2.2 Attention-Deficit/Hyperactivity Disorder

Attention-deficit/hyperactivity disorder and associated externalizing symptoms have been reported as common behavioral concerns [4]. Hyperactivity has been reported to be associated with aggression, low frustration tolerance, and oppositional defiant behavior. Oppositional symptoms leading to aggression and property destruction can be triggered by environmental stressors at home or school. Inattentive symptoms, on the other hand, may manifest as struggles to plan out tasks [22]. Children with idic(15) may have a higher rate of challenging behavior overall, not accounted for by their higher rates of epilepsy or more severe cognitive impairment [27].

8.2.3 Mood Disorders

Mood disorders, although commonly seen in idiopathic ASD, are infrequently reported in Dup15q, with no published reports of major depressive disorder. Bipolar disorder without psychotic features has generally been described as mood lability with impulsivity, not accompanied by full symptoms of an acute mood episode, although these data are limited to case reports [28, 29, 31]. A limited number of cases of schizoaffective disorder and bipolar disorder with psychotic features in

Dup15q have also been described. In these very few cases, depressive, manic, and anxiety symptoms were present [29–31].

8.2.4 Psychosis

Psychotic symptoms have not been extensively described in this population, but there are some cases reported in the literature. Maternal idic(15) has been reported in schizophrenia cohorts, but schizophrenia is not described to be a common comorbidity in Dup15q. This may, however, reflect the difficulty in recognizing and diagnosing psychotic symptoms and illnesses in those with low cognitive functioning and limited language development [15, 32]. Symptoms thus far described in Dup15q patients who have a schizophrenia spectrum disorder include bizarre behaviors, auditory hallucinations of various natures (third-person, running commentary, commenting, and commanding voices), tactile hallucinations, delusions of various natures (persecutory, grandiose, somatic, religion, and control), thought insertion, thought withdrawal, disorganized thought process, agitation, persistent negative symptoms, and descriptions of "confusion" [29, 31, 33].

8.3 Medical Comorbidities

8.3.1 Epilepsy

Epilepsy is the medical comorbidity most commonly described in Dup15q. It tends to develop in early infancy, with infantile seizures occurring at a rate of 30–40% [34–36]. Epileptic characteristics in this population range from severe infantile spasms to occasional generalized tonic-clonic seizures emerging in late childhood [26, 34]. Rates of epilepsy are around 16% in the int(15) subtype and 60–80% in the idic(15) subtype [34, 35]. Individuals with idic(15) and epilepsy tend to have focal or multifocal seizures, with many progressing to secondarily generalized epilepsy syndrome with multiple seizure types [34–36]. Electroencephalogram studies in idic(15) describe generalized background slowing, multifocal epileptiform discharges, disrupted sleep physiology, frequent spike and wave discharges, abnormal delta and alpha oscillations, and persistent beta oscillations [34–37]. A known complication of epilepsy syndromes is sudden unexpected death in epilepsy (SUDEP), of which the mechanism remains poorly understood. This occurs in 9% of individuals with epilepsy [15]. Approximately 50% of seizure-related deaths are not due to SUDEP, but rather, other causes including status epilepticus, drowning, falls, and accidents [38]. There is still no data on the exact incidence of SUDEP in Dup15, but it seems to affect a minority of this patient population [15, 39–41]. Sudden unexpected death in epilepsy almost always occurs during sleep and mostly in teenagers and young adults. Risk factors appear to be nonambulatory status and poor seizure control [41].

Poorly controlled epilepsy comes with notable developmental issues and functional impairment. Youth with Dup15q who have epilepsy have more severely affected cognitive and adaptive functioning compared to those without epilepsy [26]. Greater impairment is particularly seen in those with epileptic encephalopathy, infantile spasms, or Lennox-Gastaut syndrome [27]. No prospective or randomized controlled trial data has been published on the effectiveness of anti-seizure medication in Dup15q [15].

8.3.2 Gastrointestinal Problems

Gastrointestinal (GI) problems are commonly found in Dup15q patients. Feeding difficulties in the neonatal period have been reported [2, 42, 43]. Common GI symptoms include constipation and gastroesophageal reflux disease (GERD). Irritability and aggression may improve once GI symptoms are treated. Other less common GI issues include loose stools, vomiting, poor appetite, failure to thrive, incontinence, diarrhea, texture sensitivity, and dysphagia. GI issues were present in 76.7% of individuals with idic(15) and 87.5% of those with int(15) [44].

8.4 Assessment

8.4.1 Genetic Testing

The diagnosis of Dup15q is based on genetic testing. At least one extra maternally derived copy of the PWACR on chromosome 15 is detected on chromosomal microarray (CMA) [13]. Chromosomal microarray detects an increased number of copy repeats of 15q11.2–q13.1 but cannot distinguish between the int(15) and idic(15) subtypes [15]. Targeted duplication analysis includes methods such as fluorescent in situ hybridization (FISH), and is required to differentiate between the two forms of duplication. Targeted duplication analysis can either be done for probands in which Dup15q was detected on CMA or to identify this cytogenetic anomaly in their relatives [15].

The question of testing relatives once Dup15q has been detected in an individual is an important one. It is recommended to do genetic testing on the mother to determine if she has the genetic alteration present in both int(15) and idic(15) [15]. Testing siblings should be considered for individuals with int(15), while recurrence is extremely rare in the siblings of a proband with idic(15). All probands reported to date with idic(15) whose parents have undergone genomic testing have had the disorder due to a de novo genetic alteration; thus, genetic testing of their siblings is not warranted [15].

8.4.2 Multidisciplinary Evaluations

After the initial diagnosis, multidisciplinary assessments and follow-up visits are recommended to detect and treat frequent comorbidities, as well as to provide recommendations for behavioral support and early intervention. Growth, nutritional status, and safe oral intake should be evaluated at each follow-up visit. The decision to pursue a clinical feeding evaluation and/or radiographic swallowing study should be based on the presence of poor weight gain, choking during feeds, recurrent respiratory infections, unexplained refusal to eat, and clinical symptoms of dysphagia. At each clinical visit, other items that should be assessed are development, learning, anxiety, aggression, self-injurious behavior, self-help functioning, and the need for family social work support. Gross motor and fine motor deficits benefit from physiotherapy and occupational therapy, respectively. For patients with seizures, the presence of increased seizure frequency and new-onset motor symptoms should be assessed at each clinic visit [15].

8.5 Psychosocial Treatment

As ASD features are quite common in Dup15q, patients may need treatments indicated for ASD, such as Applied Behavioral Analysis (ABA) [15]. Integrating the practice of motor skills with pragmatic communication teaching can target areas of weakness while building on the relative strength of social interest in youth with this syndrome [26]. Being connected to a greater support system may also decrease psychosocial burden. As such, clinicians should assess the family's need to be connected with a social worker for parental support, home nursing referrals, and online resources [15].

8.6 Biological Treatment

8.6.1 Seizure Management

Seizure management is important to prevent secondary complications related to epilepsy, such as brain damage, developmental regression, and SUDEP [39]. Children with epilepsy can develop significant cognitive deficits; therefore, aggressively treating seizures is warranted [26]. Epilepsy treatment with standard antiseizure medication, vagus nerve stimulators, or a ketogenic diet is recommended and should be directed by a neurologist. It is also important to avoid seizure triggers, such as sleep deprivation, stress, and medication noncompliance [15].

8.6.2 Management of Gastrointestinal Issues

Consideration and treatment of GI issues are also important, particularly since untreated symptoms may cause discomfort, leading to irritability and aggression. Polyethylene glycol (PEG), bisacodyl, and proton pump inhibitors (PPI) have effectively treated GI symptoms in most patients with Dup15q [44].

8.6.3 Psychopharmacology

There is still very little that is published on the psychopharmacological treatment of psychiatric and behavioral comorbidities seen in Dup15q. Only a handful of publications have described case reports of patient responses to psychotropic medication trials [28–31, 45]. Hence, evidence on medication treatment to address behavioral concerns and psychiatric illnesses in this patient population remains extremely limited and is an area that requires further research. When considering the use of psychotropic medication, clinicians should consider the side effect burden, especially since patients with Dup15q may be unable to verbalize the presence of side effects.

8.6.4 Attention-Deficit/Hyperactivity Disorder

Carbamazepine at dosages of up to 800 mg twice daily decreased hyperactivity in a small number of subjects. It is still unclear how effective treatment with psychostimulants or alpha-agonists are for hyperactivity in Dup15q patients. Carbamazepine alone or in combination with guanfacine extended-release and amphetamine-dextroamphetamine mixed salts has helped decrease aggression in some patients [28].

Although inattention was described as accompanying hyperactivity in some case descriptions, to our knowledge, no publications have addressed the treatment of inattention specifically in this population [22].

8.6.5 Bipolar Disorder

Mood disorders are still not yet clearly described in Dup15, and what we know of affective disturbances are mostly isolated signs or symptom clusters [28–31]. No cases of depressive disorders have been published and symptoms of depression have only been described in a small number of patients who were ultimately diagnosed with bipolar disorder or schizophrenia spectrum disorders. Carbamazepine in dosages of up to 800 mg twice daily has been reported to be helpful in decreasing mood lability in cases described as having bipolar disorder. The effect of selective serotonin reuptake inhibitors (SSRIs), traditionally used for the treatment of depression and anxiety, have not been particularly helpful, but data is limited to case-reports [28]. No data are available on the use of serotonin norepinephrine reuptake inhibitors (SNRIs), mirtazapine, or bupropion.

No scales or standardized measures have been used to track affective or anxious symptoms in this population. However, it has been hypothesized that sustained mood stability could have a positive effect on the treatment of anxiety symptoms, and carbamazepine at dosages of 600–800 mg twice daily has been reported to decrease anxiety in a few patients [28].

8.6.6 Schizophrenia Spectrum and Other Psychotic Disorders

Although psychosis has not been described in a large number of cases within the Dup15q population, the clinical use of various antipsychotics has been reported in a small number of patients. Both first- and second-generation antipsychotics have been used, including risperidone, aripiprazole, and clozapine [29, 31, 45]. Clinical responses to antipsychotic treatment ranged from treatment-resistant psychosis to complete symptom remission [29–31].

Key Points

- The exact prevalence of Dup15q in the general population remains unknown but ranges from 0.2% to 3% in the ASD population.
- Psychiatric comorbidities are still infrequently detailed in the literature, but behavioral symptoms reported include irritability, aggression, self-injurious behavior, stereotypies, inattention, hyperactivity, and anxiety.
- Epilepsy and gastrointestinal issues such as hypotonia-related feeding difficulties, gastroesophageal reflux disease, and constipation are common medical comorbidities.
- Multidisciplinary evaluations from the time of diagnosis are recommended to assess development, identify medical and psychiatric comorbidities, and monitor progress.
- There is still relatively little that is published on the psychopharmacological treatment of behavioral and psychiatric comorbidities seen in Dup15q.
- Carbamazepine has been helpful to treat mood lability, hyperactivity, self-injury, aggression, and anxiety in a handful of patients with Dup15q.
- Few cases of psychotic symptoms in Dup15q have been described, but trials of first- and second-generation antipsychotics, including aripiprazole, risperidone, and clozapine, can be helpful and have led to symptom remission in a small number of cases.

Photographs of Individuals with the Syndrome

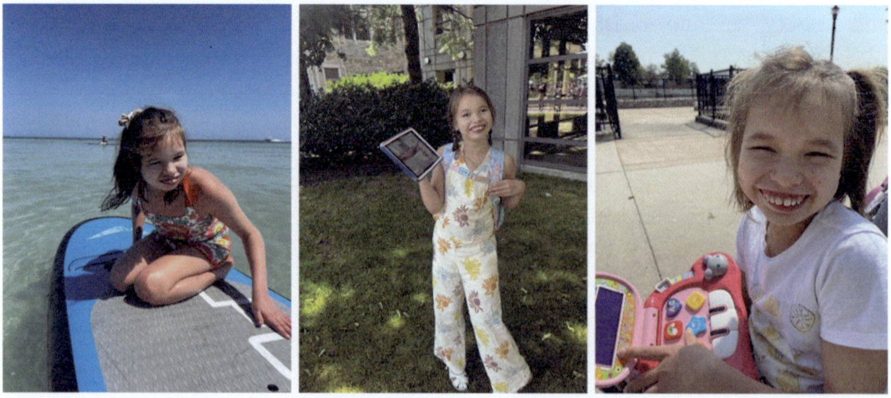

References

1. Cook EH Jr, Lindgren V, Leventhal BL, Courchesne R, Lincoln A, Shulman C, Lord C, Courchesne E. ASD or atypical ASD in maternally but not paternally derived proximal 15q duplication. Am J Hum Genet. 1997;60(4):928–34.
2. Schroer RJ, Phelan MC, Michaelis RC, Crawford EC, Skinner SA, Cuccaro M, Simensen RJ, Bishop J, Skinner C, Fender D, Stevenson RE. ASD and maternally derived aberrations of chromosome 15q. Am J Med Genet. 1998;76(4):327–36. https://doi.org/10.1002/(sici)1096-8628(19980401)76:4<327::aid-ajmg8>3.0.co;2-m.
3. Depienne C, Moreno-De-Luca D, Heron D, Bouteiller D, Gennetier A, Delorme R, Chaste P, Siffroi JP, Chantot-Bastaraud S, Benyahia B, Trouillard O, Nygren G, Kopp S, Johansson M, Rastam M, Burglen L, Leguern E, Verloes A, Leboyer M, Brice A, Gillberg C, Betancur C. Screening for genomic rearrangements and methylation abnormalities of the 15q11-q13 region in ASD spectrum disorders. Biol Psychiatry. 2009;66(4):349–59. https://doi.org/10.1016/j.biopsych.2009.01.025.
4. Leader G, Forde J, Naughton K, Maher L, Arndt S, Mannion A. Relationships among gastro-intestinal symptoms, sleep problems, challenging behaviour, comorbid psychopathology and ASD spectrum disorder symptoms in children and adolescents with 15q duplication syndrome. J Intellect Disabil Res. 2021;65(1):32–46. https://doi.org/10.1111/jir.12789.
5. Christian SL, Fantes JA, Mewborn SK, Huang B, Ledbetter DH. Large genomic duplicons map to sites of instability in the Prader-Willi/Angelman syndrome chromosome region (15q11-q13). Hum Mol Genet. 1999;8(6):1025–37. https://doi.org/10.1093/hmg/8.6.1025.
6. Pujana MA, Nadal M, Guitart M, Armengol L, Gratacòs M, Estivill X. Human chromosome 15q11-q14 regions of rearrangements contain clusters of LCR15 duplicons. Eur J Hum Genet. 2002;10(1):26–35. https://doi.org/10.1038/sj.ejhg.5200760.
7. Makoff AJ, Flomen RH. Detailed analysis of 15q11-q14 sequence corrects errors and gaps in the public access sequence to fully reveal large segmental duplications at breakpoints for Prader-Willi, Angelman, and inv dup(15) syndromes. Genome Biol. 2007;8(6):R114. https://doi.org/10.1186/gb-2007-8-6-r114.
8. Hogart A, Nagarajan RP, Patzel KA, Yasui DH, Lasalle JM. 15q11-13 GABAA receptor genes are normally biallelically expressed in brain yet are subject to epigenetic dysregulation in ASD-spectrum disorders. Hum Mol Genet. 2007;16(6):691–703. https://doi.org/10.1093/hmg/ddm014.
9. Urraca N, Cleary J, Brewer V, Pivnick EK, McVicar K, Thibert RL, Schanen NC, Esmer C, Lamport D, Reiter LT. The interstitial duplication 15q11.2-q13 syndrome includes ASD, mild facial anomalies and a characteristic EEG signature. ASD Res. 2013;6(4):268–79. https://doi.org/10.1002/aur.1284.
10. Reiter L, Cleary J, Brewer V, Jabbour JT, Schanen NC, Urraca N. Maternal, but not paternal, interstitial duplications of chromosome 15q11.2-q13 are associated with ASD in 7 individuals. In: Presented at the 59th Annual Meeting of the American Society of Human Genetics, October 23, 2009, Honolulu, Hawaii; 2009.
11. Battaglia A. The inv dup(15) or idic(15) syndrome: a clinically recognisable neurogenetic disorder. Brain Dev. 2005;27(5):365–9. https://doi.org/10.1016/j.braindev.2004.08.006.
12. Kalsner L, Chamberlain SJ. Prader-Willi, Angelman, and 15q11-q13 Duplication syndromes. Pediatr Clin North Am. 2015 Jun;62(3):587–606. https://doi.org/10.1016/j.pcl.2015.03.004.
13. Finucane BM, Lusk L, Arkilo D, Chamberlain S, Devinski O, Dindot S, et al. 15 duplication syndrome and related disorders. In: Adam MP, Ardinger HH, Pagon RA, Wallace SE, Bean LJH, Stephens K, Amemiya A, editors. GeneReviews. Seattle, WA: University of Washington, Seattle; 2016.
14. Battaglia A. The inv dup (15) or idic (15) syndrome (Tetrasomy 15q). Orphanet J Rare Dis. 2008;3:30. https://doi.org/10.1186/1750-1172-3-30.
15. Lusk L, Vogel-Farley V, DiStefano C, Jeste S. Maternal 15q Duplication syndrome. 2016 Jun 16 [updated 2021 Jul 15]. In: Adam MP, Feldman J, Mirzaa GM, Pagon RA, Wallace SE, LJH B, Gripp KW, Amemiya A, editors. GeneReviews®. Seattle (WA): University of Washington, Seattle; 2021. 1993–2024.

16. Copping NA, Christian SGB, Ritter DJ, Islam MS, Buscher N, Zolkowska D, Pride MC, Berg EL, LaSalle JM, Ellegood J, Lerch JP, Reiter LT, Silverman JL, Dindot SV. Neuronal overexpression of Ube3a isoform 2 causes behavioral impairments and neuroanatomical pathology relevant to 15q11.2-q13.3 duplication syndrome. Hum Mol Genet. 2017;26(20):3995–4010. https://doi.org/10.1093/hmg/ddx289.
17. ASD Genome Project Consortium, Szatmari P, Paterson AD, Zwaigenbaum L, Roberts W, Brian J, Liu XQ, Vincent JB, Skaug JL, Thompson AP, Senman L, Feuk L, Qian C, Bryson SE, Jones MB, Marshall CR, Scherer SW, Vieland VJ, Bartlett C, Mangin LV, Goedken R, Segre A, Pericak-Vance MA, Cuccaro ML, Gilbert JR, Wright HH, Abramson RK, Betancur C, Bourgeron T, Gillberg C, Leboyer M, Buxbaum JD, Davis KL, Hollander E, Silverman JM, Hallmayer J, Lotspeich L, Sutcliffe JS, Haines JL, Folstein SE, Piven J, Wassink TH, Sheffield V, Geschwind DH, Bucan M, Brown WT, Cantor RM, Constantino JN, Gilliam TC, Herbert M, Lajonchere C, Ledbetter DH, Lese-Martin C, Miller J, Nelson S, Samango-Sprouse CA, Spence S, State M, Tanzi RE, Coon H, Dawson G, Devlin B, Estes A, Flodman P, Klei L, McMahon WM, Minshew N, Munson J, Korvatska E, Rodier PM, Schellenberg GD, Smith M, Spence MA, Stodgell C, Tepper PG, Wijsman EM, Yu CE, Rogé B, Mantoulan C, Wittemeyer K, Poustka A, Felder B, Klauck SM, Schuster C, Poustka F, Bölte S, Feineis-Matthews S, Herbrecht E, Schmötzer G, Tsiantis J, Papanikolaou K, Maestrini E, Bacchelli E, Blasi F, Carone S, Toma C, Van Engeland H, de Jonge M, Kemner C, Koop F, Langemeijer M, Hijmans C, Staal WG, Baird G, Bolton PF, Rutter ML, Weisblatt E, Green J, Aldred C, Wilkinson JA, Pickles A, Le Couteur A, Berney T, McConachie H, Bailey AJ, Francis K, Honeyman G, Hutchinson A, Parr JR, Wallace S, Monaco AP, Barnby G, Kobayashi K, Lamb JA, Sousa I, Sykes N, Cook EH, Guter SJ, Leventhal BL, Salt J, Lord C, Corsello C, Hus V, Weeks DE, Volkmar F, Tauber M, Fombonne E, Shih A, Meyer KJ. Mapping ASD risk loci using genetic linkage and chromosomal rearrangements. Nat Genet. 2007;39(3):319–28. https://doi.org/10.1038/ng1985. Erratum in: Nat Genet. 2007 Oct;39(10):1285. Meyer, Kacie J [added]; Koop, Frederike [corrected to Koop, Frederieke]; Langemeijer, Marjolijn [corrected to Langemeijer, Marjolein]; Hijimans, Channa [corrected to Hijmans, Channa]
18. Marshall CR, Noor A, Vincent JB, Lionel AC, Feuk L, Skaug J, Shago M, Moessner R, Pinto D, Ren Y, Thiruvahindrapduram B, Fiebig A, Schreiber S, Friedman J, Ketelaars CE, Vos YJ, Ficicioglu C, Kirkpatrick S, Nicolson R, Sloman L, Summers A, Gibbons CA, Teebi A, Chitayat D, Weksberg R, Thompson A, Vardy C, Crosbie V, Luscombe S, Baatjes R, Zwaigenbaum L, Roberts W, Fernandez B, Szatmari P, Scherer SW. Structural variation of chromosomes in ASD spectrum disorder. Am J Hum Genet. 2008;82(2):477–88. https://doi.org/10.1016/j.ajhg.2007.12.009.
19. Menold MM, Shao Y, Wolpert CM, Donnelly SL, Raiford KL, Martin ER, Ravan SA, Abramson RK, Wright HH, Delong GR, Cuccaro ML, Pericak-Vance MA, Gilbert JR. Association analysis of chromosome 15 gabaa receptor subunit genes in autistic disorder. J Neurogenet. 2001;15(3–4):245–59. https://doi.org/10.3109/01677060109167380.
20. Samaco RC, Hogart A, LaSalle JM. Epigenetic overlap in ASD-spectrum neurodevelopmental disorders: MECP2 deficiency causes reduced expression of UBE3A and GABRB3. Hum Mol Genet. 2005;14(4):483–92. https://doi.org/10.1093/hmg/ddi045.
21. Frohlich J, Reiter LT, Saravanapandian V, DiStefano C, Huberty S, Hyde C, Chamberlain S, Bearden CE, Golshani P, Irimia A, Olsen RW, Hipp JF, Jeste SS. Mechanisms underlying the EEG biomarker in Dup15q syndrome. Mol ASD. 2019;10:29. https://doi.org/10.1186/s13229-019-0280-6. Erratum in: Mol ASD. 2019 Nov 6;10:37. PMID: 31312421; PMCID: PMC6609401
22. Battaglia A, Gurrieri F, Bertini E, Bellacosa A, Pomponi MG, Paravatou-Petsotas M, Mazza S, Neri G. The inv dup(15) syndrome: a clinically recognizable syndrome with altered behavior, mental retardation, and epilepsy. Neurology. 1997;48(4):1081–6. https://doi.org/10.1212/wnl.48.4.1081.
23. Borgatti R, Piccinelli P, Passoni D, Dalprà L, Miozzo M, Micheli R, Gagliardi C, Balottin U. Relationship between clinical and genetic features in "inverted duplicated chromosome 15" patients. Pediatr Neurol. 2001;24(2):111–6. https://doi.org/10.1016/s0887-8994(00)00244-7.

24. Battaglia A, Parrini B, Tancredi R. The behavioral phenotype of the idic(15) syndrome. Am J Med Genet C Semin Med Genet. 2010;154C(4):448–55. https://doi.org/10.1002/ajmg.c.30281.
25. Al Ageeli E, Drunat S, Delanoë C, Perrin L, Baumann C, Capri Y, Fabre-Teste J, Aboura A, Dupont C, Auvin S, El Khattabi L, Chantereau D, Moncla A, Tabet AC, Verloes A. Duplication of the 15q11-q13 region: clinical and genetic study of 30 new cases. Eur J Med Genet. 2014;57(1):5–14. https://doi.org/10.1016/j.ejmg.2013.10.008.
26. DiStefano C, Gulsrud A, Huberty S, Kasari C, Cook E, Reiter LT, Thibert R, Jeste SS. Identification of a distinct developmental and behavioral profile in children with Dup15q syndrome. J Neurodev Disord. 2016;8:19. https://doi.org/10.1186/s11689-016-9152-y.
27. DiStefano C, Wilson RB, Hyde C, Cook EH, Thibert RL, Reiter LT, Vogel-Farley V, Hipp J, Jeste S. Behavioral characterization of dup15q syndrome: toward meaningful endpoints for clinical trials. Am J Med Genet A. 2020;182(1):71–84. https://doi.org/10.1002/ajmg.a.61385.
28. Viamontes CG, Castillo Gonzalez J, Najjar F, Cook EH. Maternal Duplication 15q11-13 syndrome with ASD spectrum disorder: mood stabilization by carbamazepine. J Child Adolesc Psychopharmacol. 2022;32(2):122–6. https://doi.org/10.1089/cap.2021.0046.
29. Ingason A, Kirov G, Giegling I, Hansen T, Isles AR, Jakobsen KD, Kristinsson KT, le Roux L, Gustafsson O, Craddock N, Möller HJ, McQuillin A, Muglia P, Cichon S, Rietschel M, Ophoff RA, Djurovic S, Andreassen OA, Pietiläinen OP, Peltonen L, Dempster E, Collier DA, St Clair D, Rasmussen HB, Glenthøj BY, Kiemeney LA, Franke B, Tosato S, Bonetto C, Saemundsen E, Hreidarsson SJ, GROUP Investigators, Nöthen MM, Gurling H, O'Donovan MC, Owen MJ, Sigurdsson E, Petursson H, Stefansson H, Rujescu D, Stefansson K, Werge T. Maternally derived microduplications at 15q11-q13: implication of imprinted genes in psychotic illness. Am J Psychiatry. 2011;168(4):408–17. https://doi.org/10.1176/appi.ajp.2010.09111660.
30. Liao HM, Chao YL, Huang AL, Cheng MC, Chen YJ, Lee KF, Fang JS, Hsu CH, Chen CH. Identification and characterization of three inherited genomic copy number variations associated with familial schizophrenia. Schizophr Res. 2012;139(1-3):229–36. https://doi.org/10.1016/j.schres.2012.05.015.
31. Colijn MA, Smith CS, Thomas MA. Maternal 15q11.2-q13.1 duplication syndrome-associated psychosis and mania: a new case and review of the literature. Psychiatr Genet. 2024;34(1):1–7. https://doi.org/10.1097/YPG.0000000000000354.
32. Rees E, Walters JT, Georgieva L, Isles AR, Chambert KD, Richards AL, Mahoney-Davies G, Legge SE, Moran JL, McCarroll SA, O'Donovan MC, Owen MJ, Kirov G. Analysis of copy number variations at 15 schizophrenia-associated loci. Br J Psychiatry. 2014;204(2):108–14. https://doi.org/10.1192/bjp.bp.113.131052.
33. Michelson M, Eden A, Vinkler C, Leshinsky-Silver E, Kremer U, Lerman-Sagie T, Lev D. Familial partial trisomy 15q11-13 presenting as intractable epilepsy in the child and schizophrenia in the mother. Eur J Paediatr Neurol. 2011;15(3):230–3. https://doi.org/10.1016/j.ejpn.2010.11.001.
34. Conant KD, Finucane B, Cleary N, Martin A, Muss C, Delany M, Murphy EK, Rabe O, Luchsinger K, Spence SJ, Schanen C, Devinsky O, Cook EH, LaSalle J, Reiter LT, Thibert RL. A survey of seizures and current treatments in 15q duplication syndrome. Epilepsia. 2014;55(3):396–402. https://doi.org/10.1111/epi.12530.
35. Battaglia A, Bernardini L, Torrente I, Novelli A, Scarselli G. Spectrum of epilepsy and electroencephalogram patterns in idic (15) syndrome. Am J Med Genet A. 2016;170(10):2531–9. https://doi.org/10.1002/ajmg.a.37844.
36. Verrotti A, Sertorio F, Matricardi S, Ferrara P, Striano P. Electroclinical features of epilepsy in patients with InvDup(15). Seizure. 2017;47:87–91. https://doi.org/10.1016/j.seizure.2017.03.006.
37. Frohlich J, Senturk D, Saravanapandian V, Golshani P, Reiter LT, Sankar R, Thibert RL, DiStefano C, Huberty S, Cook EH, Jeste SS. A quantitative electrophysiological biomarker of duplication 15q11.2-q13.1 syndrome. PLoS One. 2016;11(12):e0167179. https://doi.org/10.1371/journal.pone.0167179.
38. Ryvlin P, Nashef L, Tomson T. Prevention of sudden unexpected death in epilepsy: a realistic goal? Epilepsia. 2013;54(Suppl. 2):23–8. https://doi.org/10.1111/epi.12180.

39. Devinsky O, Hesdorffer DC, Thurman DJ, Lhatoo S, Richerson G. Sudden unexpected death in epilepsy: epidemiology, mechanisms, and prevention. Lancet Neurol. 2016;15(10):1075–88. https://doi.org/10.1016/S1474-4422(16)30158-2.
40. Wegiel J, Schanen NC, Cook EH, Sigman M, Brown WT, Kuchna I, Nowicki K, Wegiel J, Imaki H, Ma SY, Marchi E, Wierzba-Bobrowicz T, Chauhan A, Chauhan V, Cohen IL, London E, Flory M, Lach B, Wisniewski T. Differences between the pattern of developmental abnormalities in ASD associated with duplications 15q11.2-q13 and idiopathic ASD. J Neuropathol Exp Neurol. 2012;71(5):382–97. https://doi.org/10.1097/NEN.0b013e318251f537.
41. Friedman D, Thaler A, Thaler J, Rai S, Cook E, Schanen C, Devinsky O. Mortality in isodicentric chromosome 15 syndrome: the role of SUDEP. Epilepsy Behav. 2016;61:1–5. https://doi.org/10.1016/j.yebeh.2016.04.001.
42. Shohat M, Shohat T, Rimoin DL, Mohandas T, Heckenlively J, Magenis RE, Davidson MB, Korenberg JR. Rearrangement of chromosome 15 in the region q11.2----q12 in an individual with obesity syndrome and her normal mother. Am J Med Genet. 1990;37(2):173–7. https://doi.org/10.1002/ajmg.1320370203.
43. Browne CE, Dennis NR, Maher E, Long FL, Nicholson JC, Sillibourne J, Barber JC. Inherited interstitial duplications of proximal 15q: genotype-phenotype correlations. Am J Hum Genet. 1997;61(6):1342–52. https://doi.org/10.1086/301624.
44. Shaaya EA, Pollack SF, Boronat S, Davis-Cooper S, Zella GC, Thibert RL. Gastrointestinal problems in 15q duplication syndrome. Eur J Med Genet. 2015;58(3):191–3. https://doi.org/10.1016/j.ejmg.2014.12.012.
45. Han JY, Lee HJ, Lee YM, Park J. Complete penetrance but different phenotypes in a Korean family with maternal interstitial duplication at 15q11.2-q13.1: a case report. Children (Basel). 2021;8(4):313. https://doi.org/10.3390/children8040313.

DiGeorge Syndrome

9

Dena Oaklander, Khalid I. Afzal, and Karam Radwan

9.1 Overview of the Neurodevelopmental Disorder

The 22q11.2 deletion syndrome occurs due to a deletion of approximately three million base pairs in the q11.2 region of chromosome 22. About 90% of cases occur due to a new (de novo) deletion, with the remaining 10% inherited from a parent with the deletion. This deletion results in abnormal development of several body systems, leading to various health problems, including heart defects, immune system deficiencies, cleft palate, complications related to low levels of calcium in the blood, and delayed development with behavioral and emotional problems. The exact prevalence is difficult to determine due to the wide range of phenotypic expressions and lack of diagnosis of mild cases. It is one of the most common genetic disorders, with an estimated prevalence of 1 in 2000–4000 live births. 22q11.2 deletion syndrome affects both sexes equally and has been reported across all ethnicities and geographical regions. The primary risk factor for 22q11.2 deletion syndrome is having a parent with the deletion. However, because most cases are de novo mutations, no known behavioral or environmental risk factors exist. People with 22q11.2 deletion syndrome require multidisciplinary care to manage the wide array of health problems associated with the condition. Regular monitoring and treatment are essential for managing heart defects, immune system problems, calcium levels, atypical speech and other areas of development, and additional associated conditions. Life expectancy can vary because of the syndrome's complexity and variability. With early diagnosis and appropriate care, many individuals with DiGeorge syndrome can lead healthy, productive lives. Advances in medical care

D. Oaklander (✉) · K. I. Afzal · K. Radwan
Department of Psychiatry and Behavioral Neuroscience, The University of Chicago, Chicago, IL, USA
e-mail: rkv6443@uchicagomedicine.org; kafzal@uchicago.edu; Radwan@uchicago.edu

R. P. Thom, C. J. McDougle (eds.), *Neuropsychiatric Care for Genetic Syndromes and Other Neurodevelopmental Disorders*,
https://doi.org/10.1007/978-3-031-76269-7_9

and interventions have improved the prognosis for many individuals affected by the syndrome.

9.2 Common Clinical Features

Common clinical features include congenital heart defects, palatal abnormalities, facial dysmorphisms, immune deficiencies, and neurodevelopmental delays. The underlying genetic and neurobiological mechanisms involve haploinsufficiency of multiple genes within the deleted region, leading to disrupted development of various organs and systems.

A useful mnemonic for remembering the clinical features of the syndrome is "CATCH-22": **C**onotruncal cardiac anomalies, **A**bnormal facies, **T**hymic hypoplasia, **C**left palate, **H**ypocalcemia, **22**q11.2 microdeletion [1].

9.3 Signs and Symptoms of Common Psychiatric Comorbidities

Individuals with 22q11.2 deletion syndrome commonly experience psychiatric comorbidities, including schizophrenia spectrum disorders, attention-deficit/hyperactivity disorder (ADHD), anxiety disorders, mood disorders, autism spectrum disorder (ASD), and intellectual disability (ID). Symptoms may present differently across the lifespan, with early-onset psychosis being a hallmark feature in adolescence and young adulthood.

9.3.1 Attention-Deficit/Hyperactivity Disorder

Attention-deficit/hyperactivity disorder is the most common comorbid psychiatric condition in children with 22q11.2 deletion syndrome. The clinical presentation of ADHD in children with 22q11.2 deletion syndrome is similar to ADHD in the general population [2]. Hyperactive/impulsive symptoms are more common in children with 22q11.2 deletion syndrome, likely due to lower rates of stimulant medication use. The rate of ADHD diagnosis in individuals with 22q11.2 deletion syndrome decreases with age from 37% in early childhood (6–12 years), to 23.8% in adolescence (13–17 years), and to 15.5% in adulthood (>18 years) [3]. Although the rate of ADHD is lower in adults (15.5%), this is higher than that in adults in the general population (4.40%) [3]. The decline in ADHD rates into adulthood may reflect difficulty diagnosing ADHD in the adult population, particularly in the presence of other psychiatric comorbidities like psychotic disorders or may reflect a unique evolution of ADHD symptomatology in 22q11.2 deletion syndrome [4]. Screening assessments for ADHD include the Vanderbilt ADHD rating scale and Conners rating scale [5].

9.3.2 Schizophrenia

Neuropsychiatric deficits in individuals with 22q11.2 deletion syndrome seem to follow a developmental pattern [4]. Rates of psychotic disorders, including schizophrenia, schizoaffective disorder, schizophreniform disorder, brief psychotic disorder, psychotic disorder not otherwise specified, and delusional disorder in individuals with 22q11.2 deletion syndrome gradually increase from childhood (0%), to adolescence (3.8%), to young adults (22.2%), and to adulthood (31%) [4]. Given the clinical trajectory and high incidence of psychotic disorders, 22q11.2 deletion syndrome is considered a neurogenetic model for psychosis [6, 7]. Symptoms are similar in presentation to idiopathic psychosis, including the age of onset (~20 years), positive symptoms of psychosis, and negative symptoms of psychosis [6]. However, psychosis in individuals with 22q11.2 deletion syndrome is associated with lower levels of substance use, higher levels of ADHD, avolition, and impaired stress tolerance compared to idiopathic psychosis [7]. In addition, a decline in verbal IQ scores from childhood to early adulthood is strongly correlated with the severity of psychotic symptoms [8].

9.3.3 Anxiety Disorders

Anxiety disorders are common in children with 22q11.2 deletion syndrome. The prevalence of anxiety disorders in individuals with 22q11.2 deletion syndrome, including separation anxiety, specific phobias, social phobia, panic disorder, post-traumatic stress disorder, obsessive-compulsive disorder (OCD), generalized anxiety disorder (GAD), and anxiety disorder not otherwise specified, is approximately 24% in childhood and adulthood [3]. Common anxiety disorders throughout childhood include specific phobias (21.94%), social phobia (10.34%), GAD (8.28%), separation anxiety (6.33%), and OCD (5.52%) [9]. Panic disorder is the only subtype to increase in prevalence over the lifespan, from 1.2% in childhood to 14.41% in adulthood [3]. Anxiety disorders are more frequent in females (57.22%) than in males, though this difference was only significant in adults [3]. Approximately 69.11% of subjects met the diagnostic criteria for one anxiety disorder, 22.03% for two, and 9.11% for three or more anxiety disorders [3]. Symptoms of anxiety in individuals with 22q11.2 deletion syndrome appear similar to those who do not have the syndrome. Screening assessments for anxiety disorders include the Multidimensional Anxiety Scale for Children, Second Edition (MASC-2) and Screen for Child Anxiety Related Emotional Disorders (SCARED).

9.3.4 Mood Disorders

Mood disorders are common in 22q11.2 deletion syndrome. The prevalence of mood disorders, including major depressive disorder, dysthymia, bipolar disorder/hypomanic episodes, and mood disorder not otherwise specified, increases from childhood

(3.29%,) to adolescence (11.85%), and to young adulthood (18.27%) [3]. The highest rate of mood disorders includes major depressive disorder (2.19–10.84%) compared to lower rates of dysthymia (1.1–5%) and bipolar/hypomanic episodes (0–3.94%) [3]. Unipolar mood disorders (major depressive disorder and dysthymia) were more frequent in females (61.18%) than in males, though the difference was only significant in adults [3]. In a study of 74 children and adolescents with 22q11.2 deletion syndrome ages 6–18 years, researchers found that increased rates of depression occurred at important developmental periods that require increased autonomy, independence, communication, and cognition—areas that are challenging for individuals with 22q11.2 deletion syndrome [10]. Social isolation, poor grades, and peer rejection affect self-esteem and increase the risk of these individuals developing depression [10]. Screening for mood disorders includes rapport building and confidential assessment, evaluation based on the Diagnostic and Statistical Manual of Mental Disorders (DSM) symptomatology, including rating scales such as the PHQ-9, and evaluation of the risk of harm to self or others, including rating scales such as the Columbia-Suicidal Severity Rating Scale (CSSRS) [11]. Screening for bipolar disorder based on DSM symptomatology is also important. Structured diagnostic interviews and questionnaires such as the Kiddie Schedule for Affective Disorders and Schizophrenia (K-SADS) and Washington University at St. Louis Kiddie Schedule for Affective Disorders and Schizophrenia (WASH-U-KSADS) may help diagnose bipolar disorder. Similarly, the Young Mania Rating Scale (YMRS) may be used to assess the severity of manic symptoms and treatment response [12].

9.3.5 Autism Spectrum Disorder

The prevalence of ASD, including autism disorder, Asperger's disorder, and pervasive developmental disorder not otherwise specified, differed among age groups and was lowest in childhood (12.77%), highest in adolescence (26.54%), and then reduced in adulthood (16.1%) [3]. Gender differences were not present [3]. A 2006 study of 60 individuals ages 9–18 years with 22q11.2 deletion syndrome found high rates of ASD (50%) [13]. Similarly, a small 2007 study of 41 individuals ages 6.5–15.8 years with 22q11.2 deletion syndrome found that 40% met the criteria for ASD [14]. The diagnosis of ASD in 22q11.2 deletion syndrome can be challenging to make, given the high level of phenotypic overlap between the two conditions, and clinicians must be careful not to overdiagnose ASD [15]. The presence of rituals, motor stereotypies, repetitive use of objects, deficits in nonverbal communication and peer relations, and delayed or absent make-believe play most likely suggest comorbid ASD [15]. In contrast, difficulties with shared attention, deficits in gestural communication, difficulties initiating conversation, and restricted interests appear to be phenotypic features of 22q11.2 deletion syndrome [15]. In addition, there is a higher rate of psychiatric comorbidity in individuals with 22q11.2 deletion syndrome and ASD than in those with 22q11.2 deletion syndrome alone [14]. Screening assessments for ASD include the Modified Checklist for Autism in Toddlers (M-CHAT) and the Autism Screening Questionnaire (ASQ) for older children. Diagnostic assessments include the Autism Diagnostic Interview, Revised (ADI-R) and the Autism Diagnostic Observation Schedule, Second Edition (ADOS-2).

9.3.6 Intellectual and Learning Disabilities

Beginning in infancy, developmental delays, including motor, speech, and language deficits, are commonly observed in 22q11.2 deletion syndrome [16]. In preschool and early childhood, learning disabilities are very common [3, 17]. Children with 22q11 deletion syndrome have more difficulty with mathematics compared to reading, which may partially be related to impairments in procedural calculation, word problem-solving, and visuo-spatial attention [18]. Approximately 45% of patients with 22q11.2 deletion syndrome have borderline intellectual functioning (full-scale IQ 70–85), and about 40% have mild-to-moderate ID [18]. Neuropsychological and learning profiles characteristic of 22q11.2 deletion syndrome include deficits in visual-spatial skills, processing new and complex information, abstract reasoning, and visual attention [16]. Relative areas of strength include auditory memory and language skills [16]. Variability in cognitive functioning appears partially related to the mode of inheritance, given that individuals with familially inherited deletions are more severely affected cognitively than those with de novo deletions [18]. Severe or profound ID is rare in children with 22q11.2 deletion syndrome, though it is more frequent in adults [19]. Assessment tools include evaluating for developmental delays (Ages and Stages Questionnaire (ASQ-3)), intellectual functioning (Bayley Scales of Infant and Toddler Development; Stanford-Binet Intelligence Scales; Wechsler Preschool and Primary Scale of Intelligence, Revised; and Wechsler Intelligence Scale for Children, Fourth Edition), nonverbal intelligence (Leiter International Performance Scale), and adaptive functioning (Vineland Adaptive Behavior Scales, Third Edition) [20].

9.4 Assessment

Prenatal screening for 22q11.2 deletion syndrome is possible through tests that look for deletions in chromosome 22. After birth, a diagnosis is typically made using a blood test called a fluorescence in situ hybridization (FISH) test to look for the deletion of a part of chromosome 22.

A *definitive diagnosis* of 22q11.2 deletion syndrome includes the presence of low CD3+ T cells (<500/mm^3), paired with typical clinical symptoms (e.g., congenital conotruncal cardiac abnormalities and hypocalcemia lasting more than 3 weeks and requiring treatment) and a confirmed genetic test with a deletion in chromosome 22q11.2. Criteria for a *probable diagnosis* consist of reduced CD3+ T cells (<1500/mm^3) and a deletion of chromosome 22q11.2. Patients with reduced CD3+ T cells (<1500/mm^3), along with a cardiac defect, hypocalcemia of more than 3 weeks duration that requires therapy, or dysmorphic facies or palatal abnormalities are diagnosed with a *possible diagnosis* of 22q11.2 deletion syndrome [21].

Diagnostic tests may include cardiac evaluation and echocardiogram, serum calcium and phosphorus levels, complete blood cell count with differential to evaluate for lymphopenia, chest radiograph to evaluate for the absence of a thymic shadow, renal ultrasound to assess for structural genitourinary tract abnormalities, T and B cell phenotyping using flow cytometry, and immunoglobulin levels. The most common full-scale IQ in 22q11.2 deletion syndrome is in the borderline range of intellectual functioning (70–85) [22]. Severe ID is rare; however, ID and communication limitations may warrant specialized psychological testing for cognitive and adaptive functioning. Developmental assessments and psychiatric evaluations facilitate establishing a baseline cognitive profile, identifying co-occurring conditions, and planning treatment.

9.5 Psychosocial Treatments

Individuals with 22q11.2 deletion syndrome have lifelong needs that require considerable support [23]. Due to difficulties with fine/gross motor skills and speech and language delays during infancy and toddlerhood, therapeutic interventions include physical therapy, occupational therapy, and speech therapy [24]. Establishing care with a developmental-behavioral pediatrician is important. When the child is school-aged, the focus shifts toward providing appropriate educational support and fostering social interactions [24]. Cognitive difficulties and learning disabilities warrant neuropsychological evaluation, cognitive remediation, and school accommodations [24]. Social cognition training helps improve social cognition and social skills [25]. In addition, Applied Behavior Analysis (ABA) may be helpful for those with comorbid ASD and deficits in social reciprocity and communication skills [26]. Treatable psychiatric conditions may emerge throughout childhood, adolescence, and adulthood, which warrant further evaluation by a psychiatrist [24]. A modified cognitive behavioral therapy (CBT) approach to treating anxiety and depression is helpful, as well as interpersonal therapy for depression. Although CBT is not indicated for schizophrenia in the general population, CBT is an effective psychosocial intervention to address psychotic symptoms such as amotivation, anhedonia, social avoidance, or withdrawal in individuals with 22q11.2 deletion syndrome [27]. Caregiver guidance is also essential, focusing on behavioral parenting techniques, promoting independence, and fostering social skills [28].

In summary, psychosocial treatments for 22q11.2 deletion syndrome focus on addressing developmental delays, behavioral challenges, and social difficulties. Treatments may include early intervention services, special education programs, behavioral therapies, social skills training, and family support services.

9.6 Biological Treatments

According to clinical practice guidelines, the general recommendation is standard psychopharmacological management of psychiatric disorders in 22q11.2 deletion syndrome [29–31]. The medications target specific symptoms and co-occurring disorders such as psychosis, anxiety, mood, or ADHD. The starting dose of medications should be lower than the FDA-recommended starting dose, and the dose titration must be slower than the generally accepted guidelines utilizing the "start low, go slow" approach while carefully monitoring side effects [30].

Antipsychotics are used to address psychotic symptoms in 22q11.2 deletion. Common side effects include: (1) akathisia and/or parkinsonism (higher risk with haloperidol and other first-generation antipsychotics), (2) metabolic syndrome (all second-generation antipsychotics), (3) drowsiness, (4) appetite changes, (5) convulsions, (6) hyperprolactinemia (especially with risperidone), (7) menstrual irregularities, (8) hypersalivation (associated with clozapine), (9) QTc interval prolongation, (10) elevated liver enzymes, and (11) agranulocytosis (especially with clozapine) [32]. Clozapine and olanzapine are linked with the most weight gain, followed by risperidone, quetiapine, ziprasidone, and aripiprazole [33]. Aripiprazole is weight-neutral in adults but not in children and adolescents. Clozapine requires special monitoring due to the risk of agranulocytosis. White blood cell (WBC) count, differential count, and absolute neutrophil count (ANC) are checked weekly for 6 months, fortnightly for up to 6 months, and then monthly [33]. The clozapine level should be checked every 3 months [34]. Clozapine lowers the seizure threshold, and the prophylactic addition of anticonvulsants such as valproic acid may prevent an unwarranted side effect of an effective treatment [35].

Metabolic syndrome is considered if three or more of the following are present: (1) waist circumference (men >40 inches and women ≥35 inches; (2) triglycerides ≥150 mg/dL; (3) HDL: men <40 mg/dL, women <50 mg/dL, or receiving treatment for reduced HDL; (4) blood pressure: ≥130 mm Hg systolic blood pressure, ≥85 mm Hg diastolic blood pressure, or receiving antihypertensive drug treatment; and (5) fasting glucose: ≥100 mg/dL or receiving treatment for elevated glucose [36]. Table 9.1 details the recommendations for metabolic monitoring.

Table 9.1 Metabolic monitoring for antipsychotics [32]

	Baseline	4 Weeks	8 Weeks	12 Weeks	6 Months	Annual
Weight/body mass index	X	X	X	X	X	X
Fasting plasma glucose/ hemoglobin A1c	X			X	X	X
Lipids	X			X	X	X
Blood pressure	X			X	X	X

Revisit all monitoring when clinically relevant if there is a change in antipsychotic medication. Ideally, monitor weekly for the first 4–6 weeks and then every 2–4 weeks up to 12 weeks. Hemoglobin A1c should be used to monitor long-term blood glucose, but fasting plasma glucose may be more appropriate in the early weeks of treatment.

The evidence-based treatments for anxiety, depression, and OCD consist of antidepressants, namely selective serotonin reuptake inhibitors (SSRIs) and serotonin-norepinephrine reuptake inhibitors (SNRIs). Antidepressants are generally safe and well-tolerated. The common side effects are nausea, headache, diarrhea, dizziness, sedation, irritable mood, risk of mania, and suicidal ideation (13–25-year-old age group). The suicide risk increases when starting at a higher dose or with fast medication titration. Cognitive behavioral therapy is effective in addressing depression and anxiety disorders and must be recommended concomitantly with medication.

Attention-deficit/hyperactivity disorder is treated with stimulants or non-stimulants. A baseline electrocardiogram (EKG) and consulting a cardiologist are recommended before initiating treatment with stimulants due to the cardiac anomalies associated with 22q11.2 deletion syndrome. The most common side effects include loss of appetite, irritability, anxiety, insomnia, worsening of psychosis, high blood pressure, and growth stunting [37]. Non-stimulants such as guanfacine, clonidine, atomoxetine, and viloxazine do not affect appetite and may be used to address co-occurring anxiety. A comprehensive clinical evaluation by a pediatric cardiologist at baseline includes a physical examination, family history, echocardiogram, EKG, heart rate, and blood pressure [37]. Electrocardiogram, heart rate, and blood pressure must be monitored every 3 or 6 months after that [34].

Mood stabilizers such as divalproex and lithium have been used in 22q11.2 deletion syndrome to address mood symptoms and co-occurring bipolar disorder. Divalproex can lead to weight gain, hyperglycemia, and hepatic toxicity, warranting close monitoring for metabolic syndrome, as noted above. In addition, Divalproex serum level and liver function tests twice a year are recommended. The optimal divalproex blood level is 60–100 mg/dL. Lithium is a salt that can affect kidney, thyroid, and cardiac functions. Lithium requires optimal monitoring of the blood level every 3–6 months, along with thyroid function tests, and renal function monitoring with blood urea nitrogen and creatinine [38, 39].

There are no recognized preventive measures for any psychiatric disorder. However, reducing stress and avoiding alcohol and drugs, particularly early and persistent marijuana use, are recommended to reduce the risk of mood and psychotic disorders [40]. Tailored standard nonpharmacologic treatments, as noted in the psychosocial section, must be considered to address the specific needs of the affected individuals [41].

9.7 Common Medical Comorbidities

22q11.2 deletion syndrome is the most common microdeletion disorder in humans and results in haploinsufficiency of 46 protein-coding genes, 7 microRNAs, 10 non-coding RNAs, and 27 pseudogenes in those with the standard 3-Mb LCR22A–LCR22D deletion [42]. This deletion leads to a variety of symptoms that affect multiple organs, including several birth defects, numerous medical issues, developmental and cognitive differences, and psychiatric illnesses. Pediatricians and specialists across various medical fields must be familiar with the syndrome's extensive phenotypic range. Diverse symptoms, including cardiovascular abnormalities, thymic dysgenesis, and immune deficiencies, characterize this condition [43]. Approximately 60–80% of children with 22q11.2 deletion syndrome exhibit congenital heart disease, with significant issues such as tetralogy of Fallot, interrupted aortic arch, and ventricular septal defects [44]. The syndrome's impact on the immune system, through thymic hypoplasia or aplasia, increases infection risks. Moreover, the syndrome involves renal and skeletal anomalies and influences physical and cognitive development. The literature underscores the necessity of multidisciplinary approaches for the comprehensive care of those affected, advocating for prompt diagnosis and intervention to enhance prognoses.

The syndrome's wide clinical variability and the significant differences in symptoms among individuals complicate its nomenclature. Notably, 22q11.2 deletion syndrome is a leading cause of syndromic palatal anomalies, velopharyngeal dysfunction, and schizophrenia and is second only to Down syndrome in causing developmental delays and congenital heart disease [45]. It is also a frequent cause of conotruncal heart anomalies. The congenital heart defects associated with 22q11.2 deletion syndrome demand specialized perioperative care due to the increased mortality risks from factors like vasomotor instability, airway hyperresponsiveness, and infection, especially fungal, which adversely affect early surgical outcomes and potentially impair cognitive and mental health. Cardiovascular issues are a primary cause of early mortality in adults with the syndrome.

Moreover, 22q11.2 deletion syndrome is linked with neurological conditions such as epilepsy and a higher seizure incidence, which may stem from various factors, including hypoxia from heart defects and surgeries, hypocalcemia, thyroid issues, infections, and fever. The syndrome also increases the likelihood of movement disorders, including catatonia and Parkinson's disease [46]. Endocrine abnormalities, notably hypoparathyroidism, thyroid dysfunction, and growth retardation, are significant aspects of 22q11.2 deletion syndrome. Hypocalcemia, a classic sign, arises from low parathormone levels and possible 25(OH)D3 deficiency, presenting variably from silent neonatal conditions to overt hypoparathyroidism. Thyroid dysfunction, often manifesting as autoimmune thyroiditis, typically appears in later childhood or adulthood. The developmental issues of the thymus, parathyroid glands, and heart's conotruncal regions in 22q11.2 deletion syndrome are attributed to disrupted neural crest cell migration into the pouch ectoderm [43].

The ten most common medical systems associated with 22q11.2 deletion syndrome are included in Table 9.2.

Key Points to Remember

- 22q11.2 deletion syndrome is a genetic disorder with a wide range of clinical manifestations, including neurodevelopmental delays and psychiatric comorbidities.
- Assessment should include genetic testing, comprehensive medical evaluations, and psychiatric assessment.

Table 9.2 Medical complications associated with 22q11.2 deletion syndrome

Medical problem	Description
Congenital heart defects	Various heart issues, e.g., tetralogy of Fallot and interrupted aortic arch
Immunodeficiency	Reduced T cell production due to thymic hypoplasia or aplasia, ectopic thymus, juvenile idiopathic arthritis, and autoimmune cytopenia [47]
Endocrine	Hypocalcemia, Hashimoto thyroiditis, Grave's disease, diabetes, hypertriglyceridemia, obesity, and growth hormone deficiency [48]
Developmental delays	Speech and learning difficulties
Otolaryngologic problems	Pharyngeal dysfunction, laryngeal atresia due to a glottic web or partial laryngeal stenosis, laryngomalacia, laryngeal cleft, vocal fold abnormalities, and obstructive sleep apnea (OSA) [45]
Neurological disorders	Epilepsy, catatonia, Parkinson's disease, cerebral atrophy, polymicrogyria, atrophy of the hippocampus, and cerebellar atrophy [46]
Feeding difficulties and gastrointestinal problems	Reflux, swallowing difficulties, failure to thrive in infancy, esophageal atresia, imperforate anus, celiac disease, and inflammatory bowel disease
Renal anomalies	Structural kidney abnormalities, multicystic dysplastic kidney, hydronephrosis, duplicated collecting system
Hearing loss	Both conductive and sensorineural types
Skeletal differences	Spine abnormalities (scoliosis), cleft palate, and other skeletal irregularities

- Treatment approaches should be multidisciplinary, incorporating psychosocial interventions and biological treatments tailored to individual needs.
- Clinicians should be familiar with the common medical comorbidities to ensure safe and effective pharmacotherapy.

Photographs of Individuals with the Syndrome

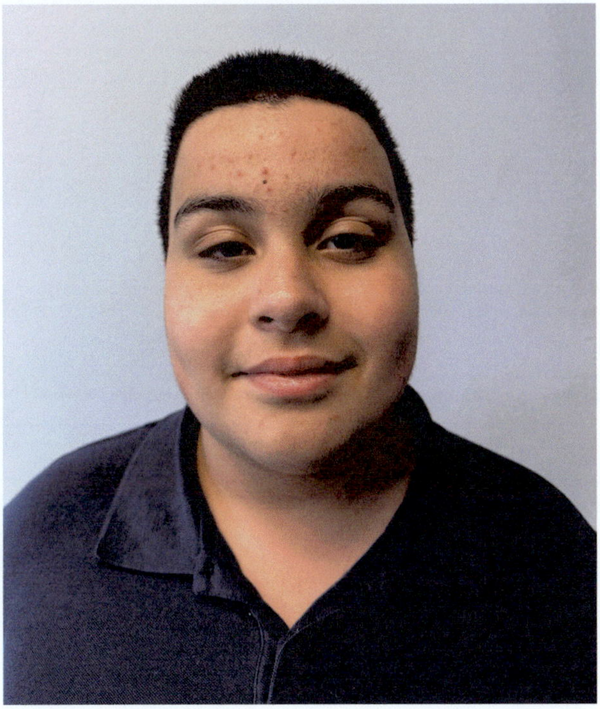

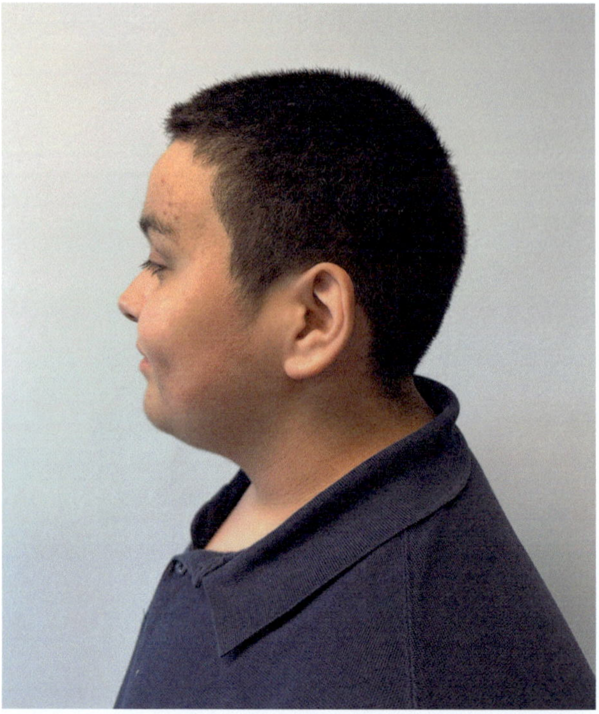

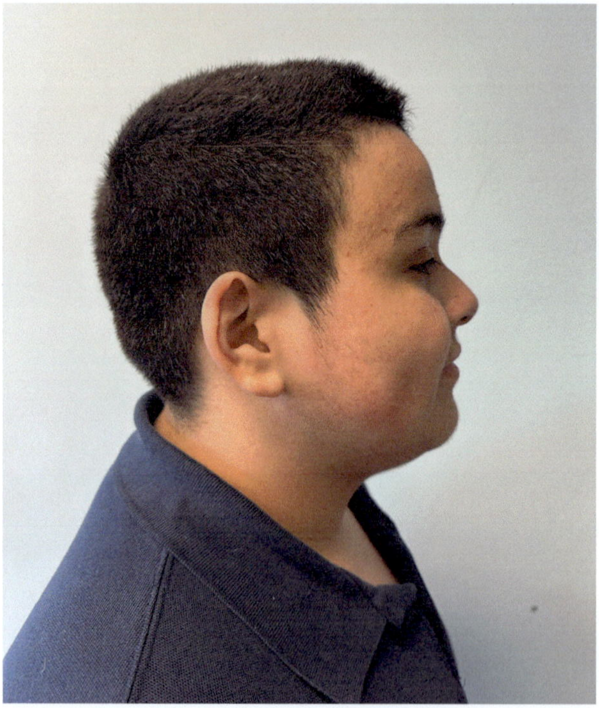

References

1. Lackey AE, Muzio MR. DiGeorge syndrome. Treasure Island (FL): StatPearls Publishing; 2023 [updated 2023 Aug 8]. Available from: https://www.ncbi.nlm.nih.gov/books/NBK549798/
2. Antshel KM, Hendricks K, Shprintzen R, et al. The longitudinal course of attention deficit/hyperactivity disorder in velo-cardio-facial syndrome. J Pediatr. 2013;163(1):187–93.e1.
3. Schneider M, Debbané M, Bassett AS, et al. Psychiatric disorders from childhood to adulthood in 22q11.2 deletion syndrome: results from the International Consortium on Brain and Behavior in 22q11.2 deletion syndrome. Am J Psychiatry. 2014;171(6):627–39.
4. Green T, Gothelf D, Glaser B, et al. Psychiatric disorders and intellectual functioning throughout development in velocardiofacial (22q11.2 deletion) syndrome. J Am Acad Child Adolesc Psychiatry. 2009;48(11):1060–8.
5. Pliszka S. Practice parameter for the assessment and treatment of children and adolescents with attention-deficit/hyperactivity disorder. J Am Acad Child Adolesc Psychiatry. 2007;46(7):894–921.
6. Tang SX, Moore TM, Calkins ME, et al. The psychosis spectrum in 22q11.2 deletion syndrome is comparable to that of nondeleted youths. Biol Psychiatry. 2017;82(1):17–25.
7. Jhawar N, Brown MJ, Cutler-Landsman D, Kates WR, Angkustsiri K, Antshel KM. Longitudinal psychiatric and developmental outcomes in 22q11.2 deletion syndrome: a systematic review. J Dev Behav Pediatr. 2021;42(5):415–27.
8. Gothelf D, Eliez S, Thompson T, et al. COMT genotype predicts longitudinal cognitive decline and psychosis in 22q11.2 deletion syndrome. Nat Neurosci. 2005;8(11):1500–2.
9. Schneider SE, Phillips WM. Depression and anxiety in medical, surgical, and pediatric interns. Psychol Rep. 1993;72(3 Pt 2):1145–6.
10. Fabbro A, Rizzi E, Schneider M, Debbane M, Eliez S. Depression and anxiety disorders in children and adolescents with velo-cardio-facial syndrome (VCFS). Eur Child Adolesc Psychiatry. 2012;21(7):379–85.
11. Birmaher B, Brent D, Bernet W, et al. Practice parameter for the assessment and treatment of children and adolescents with depressive disorders. J Am Acad Child Adolesc Psychiatry. 2007;46(11):1503–26.
12. McClellan J, Kowatch R, Findling RL. Practice parameter for the assessment and treatment of children and adolescents with bipolar disorder. J Am Acad Child Adolesc Psychiatry. 2007;46(1):107–25.
13. Vorstman JAS, Morcus MEJ, Duijff SN, et al. The 22q11.2 deletion in children: high rate of autistic disorders and early onset of psychotic symptoms. J Am Acad Child Adolesc Psychiatry. 2006;45(9):1104–13.
14. Antshel KM, Aneja A, Strunge L, et al. Autistic spectrum disorders in velo-cardio facial syndrome (22q11.2 deletion). J Autism Dev Disord. 2007;37(9):1776–86.
15. Kates WR, Antshel KM, Fremont WP, et al. Comparing phenotypes in patients with idiopathic autism to patients with velocardiofacial syndrome (22q11 DS) with and without autism. Am J Med Genet A. 2007;143a(22):2642–50.
16. Swillen A, Vandeputte L, Cracco J, et al. Neuropsychological, learning and psychosocial profile of primary school aged children with the velo-cardio-facial syndrome (22q11 deletion): evidence for a nonverbal learning disability? Child Neuropsychol. 1999;5(4):230–41.
17. De Smedt B, Swillen A, Verschaffel L, Ghesquière P. Mathematical learning disabilities in children with 22q11.2 deletion syndrome: a review. Dev Disabil Res Rev. 2009;15(1):4–10.
18. De Smedt B, Devriendt K, Fryns JP, Vogels A, Gewillig M, Swillen A. Intellectual abilities in a large sample of children with velo-cardio-facial syndrome: an update. J Intellect Disabil Res. 2007;51(Pt 9):666–70.
19. Evers LJ, De Die-Smulders CE, Smeets EE, Clerkx MG, Curfs LM. The velo-cardio-facial syndrome: the spectrum of psychiatric problems and cognitive deterioration at adult age. Genet Couns. 2009;20(4):307–15.

20. Volkmar F, Siegel M, Woodbury-Smith M, King B, McCracken J, State M. Practice parameter for the assessment and treatment of children and adolescents with autism spectrum disorder. J Am Acad Child Adolesc Psychiatry. 2014;53(2):237–57.
21. Conley ME, Notarangelo LD, Etzioni A. Diagnostic criteria for primary immunodeficiencies. Representing PAGID (Pan-American Group for Immunodeficiency) and ESID (European Society for Immunodeficiencies). Clin Immunol. 1999;93(3):190–7.
22. Everaert E, Selten I, Boerma T, et al. The language profile of preschool children with 22q11.2 deletion syndrome and the relationship with speech intelligibility. Am J Speech Lang Pathol. 2023;32(1):128–44.
23. Cosman T, Finless A, Rideout AL, et al. An online survey to understand the needs of caregivers of family members with 22q11 deletion syndrome. J Intellect Disabil Res. 2023;67(9):860–8.
24. Bassett AS, McDonald-McGinn DM, Devriendt K, et al. Practical guidelines for managing patients with 22q11.2 deletion syndrome. J Pediatr. 2011;159(2):332–9.e1.
25. Shashi V, Harrell W, Eack S, et al. Social cognitive training in adolescents with chromosome 22q11.2 deletion syndrome: feasibility and preliminary effects of the intervention. J Intellect Disabil Res. 2015;59(10):902–13.
26. Tang KL, Antshel KM, Fremont WP, Kates WR. Behavioral and psychiatric phenotypes in 22q11.2 deletion syndrome. J Dev Behav Pediatr. 2015;36(8):639–50.
27. Demily C, Franck N. Cognitive behavioral therapy in 22q11.2 microdeletion with psychotic symptoms: what do we learn from schizophrenia? Eur J Med Genet. 2016;59(11):596–603.
28. Cutler-Landsman D. Educating children with velo-cardio-facial syndrome, 22q11.2 deletion syndrome, and DiGeorge syndrome. 3rd ed. Plural Publishing; 2020. 387p.
29. Boot E, Óskarsdóttir S, Loo JCY, et al. Updated clinical practice recommendations for managing adults with 22q11.2 deletion syndrome. Genet Med. 2023;25(3):100344.
30. Boot E, Butcher NJ, Vorstman JA, van Amelsvoort TA, Fung WL, Bassett AS. Pharmacological treatment of 22q11.2 deletion syndrome-related psychoses. Pharmacopsychiatry. 2015;48(6):219–20.
31. Dori N, Green T, Weizman A, Gothelf D. The effectiveness and safety of antipsychotic and antidepressant medications in individuals with 22q11.2 deletion syndrome. J Child Adolesc Psychopharmacol. 2017;27(1):83–90.
32. DeJongh BM. Clinical pearls for the monitoring and treatment of antipsychotic induced metabolic syndrome. Ment Health Clin. 2021;11(6):311–9.
33. Kar N, Barreto S, Chandavarkar R. Clozapine monitoring in clinical practice: beyond the mandatory requirement. Clin Psychopharmacol Neurosci. 2016;14(4):323–9.
34. Mosheva M, Korotkin L, Gur RE, Weizman A, Gothelf D. Effectiveness and side effects of psychopharmacotherapy in individuals with 22q11.2 deletion syndrome with comorbid psychiatric disorders: a systematic review. Eur Child Adolesc Psychiatry. 2020;29(8):1035–48.
35. Colijn MA. Clozapine use in 22q11.2 deletion syndrome: a systematic review of the literature. J Clin Psychopharmacol. 2024;44(2):168–78.
36. Cooper SJ, Reynolds GP, Barnes T, et al. BAP guidelines on the management of weight gain, metabolic disturbances and cardiovascular risk associated with psychosis and antipsychotic drug treatment. J Psychopharmacol. 2016;30(8):717–48.
37. Basel D, Mosheva M, Maeder J, et al. Stimulant treatment effectiveness, safety and risk for psychosis in individuals with 22q11.2 deletion syndrome. Eur Child Adolesc Psychiatry. 2022;31(9):1367–75.
38. Damba JJ, Bodenstein K, Lavin P, et al. Psychotropic drugs and adverse kidney effects: a systematic review of the past decade of research. CNS Drugs. 2022;36(10):1049–77.
39. Shetty SS, AnnajiGowda HH, Dahale AB. Valproate-induced hyperammonemia, neuroleptic sensitivity, and cerebellar atrophy - a clinical conundrum in the management of bipolar disorder. Bipolar Disord. 2024;26(2):200–3.
40. Khokhar JY, Dwiel LL, Henricks AM, Doucette WT, Green AI. The link between schizophrenia and substance use disorder: a unifying hypothesis. Schizophr Res. 2018;194:78–85.

41. Buijs PC, Bassett AS, Gold DA, Boot E. Cognitive behavioral therapy in 22q11.2 deletion syndrome: a case study of two young adults with an anxiety disorder. J Intellect Disabil. 2021;25(4):695–704.
42. Kobrynski LJ, Sullivan KE. Velocardiofacial syndrome, DiGeorge syndrome: the chromosome 22q11.2 deletion syndromes. Lancet. 2007;370(9596):1443–52.
43. Szczawińska-Popłonyk A, Schwartzmann E, Chmara Z, et al. Chromosome 22q11.2 deletion syndrome: a comprehensive review of molecular genetics in the context of multidisciplinary clinical approach. Int J Mol Sci. 2023;24(9):8317.
44. Unolt M, Versacci P, Anaclerio S, et al. Congenital heart diseases and cardiovascular abnormalities in 22q11.2 deletion syndrome: from well-established knowledge to new frontiers. Am J Med Genet A. 2018;176(10):2087–98.
45. Seselgyte R, Swan MC, Birch MJ, Kangesu L. Velopharyngeal incompetence in children with 22q11.2 deletion syndrome: velar and pharyngeal dimensions. J Craniofac Surg. 2021;32(2):578–80.
46. Bayat M, Bayat A. Neurological manifestation of 22q11.2 deletion syndrome. Neurol Sci. 2022;43(3):1695–700.
47. Di Cesare S, Puliafito P, Ariganello P, et al. Autoimmunity and regulatory T cells in 22q11.2 deletion syndrome patients. Pediatr Allergy Immunol. 2015;26(6):591–4.
48. Levy-Shraga Y, Gothelf D, Goichberg Z, et al. Growth characteristics and endocrine abnormalities in 22q11.2 deletion syndrome. Am J Med Genet A. 2017;173(5):1301–8.

Further Reading

Bassett AS, McDonald-McGinn DM, Devriendt K, et al. Practical guidelines for managing patients with 22q11.2 deletion syndrome. J Pediatr. 2011;159(2):332–339.e1.

McDonald-McGinn DM, Sullivan KE, Marino B, et al. 22q11.2 deletion syndrome. GeneReviews® [Internet]; 2011.

Shprintzen RJ. Velo-cardio-facial syndrome: 30 years of study. Dev Disabil Res Rev. 2008;14(1):3–10.

Van L, Boot E, Bassett AS. Update on the 22q11.2 deletion syndrome and its relevance to schizophrenia. Curr Opin Psychiatry. 2017;30(3):191–6. https://doi.org/10.1097/YCO.0000000000000324.

Van L, Butcher NJ, Costain G, Ogura L, Chow EWC, Bassett AS. Fetal growth and gestational factors as predictors of schizophrenia in 22q11.2 deletion syndrome. Genet Med. 2016;18(4):350–5.

Tuberous Sclerosis Complex 10

David W. Dunn and Lydia J. Fisher

10.1 Overview of the Neurodevelopmental Disorder

Individual features of tuberous sclerosis complex (TSC) were described in the 1800s with the first description of the entity by Bourneville in 1880. He described a child with epilepsy and developmental delay who also had lesions in the brain and kidney. The genetic changes responsible for tuberous sclerosis were discovered in the 1990s. There have been over 200 variants found in *TSC1* and *TSC2* [1].

The estimated incidence of TSC is approximately 1:6000 to 1:10,000. There is no universal screening for TSC, so the exact incidence is unknown. Tuberous sclerosis complex affects both biological sexes equally and there are no known geographic differences in incidence.

The definite diagnosis of TSC can be based on the identification of pathologic variants in either the *TSC1* (chromosome 9q34) or *TSC2* (chromosome 16p13.3) gene, with or without clinical features of TSC. Diagnosis can also be made by identifying core clinical features. The International Tuberous Sclerosis Complex Consensus Group recommends a *definite clinical diagnosis* when there are two major criteria or one major criterion accompanied by two minor criteria present. A possible diagnosis occurs when there is one major or two or more minor criteria present [2] which are summarized in Table 10.1.

D. W. Dunn (✉)
Department of Psychiatry, Indiana University School of Medicine, Indianapolis, IN, USA

Department of Neurology, Indiana University School of Medicine, Indianapolis, IN, USA
e-mail: ddunn@iu.edu

L. J. Fisher
Department of Psychiatry, Indiana University School of Medicine, Indianapolis, IN, USA
e-mail: lydfisch@iu.edu

R. P. Thom, C. J. McDougle (eds.), *Neuropsychiatric Care for Genetic Syndromes and Other Neurodevelopmental Disorders*,
https://doi.org/10.1007/978-3-031-76269-7_10

Table 10.1 Diagnostic criteria by age of presentation

Major criteria
Infancy and preschool years
Hypopigmented macules (three or more, at least 5 mm in diameter)
Fibrous cephalic plaque
Shagreen patch
Multiple cortical tubers and/or radial migration lines
Subependymal nodules (two or more)
Cardiac rhabdomyomas
Childhood
Subependymal giant cell astrocytoma
Multiple retinal hamartomas
Angiofibroma (three or more)
Adolescence and adulthood
Ungual fibroma (two or more)
Renal angiomyolipomas (two or more)
Lymphangiomyomatosis

Minor criteria
Childhood
Multiple renal cysts
Dental enamel pits (three or more)
Intraoral fibromas (two or more)
Retinal achromatic patch
Adolescence and adulthood
Confetti skin lesions
Sclerotic bone lesions

The most common manifestations affect the brain, skin, and kidneys. Information on clinical features has been collected by the TuberOus SClerosis registry to increase disease Awareness (TOSCA) which includes 2,093 patients of all ages. Cortical tubers were found in 82%, subependymal nodules were found in 78%, epilepsy was found in 83.5%, and intellectual disability (ID) was found in 55%. Hypomelanotic macules were seen in 67% and facial angiofibroma were seen in 57%. Forty-seven percent had renal angiomyolipoma [3].

10.2 Underlying Genetic/Neurobiological Mechanisms

The *TSC1* gene is located on chromosome 9q34, while *TSC2* is located on chromosome 16p13. *TSC1* encodes hamartin, and *TSC2* encodes tuberin. Hamartin and tuberin form a complex that acts as a tumor suppressor. Gene variants are found in 90% of individuals with TSC. Of those without identified mutations, half have mosaic or intronic variants. The disorder is inherited in an autosomal dominant manner. The mutation is completely penetrant, but the expression is highly variable. Mutations arise de novo in approximately two-thirds of affected individuals. One-third have changes in the *TSC1* gene and two-thirds have changes in *TSC2*. Those with mutations in *TSC2* have more infantile spasms, subependymal giant cell astrocytoma (SEGA), and ID compared to those with *TSC1* mutations. The manifestations of TSC are generally less severe in those with mosaicism or without an identified mutation.

The hamartin-tuberin complex inhibits RAS homolog expressed in the brain (Rheb) that in turn inhibits the mammalian target of rapamycin (mTOR). mTOR is a protein kinase that works through the protein complexes mTORC1 and mTORC2. They have a major role in cellular growth and proliferation, axonal sprouting, and synapse formation. Mutations in the *TSC1* or *TSC2* genes result in overactivation of mTOR resulting in the development of benign tumors and hamartomas in multiple organs including the brain, eyes, kidneys, lungs, heart, and other organs [4–8].

Dysregulation caused by activation of mTOR begins prenatally during the formation of the cortex. Characteristic lesions include dyslamination and abnormal cells. Cortical tubers contain dysmorphic neurons and giant cells and subependymal nodules are characterized by large abnormal astrocytes. Small areas of gray and white matter lesions can be found on neuropathological examination. There may also be a reduction in the amount of myelin and decreased oligodendrocytes. Abnormalities in GABAergic signaling causing an excitatory-inhibitory imbalance play an important role in epileptogenesis. Neuroinflammation is also found in neuropathological samples [6].

Knowledge of the neurobiological mechanisms has led to the exploration of mTOR inhibitors as potential precision treatments for many of the clinical features of TSC. The mTOR inhibitors (rapamycin, everolimus, and sirolimus) have been effective in treating cardiac rhabdomyomas, epilepsy, renal angiofibromas, and lymphangiomyomatosis (LAM) [9–12]. Trials of mTOR inhibitors targeting the cognitive and behavioral manifestations of TSC have demonstrated limited to no efficacy [13, 14].

10.3 Common Clinical Features

The characteristic features of TSC are age-related. Imaging studies have found cardiac rhabdomyoma and cortical tubers in utero. Epilepsy, developmental delay, and features of autism spectrum disorder (ASD) appear in the first year of life. By the elementary school years, facial angiofibroma and symptoms of attention-deficit/hyperactivity disorder (ADHD) are seen. Ungual fibromas, anxiety, and depression are usually first diagnosed in adolescence. Renal cysts appear as early as elementary school age and angiomyolipoma in the adolescent and young adult years. Lymphangiomyomatosis (LAM) is found in adult women [4].

Cardiac rhabdomyomas develop antenatally. They were reported in 34% of the population in the TOSCA study [3]. These lesions spontaneously regress. They are rarely symptomatic but may cause obstruction and heart failure requiring treatment.

Skin lesions are seen in most individuals with TSC. Hypomelanotic macules appear early, often at birth or in the first year of life. Facial angiofibromas develop later, typically appearing in the early elementary school years and increasing in number and size over time. They are erythematous, papular lesions that can bleed and be cosmetically problematic. Forehead plaques and shagreen patches, a thickened dimpled lesion seen most often on the back, are less common and occur in 15–25% of individuals with TSC. Ungual fibromas, nodular lesions adjacent to or below the nail beds, first appear in adolescence [15, 16]. Topical sirolimus can be used for angiofibroma with surgery or laser treatments for lesions that bleed or are disfiguring [17] (Fig. 10.1).

Renal angiomyolipomas occur in approximately half of patients with TSC, and renal cysts occur in one-fourth of patients with TSC. They are found in late childhood or early adolescence. These lesions may be painful, may grow slowly, and can hemorrhage. They may lead to hypertension and impaired renal function. Renal carcinoma occurs rarely. Everolimus is the preferred medication to reduce growth with selective embolization for lesions that continue to grow or for acute hemorrhage into a lesion [18].

Lymphangiomyomatosis consists of multiple cystic lesions in the lung. It may occur sporadically or in association with TSC. Lymphangiomyomatosis occurs almost always in women over the age of 18 years. Lymphangiomyomatosis was reported in 7% of the TOSCA sample [3]. It causes overgrowth of smooth muscle cells and cysts in the lungs and presents with dyspnea or pneumothorax. Sirolimus is approved for symptomatic LAM [19].

Several central nervous system lesions are characteristic of TSC. Cortical tubers may be observed in utero. They are hamartomas with dysplastic neurons and abnormalities of cortical lamination. Cortical tubers and the adjacent brain tissue are the locus for epileptiform activity. Subependymal nodules are found along the walls of the lateral ventricles. Both tubers and subependymal nodules are enhancing lesions on T2-weighted magnetic resonance imaging (MRI) sequences. Subependymal giant cell astrocytomas (SEGAs) grow near the foramen of Monro and may cause obstruction of cerebrospinal fluid flow and hydrocephalus. In the TOSCA study, 82% had cortical tubers, 78% had subependymal nodules, and 24% had SEGA. Everolimus has been used for growing or large tumors not causing symptoms. Surgical resection with ventricular shunting is usually required for lesions causing obstructive hydrocephalus [11, 20, 21] (Fig. 10.2).

Epilepsy occurs in approximately 80% of individuals with TSC [20]. In the TOSCA study, approximately three-fourths of patients developed seizures before 2 years of age. Focal seizures and infantile spasms are the most common seizure types [3]. Patients with epilepsy and TSC are at risk for drug-resistant epilepsy. Drug-resistant epilepsy was seen in 50–60% of the patients with TSC in early clinical case series [22–24]. A recent systematic review of epilepsy and TSC found drug-resistant epilepsy in approximately one-third of individuals with TSC. In this review, risk factors for drug-resistant epilepsy were *TSC2* mutations, early infantile spams, and higher cortical tuber load. Early onset of epilepsy, infantile spasms, and higher tuber number or higher tuber/cortex load are risk factors for cognitive impairment and ASD [25]. Vigabatrin, everolimus, and cannabidiol are TSC-specific treatments and are discussed later. Otherwise, anti-seizure medications are

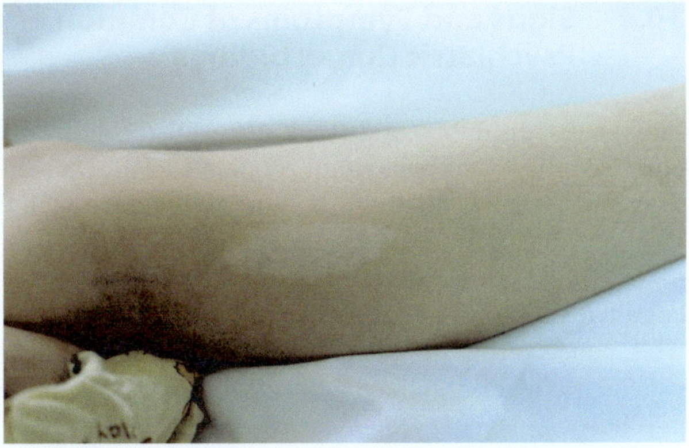

Fig. 10.1 Hypopigmented macule

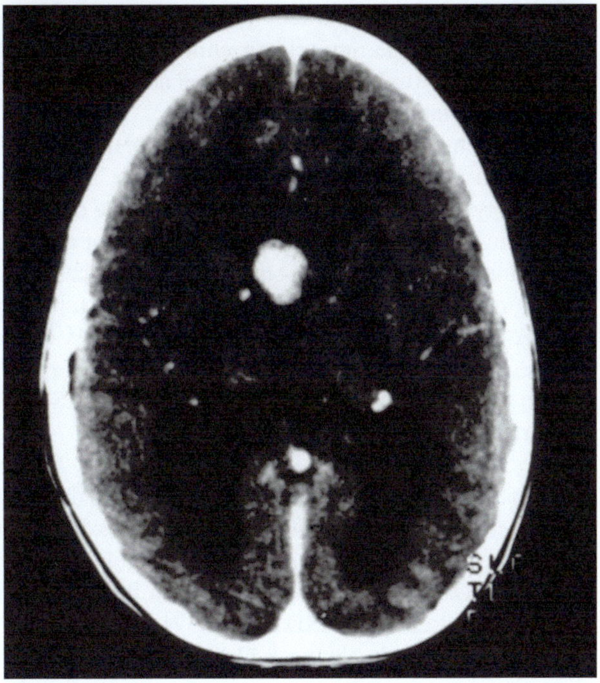

Fig. 10.2 Giant cell astrocytoma

used as in any form of epilepsy. Seizure surgery and vagal nerve stimulation are options for drug-resistant epilepsy [26].

The lesions associated with TSC may be found in multiple other organs. For example, retinal hamartoma and retinal achromatic lesions are listed in the TSC clinical criteria but seldom cause vision loss. Dental pits and hamartomas in bone, liver, and pancreas have occurred but are rarely symptomatic and do not require intervention [2].

10.4 Signs and Symptoms of Common Psychiatric Comorbidities

Intellectual disability and ASD are well-recognized manifestations of TSC, but other cognitive and behavioral problems have received less attention. For this reason, the neuropsychology group of the International Tuberous Sclerosis Complex Consensus Group devised the term TSC-associated neuropsychiatric disorders (TAND) and developed a questionnaire to screen for behavioral, emotional, and cognitive problems in people with TSC. TSC-associated neuropsychiatric disorders were conceived as an umbrella term covering six areas (levels): behavioral level, psychiatric level, intellectual level, academic level, neuropsychological level, and psychosocial level [27].

The behavioral level of TAND covers symptoms rather than diagnoses. Symptoms vary by age and the presence or absence of ID. Temper tantrums, aggression, self-injurious behaviors, hyperactivity, impulsivity, and sleep disruption are more common in children, particularly in children with ID. Aggressive behaviors tend to abate with age. Anxiety and depression are more common in adolescents and adults and are not related to ID [28–31].

The psychiatric level includes ASD ADHD, anxiety, and depression. In TSC, a diagnosis of ASD is usually made in the first 2 years of life, ADHD at school age, and anxiety and depression in late adolescence or emerging adulthood [30, 31].

Autism spectrum disorder affects 20–50% of children with TSC. Consistent predictors for ASD are the early onset of infantile spasms and cognitive delay. Probable predictors are frequent, severe seizures, higher tuber/brain ratio, and a *TSC2* mutation [32–35]. However, in the TOSCA study, de Vries et al. did not find an association between ASD and *TSC2* after controlling for intellectual ability. They found that boys with TSC were more likely to have ASD than girls [30]. Nevertheless, ASD may occur without any of the predictors.

Jeste et al. [36] found that signs of ASD in TSC can be demonstrated before 1 year of age. They found early delays in visual reception, fine motor ability, and cognitive delays at 12 months and 36 months in infants with TSC that developed ASD compared to infants with TSC without ASD. They also showed that the symptoms of ASD in children with TSC were the same as those seen in a comparison group of children with ASD alone [37]. Results from the TSC Autism Center of Excellence Research Network also found that delays could be found as early as 6 months of age in children who went on to develop ASD [38].

Children with TSC are also at risk for ADHD. In the TOSCA study, the diagnosis of ADHD was made at an average age of 7.7 years. ADHD seems to occur in 30–50% of children with TSC. Boys were more likely to have a diagnosis of ADHD than girls [3]. The prevalence of ADHD in children with epilepsy was also found to be 30–40% in a clinical series, which raises the question of whether the risk of ADHD in TSC is due to an association with epilepsy or whether there are specific features of TSC that increase the risk of ADHD [39].

Anxiety and depression have also been associated with TSC. Muzykewicz et al. [31] assessed 241 patients with TSC with an average age of 20 years. They found a mood disorder in 27% and anxiety in 30%. Mood disorder was comorbid with ADHD and anxiety, and those with anxiety had a comorbid mood disorder and no ID. In the TOSCA study, 9% had anxiety and 6% had depression. The average age of diagnosis was 18 years for anxiety and 24 years for depression. The authors of the TOSCA study noted significant missing data for TAND and suggested that their prevalence figures were probably an underestimate [3].

On the intellectual level of TAND, approximately half of the individuals with TSC have ID. In the TOSCA study, 45% of respondents were in the normal range for intellectual ability [3]. Early onset seizures, infantile spasms, and poorly controlled seizures were predictors of subsequent cognitive delay. ID seems more likely in those with mutations in *TSC2* than in those with mutations in *TSC1* [40–45].

There is less information about the academic level. Impaired school performance even in those TSC patients with normal intelligence seems to be common [28–30]. This was seen in 58% of participants in the TOSCA study. Of note, less than half had received an appropriate assessment for learning disability [3].

Findings at the neuropsychological level overlap with findings at the intellectual and academic levels. Deficits have been found in attention, executive functioning, and memory [29, 30].

Caregiver burden has been a significant concern on the psychosocial level of TAND [46]. A survey of parents and caregivers of individuals with TSC found a decrease in physical and mental health and quality of life compared to national norms. On the Hamilton Depression Inventory, 42% of caregivers scored in the mild-to-severe range for depression. Psychotropic medication use was reported in 19% of caregivers compared to a national average of 11% [47].

10.5 Assessments

Because the symptoms and clinical complications of TSC evolve over the lifespan, repeated careful monitoring is essential. At the time of diagnosis, there should be genetic testing, an electroencephalogram (EEG), and a magnetic resonance imaging (MRI) scan of the brain. The family should be offered genetic counseling. The International Tuberous Sclerosis Complex Consensus Group has published a recommendation for surveillance [2]. An EEG should be performed every 6 weeks until 12 months of age and then every 3 months until 2 years of age. An MRI of the brain should be performed every 1–3 years for patients with asymptomatic SEGA until the age of 25 years. An MRI scan of the abdomen to assess for renal lesions should be obtained every 1–3 years for life. Women with TSC need a chest computerized tomography scan every 5–7 years for asymptomatic LAM until menopause. An electrocardiogram (ECG) should be performed to monitor for cardiac conduction abnormalities every 3–5 years. Patients should have annual skin, dental, and eye exams. TSC-associated neuropsychiatric disorders screening should occur yearly with more extensive assessments during developmental periods including infancy (0–3 years), preschool (3–6 years), elementary (6–9 years), adolescence (12–16 years), and young adulthood (18–25 years).

In their initial report on TAND, the Tuberous Sclerosis Complex Neuropsychiatry Panel provided a TAND Checklist. This is a 12-item checklist for treatment teams to complete. It takes approximately 10 minutes and helps improve awareness of the multiple aspects of TAND [27]. Currently, a self-report checklist is being developed for individuals with TSC or their caregivers to complete. It has 14 sections and requires 15–20 minutes to complete. Initial studies have found the self-report form to be feasible and acceptable [48].

10.6 Psychosocial Treatments

There are no specific trials of psychosocial treatments for patients with TSC. There has been a recent international group of experts on TSC that published consensus recommendations for the evaluation and treatment of TAND. Their recommendations are based on trials for the treatment of behavioral and cognitive problems in children without TSC [49]. The clinical manifestations of ASD in children with TSC are the same as those found in non-syndromic ASD. The recommendation from the TAND group is to use standard, multimodal behavioral treatments for ASD [29]. This should include behavioral therapies such as applied behavioral analysis or functional behavior assessment. Speech and language therapy, occupational therapy, and physical therapy are often beneficial [50]. Cognitive behavioral therapy may be the first-line treatment for anxiety and depression, either alone for mild-to-moderate problems or combined with medication for more severe anxiety and depression [51]. Special education is essential for learning disabilities.

One essential part of psychosocial treatment is education about TSC and the potential for emergent problems over time. Parents, caregivers, and individuals with TSC need to be informed about TAND and should be encouraged to seek both academic and behavioral assistance when needed. Of note, less than half of individuals with TSC with academic difficulties had received an appropriate assessment [3].

Because of the complexity of the disorder, those with more severe difficulties should be referred to a TSC clinic [52]. The Tuberous Sclerosis Alliance website lists 72 TSC clinics in the United States. Families may also benefit from a referral to an organization such as the Tuberous Sclerosis Alliance. This organization provides education and support for families and lessens the isolation felt by many families.

10.7 Biological Treatments

Several specific biological treatments are available for certain individuals with TSC. For example, vigabatrin is an anti-seizure medication that has been used to treat infantile spasms. It was much more effective in treating infantile spasms in children with TSC than in children with infantile spams without TSC. Because of the association between early onset seizures and cognitive delays and ASD, it was hoped that early administration of vigabatrin at the time of epileptiform changes prior to the onset of seizures would result in a decreased incidence of cognitive and behavior problems. In the randomized EPISTOP trial of vigabatrin, patients who received early vigabatrin had no spasms, a later onset of seizures, and a decreased incidence of drug-resistant epilepsy. However, early administration of vigabatrin did not affect the incidence of ASD at 24 months [53]. In the double-blind, randomized PREVeNT trial, there was no difference in the frequency of focal seizures, drug-resistant epilepsy, or developmental outcomes at 24 months [54]. Vigabatrin remains the first-choice anti-seizure medication for infantile spasms in children with TSC. It is effective and safe but does not reduce ID or ASD.

Knowledge of the neurobiological mechanisms of TSC has led to advances in precision treatment with mTOR inhibitors to reduce the burden of epilepsy, SEGA growth, renal angiomyolipoma, and LAM. Everolimus has been FDA-approved for the treatment of partial onset seizures in patients with TSC, for SEGA, and for renal angiomyolipoma [11, 12, 55, 56]. Oral sirolimus is approved for LAM and topical sirolimus is approved for facial angiofibroma [17].

As with early use of vigabatrin, the hope was that mTOR inhibitors might improve cognition and behavior. Rapamycin (an mTOR inhibitor) was tested in a mouse model of *TSC2* and improved cognitive function. Trials in humans, however, have been similarly disappointing. Krueger et al. assessed everolimus (another mTOR inhibitor) in a double-blind placebo-controlled trial. Participants were 6–21 years of age, had a full-scale IQ >60, and had definite TSC. There was no difference between the drug and placebo on 36 of 38 measures of cognition or behavior [13]. Overwater et al. also performed a double-blind, placebo-controlled 12-month trial in 60 children with TSC, 4–17 years of age with a full-scale IQ <80. There was no effect on cognition, autism symptoms, neuropsychological measures, or behavior [14]. It is possible that giving an mTOR inhibitor at an earlier age might have made a difference.

Cannabidiol has been used for the treatment of drug-resistant epilepsy with approximately half the patients in one trial having a >50% reduction in seizure number. Diarrhea and somnolence were the most common side effects. Cannabidiol has been approved for the treatment of focal seizures in patients with TSC [57]. A placebo-controlled randomized trial conducted by Thiele et al. demonstrated that cannabidiol at doses of 25 mg/kg/day and 50 mg/kg/day was effective in reducing seizure frequency with a 50% decrease in seizure frequency seen in 36–40% of patients who received cannabidiol [58]. Factors that predict responsiveness to cannabidiol require further evaluation. The effect of cannabidiol on cognition and behavior in patients with TSC also remains unknown [59]. Randomized trials are underway to assess cannabidiol for the management of ASD symptoms in children without TSC. One 12-week randomized pilot trial in patients with ASD 5–21 years of age showed a reduction in disruptive behavior and improvement in total Social Responsiveness Scale score [60].

For those patients with TSC and drug-resistant seizures, epilepsy surgery may be an option. There was an initial concern that patients with multiple cortical tubers might not be candidates for surgery. However, those with focal seizures may have a single tuber that is the origin of most seizures. A review of seizure surgery for patients with TSC found that approximately two-thirds achieved seizure freedom [61]. The potential benefits for behavior and cognition are less certain. Prior studies of seizure surgeries in children with epilepsy but not TSC found improved cognition in those with postoperative seizure freedom but no definite improvement in behavior [62, 63]. One small study of 19 patients <2 years of age with TSC found a smaller decline in cognitive function in those who had a significant reduction in seizures compared to those with persistent refractory epilepsy [64].

Psychopharmacology for children with ASD and TSC is essentially the same as that used in children with non-TSC-associated ASD [65]. Aripiprazole and risperidone can be used for challenging behaviors without a significant risk of lowering the seizure threshold [66, 67]. There are no major drug interactions between these two medications and mTOR inhibitors. Valproic acid may help reduce irritability in children with TSC and can also help with seizure control.

For children with ADHD and TSC, stimulant medication is the first-line option based on trials for children with ADHD alone and in children with ADHD and epilepsy [39]. Atomoxetine and guanfacine are additional options. If the child with TSC has comorbid ADHD and ASD, stimulants may be effective but are less effective and have an increased risk of adverse effects such as irritability than in children with ADHD without comorbid ASD [68].

Selective serotonin reuptake inhibitors (SSRIs) are used to treat anxiety and depression in patients with TSC. They do not lower the seizure threshold. High-dose bupropion and tricyclic antidepressants may have an adverse effect on seizure control [66]. There is no significant drug interaction between SSRIs and mTOR inhibitors or vigabatrin.

10.8 Common Medical Comorbidities

A major concern for pharmacotherapy of behavior problems in the child with TSC is epilepsy. Fortunately, most psychotropic medications can be used safely in children with epilepsy. For the treatment of severe behavior problems associated with ASD, risperidone and aripiprazole have not lowered the seizure threshold. Olanzapine and quetiapine are associated with a minor increase in seizure risk. Clozapine is the most likely to increase the risk of seizures [66, 67]. Stimulant medication for ADHD is safe and effective, even in children with severe epilepsy. A consensus report from the International League Against Epilepsy concluded that methylphenidate could be used safely. Atomoxetine is probably effective and safe, and amphetamines can also be used, though the data is limited [39]. Most antidepressants can be used in children with epilepsy and might minimally improve seizure control. The exceptions are higher-dose bupropion and tricyclic antidepressants [66].

Anti-seizure medications may have adverse effects on cognition and behavior [66, 69]. Adverse effects on cognition have been seen with barbiturates, benzodiazepines, and polypharmacy. Problems with memory and attention have been associated with topiramate. Discontinuation due to adverse behavioral effects was most often seen with perampanel, followed by topiramate, levetiracetam, and zonisamide.

Depression has been associated with zonisamide, clobazam, and topiramate, and irritability has been associated with perampanel, brivaracetam, levetiracetam, and topiramate [70]. Sedation and irritability have been reported with cannabidiol [58]. There seem to be minimal behavioral and cognitive adverse effects of the mTOR inhibitors.

Key Points to Remember

- Tuberous sclerosis complex is a multi-system autosomal dominant disorder caused by mutations in the *TSC1* gene on chromosome 9q34 or in the *TSC2* gene on chromosome 16p13.3 that result in loss of tumor suppression in the mTOR pathway.
- The manifestations of TSC range from minimal to severe and disabling.
- Children with TSC are at risk for cognitive disability, autism spectrum disorder, and drug-resistant epilepsy.
- TSC-associated neuropsychiatric disorders include autism spectrum disorder, ADHD, anxiety, depression, intellectual disability, and learning disorders.
- Early onset epilepsy is associated with intellectual disability and autism spectrum disorder, but control of epilepsy has not consistently resulted in less cognitive and emotional disturbance.
- mTOR inhibitors such as sirolimus and everolimus may reduce seizure frequency and decrease the growth of SEGAs, renal angiomyolipomas, and lesions of lymphangiomyomatosis, but do not improve cognition or reduce the incidence or severity of autism spectrum disorder.

References

1. Peron A, Northrup H. Tuberous sclerosis complex. Am J Med Genet. 2018;178C:274–7.
2. Northrup H, Aronow ME, Bebin RM, et al. Updated international tuberous sclerosis diagnostic criteria and surveillance and management recommendations. Pediatr Neurol. 2021;123:50–66.
3. Kingswood JC, d'Augères GB, Belousova E, et al. TuberOus SClerosis registry to increase disease Awareness (TOSCA)-baseline data on 2093 patients. Orphanet J Rare Dis. 2017;12:2.
4. Crino PB, Nathanson KL, Henske EP. The tuberous sclerosis complex. N Engl J Med. 2006;355:345–56.
5. Wong M. Mammalian target of rapamycin (mTOR) inhibition as a potential antiepileptic therapy: from tuberous sclerosis to common acquired epilepsies. Epilepsia. 2010;51:27–36.
6. Curatolo P, Specchio N, Aonica E. Advances in the genetics and neuropathology of tuberous sclerosis complex: edging closer to targeted therapy. Lancet Neurol. 2022;21:843–56.
7. Curatolo P, Trivisano M, Specchio N. Updated genotype-phenotype correlations in TSC. Semin Pediatr Neurol. 2023;47:101086.
8. Zhao W, Kie C, Zhang X, et al. Advances in the mTOR signaling pathway and its inhibitor rapamycin in epilepsy. Brain Behav. 2023;13:e2995.
9. Ehninger D, Han S, Shilyansky C, et al. Reversal of learning deficits in a Tsc2 +/− mouse model of tuberous sclerosis. Nat Med. 2008;14:843–8.
10. Jülich K, Sahin M. Mechanism-based treatment in tuberous sclerosis complex. Pediatr Neurol. 2014;50:290–6.

11. Franz DN, Krueger DA. mTOR inhibitor therapy as a disease modifying therapy for tuberous sclerosis complex. Am J Med Genet. 2018;178C:365–73.
12. Cockerell I, Christensen J, Hoei-Hansen CE, et al. Effectiveness and safety of everolimus treatment in patients with tuberous sclerosis complex in real-world clinical practice. Orphanet J Rare Dis. 2023;18:377.
13. Krueger DA, Sadhwani A, Byars AW, et al. Everolimus for treatment of tuberous sclerosis complex-associated neuropsychiatric disorders. Ann Clin Transl Neurol. 2017;4:877–87.
14. Overwater IE, Rietman AB, Mous SE, et al. A randomized controlled trial with everolimus for IQ and autism in tuberous sclerosis complex. Neurology. 2019;93:e200–9.
15. Webb DW, Clarke A, Fyer A, Osborne JP. The cutaneous features of tuberous sclerosis: a population study. Br J Dermatol. 1996;135:1–5.
16. Teng JM, Cowen EW, Wataya-Kaneda M, et al. Dermatologic and dental aspects of the 2012 international tuberous sclerosis complex consensus statements. JAMA Dermatol. 2014;150:1095–101.
17. Koenig MK, Bell CS, Hebert AA, et al. Efficacy and safety of topical rapamycin in patients with facial angiofibromas secondary to tuberous sclerosis complex: the TREATMENT randomized clinical trial. JAMA Dermatol. 2018;154:773–80.
18. Bissler JJ, Kingswood JC. Renal manifestation of tuberous sclerosis complex. Am J Med Genet. 2018;178C:338–47.
19. Gupta N, Henske EP. Pulmonary manifestations in tuberous sclerosis complex. Am J Med Genet. 2018;178C:326–37.
20. Curatolo P, Moavero R, de Vries PJ. Neurological and neuropsychiatric aspects of tuberous sclerosis complex. Lancet Neurol. 2015;14:733–45.
21. Lu DS, Karas PJ, Krueger DA, Weiner HL. Central nervous system manifestations of tuberous sclerosis complex. Am J Med Genet. 2018;178C:291–8.
22. Chu-Shore CJ, Major P, Camposano S, Muzykewicz D, Thiele EA. The natural history of epilepsy in tuberous sclerosis complex. Epilepsa. 2010;51:1236–41.
23. Jeong A, Nakagawa JA, Wong M. Predictors of drug-resistant epilepsy in tuberous sclerosis complex. J Child Neurol. 2017;32:1092–8.
24. De Ridder J, Verhelle B, Vervisch J, et al. Early epileptiform EEG activity in infants with tuberous sclerosis complex predicts epilepsy and neurodevelopmental outcomes. Epilepsia. 2021;62:1208–19.
25. Miszewska D, Sugalska M, Jozwiak S. Risk factors associated with refractory epilepsy in patients with tuberous sclerosis complex: a systematic review. J Clin Med. 2021;10:5495.
26. Curatolo P, Nabbout R, Lagae L, et al. Management of epilepsy associated with tuberous sclerosis complex: updated clinical recommendations. Eur J Paediatr Neurol. 2018;22:738–48.
27. De Vries PJ, Whittemore VH, Leclezio L, et al. Tuberous sclerosis associated neuropsychiatric disorders (TAND) and the TAND checklist. Pediatr Neurol. 2015;52:16–24.
28. De Vries PJ, Belousova E, Benedik MP, et al. TSC-associated neuropsychiatric disorders (TAND): findings from the TOSCA natural history study. Orphanet J Rare Dis. 2018;13:157.
29. De Vries PJ, Wilde L, de Vries M, et al. A clinical update on tuberous sclerosis complex-associated neuropsychiatric disorders (TAND). Am J Genet. 2018;178C:309–20.
30. De Vries PJ, Belousova E, Benedik MP, et al. Tuberous sclerosis complex-associated neuropsychiatric disorders (TAND): new findings on age, sex, and genotype in relation to intellectual phenotype. Front Neurol. 2020;11:603.
31. Muzykewicz DA, Newberry P, Danforth N, et al. Psychiatric comorbid conditions in a clinic population of 241 patients with tuberous sclerosis complex. Epilepsy Behav. 2007;11:506–13.
32. Vignoli A, Briola FL, Peron A, et al. Autism spectrum disorder in tuberous sclerosis complex: searching for risk markers. Orphanet J Rare Dis. 2015;10:154.
33. Specchio N, Pietrafusa N, Trivisano M, et al. Autism and epilepsy in patients with tuberous sclerosis complex. Front Neurol. 2020;11:639.
34. Samanta D. An updated review of tuberous sclerosis complex-associated autism spectrum disorder. Pediatr Neurol. 2020;109:4–11.

35. Mitchell RA, Mitchell M, Williams K. The autism spectrum disorder phenotype in children with tuberous sclerosis complex: a systematic review and meta-analysis. Dev Med Child Neurol. 2002;64:1214–29.
36. Jeste SS, Wu JY, Senturk D, et al. Early developmental trajectories associated with ASD in infants with tuberous sclerosis complex. Neurology. 2014;83:160–8.
37. Jeste SS, Varcin KJ, Hellemann GS, et al. Symptom profiles of autism spectrum disorder in tuberous sclerosis complex. Neurology. 2016;87:766–72.
38. Capal JK, Williams ME, Pearson DA, et al. Profile of autism spectrum disorder in tuberous sclerosis complex: results from a longitudinal, prospective, multisite study. Ann Neurol. 2021;90:874–86.
39. Auvin S, Wirrell E, Donald KA, et al. Screening, diagnosis, and management of ADHD in children with epilepsy. Consensus paper of the task force on comorbidities of the ILAE pediatric commission. Epilepsia. 2018;59:1867–80.
40. Cusmai R, Moavero R, Bombardieri R, Vigevano F, Curatolo P. Long-term neurological outcome in children with early-onset epilepsy associated with tuberous sclerosis. Epilepsy Behav. 2011;22:735–9.
41. Van Eeghen AM, Chu-Shore C, Pulsifer MB, et al. Cognitive and adaptive development of patients with tuberous sclerosis complex: a retrospective, longitudinal investigation. Epilepsy Behav. 2012;23:10–5.
42. Capal JK, Bernandino-Cuesta B, Horn PS, et al. Influence of seizures on early development in tuberous sclerosis complex. Epilepsy Behav. 2017;70:245–52.
43. Tye C, McEwen FS, Liang H, et al. Long-term cognitive outcomes in tuberous sclerosis complex. Dev Med Child Neurol. 2020;62:322–9.
44. De Ridder J, Lavanga M, Verhelle B, et al. Prediction of neurodevelopment in infants with tuberous sclerosis complex using early EEG characteristics. Front Neurol. 2020;11:582891.
45. Hulshof HM, Kuijf H, Kotulska K. Association of early MRI characteristics with subsequent epilepsy and neurodevelopmental outcomes in children with tuberous sclerosis complex. Neurology. 2022;98:e1216–25.
46. Zöllner JP, Franz DN, Hertzberg C, et al. A systematic review on the burden of illness in individuals with tuberous sclerosis complex (TSC). Orphanet J Rare Dis. 2020;15:23.
47. Rentz AM, Skalicky AM, Pashos CL, et al. Caring for children with tuberous sclerosis: what is the physical and mental health impact on caregivers? J Child Neurol. 2015;30:1574–81.
48. Heunis T, Chambers N, Vanclooster S, et al. Development and feasibility of the self-report quantified tuberous sclerosis complex-associated neuropsychiatric disorders checklist (TAND-SQ). Pediatr Neurol. 2023;147:101–23.
49. De Vries PJ, Heunis T, Vanclooster S, et al. International consensus recommendations for the identification and treatment of tuberous sclerosis complex-associated neuropsychiatric disorders (TAND). J Neurodev Disord. 2023;15:32.
50. Will MN, Currans K, Smith J, et al. Evidence-based interventions for children with autism spectrum disorder. Curr Probl Pediatr Adolsec Health Care. 2018;48:234–49.
51. Walter HJ, Bukstein OG, Abright AR, et al. Clinical practice guideline for the assessment and treatment of children ad adolescents with anxiety disorders. J Am Acad Child Adolesc Psychiatry. 2020;59:1107–24.
52. Annear NMP, Appleton RE, Bassi Z, et al. Tuberous sclerosis complex (TSC): expert recommendations for provision of coordinated care. Front Neurol. 2019;10:1116.
53. Kotulska K, Kwiatkowski DJ, Curatolo P, et al. Prevention of epilepsy in infants with tuberous sclerosis in the EPISTOP trial. Ann Neurol. 2021;89:304–14.
54. Bebin EM, Peters JM, Porter BE, et al. Early treatment with vigabatrin does not decrease focal seizures or improve cognition in tuberous sclerosis complex: the prevent trial. Ann Neurol. 2024;95:15–26.
55. Franz DN, Lawson JA, Yapici Z, et al. Adjunctive everolimus therapy for tuberous sclerosis complex-associated refractory seizures: results from the postextension phase of EXIST-3. Epilepsia. 2021;62:3029–41.

56. Davies M, Saxena A, Kingswood JC. Management of everolimus-associated adverse events in patients with tuberous sclerosis complex: a practical guide. Orphanet J Rare Dis. 2017;12:35.
57. Szaflarski JP, Bebin EM, Comi AM, et al. Long-term safety and treatment effects of cannabidiol in children and adults with treatment-resistant epilepsies: expanded access program results. Epilepsia. 2018;59:1540–8.
58. Thiele EA, Bebin EM, Bhathal H, et al. Add-on cannabidiol treatment for drug-resistant seizures in tuberous sclerosis complex. A placebo-controlled randomized clinical trial. JAMA Neurol. 2021;78:285–92.
59. Samanta D. A scoping review of cannabidiol therapy in tuberous sclerosis: current evidence and perspectives for future development. Epilepsy Behav. 2022;128:108577.
60. Aran A, Harel M, Cassuto H, et al. Cannabinoid treatment for autism: a proof-of-concept randomized trial. Mol Autism. 2021;12:6.
61. Specchio N, Pepi C, de Palma L, et al. Surgery for drug-resistant tuberous sclerosis complex-associated epilepsy: who, when, and what. Epileptic Disord. 2021;23:53–73.
62. Stefanos-Yakoub I, Wingeier K, Held U, et al. Long-term intellectual and developmental outcomes after pediatric epilepsy: a systematic review and meta-analysis. Epilepsia. 2024;65:251–65.
63. Reilly C, Baldeweg T, Stewart N, et al. Do behavior and emotions improve after pediatric epilepsy surgery? A systematic review. Epilepsia. 2019;60:885–97.
64. Grayson LE, Peters JM, McPherson T, et al. Pilot study of neurodevelopmental impact of early epilepsy surgery in tuberous sclerosis complex. Pediatr Neurol. 2020;109:39–46.
65. Lamy M, Erickson CA. Pharmacological management of behavioral disturbances in children and adolescents with autism spectrum disorders. Curr Probl Pediatr Adolesc Health Care. 2018;48:250–64.
66. Alper K, Schwartz KA, Kolts RL, Khan A. Seizure incidence in psychopharmacological clinical trials: an analysis of Food and Drug Administration (FDA) summary basis of approval rights. Biol Psychiatry. 2007;62:345–54.
67. Kanner AM. Management of psychiatric and neurological comorbidities in epilepsy. Nat Rev Neurol. 2016;12:106–16.
68. Joshi G, Wilens TE. Pharmacotherapy of attention-deficit/hyperactivity disorder in individuals with autism spectrum disorder. Child Adolesc Psychiatr Clin N Am. 2022;31:449–68.
69. Afzal KI, Anam S, Hunter SJ. The effects of antiepileptic drugs on pediatric cognition, mood, and behavior. J Pediatr Epilepsy. 2017;6:3–18.
70. Stephen LJ, Wishart A, Brodie MJ. Psychiatric side effects and antiepileptic drugs: observations from prospective audits. Epilepsy Behav. 2017;71:73–8.

Further Reading

Crino PB, Nathanson KL, Henske EP. The tuberous sclerosis complex. N Engl J Med. 2006;355:345–56.

Curatolo P, Nabbout R, Lagae L, et al. Management of epilepsy associated with tuberous sclerosis complex: updated clinical recommendations. Eur J Paediatr Neurol. 2018;22:738–48.

Curatolo P, Specchio N, Aonica E. Advances in the genetics and neuropathology of tuberous sclerosis complex: edging closer to targeted therapy. Lancet Neurol. 2022;21:843–56.

De Vries PJ, Heunis T, Vanclooster S, et al. International consensus recommendations for the identification and treatment of tuberous sclerosis complex-associated neuropsychiatric disorders (TAND). J Neurodev Disord. 2023;15:32.

Kingswood JC, d'Augeres GB, Belousova E, et al. TuberOus Sclerosis registry to increase disease Awareness (TOSCA)-baseline data on 2093 patients. Orphanet J Rare Dis. 2017;12:2.

Northrup H, Aronow ME, Bebin RM, et al. Updated international tuberous sclerosis diagnostic criteria and surveillance and management recommendations. Pediatr Neurol. 2021;123:50–66.

Specchio N, Pietrafusa N, Trivisano M, et al. Autism and epilepsy in patients with tuberous sclerosis. Front Neurol. 2020;11:639.

11 Turner Syndrome

W. Philip Bartel, Robert Accordino, Bushra Awidi,
and Laura M. Prager

11.1 Overview of Turner Syndrome

11.1.1 Common Clinical Features

Turner syndrome (TS) can be diagnosed at any age, from before birth to adulthood. However, most individuals are diagnosed during childhood, with the highest percentage of diagnoses occurring during middle childhood. As TS can present with a broad array of phenotypes, initiating diagnostic testing depends upon the clinical recognition of specific patterns of symptoms in female patients. Among the most recognizable features are short stature, left-sided cardiovascular anomalies, a "shield chest" with widely spaced nipples, delayed puberty, delayed breast development, amenorrhea, lymphedema, and a webbed neck. Distinctive facial features include the presence of epicanthal folds, a low posterior hairline, and rotated ears. In addition to the cardiovascular anomalies, TS can also manifest with renal anomalies, autoimmune dysfunction, liver dysfunction, and hearing loss. A minority of

W. P. Bartel
University of Pittsburgh School of Medicine, Pittsburgh, PA, USA
e-mail: william_bartel@alumni.brown.edu

R. Accordino
Department of Psychiatry, Weill Cornell Medicine, New York, USA
e-mail: rea9041@med.cornell.edu

B. Awidi
Department of Psychiatry, Massachusetts General Hospital, Boston, MA, USA
e-mail: bawidi@mgh.harvard.edu

L. M. Prager (✉)
Department of Psychiatry and Behavioral Science, Boston Children's Hospital, Boston, MA, USA
e-mail: laura.prager@childrens.harvard.edu

R. P. Thom, C. J. McDougle (eds.), *Neuropsychiatric Care for Genetic Syndromes and Other Neurodevelopmental Disorders*,
https://doi.org/10.1007/978-3-031-76269-7_11

women with TS will present with developmental delay, but many present with an uneven neuropsychological profile and comorbid psychiatric disorders. These conditions are reviewed in depth in subsequent sections on neurocognitive dysfunction and other common comorbidities. Finally, it is important to be aware of other musculoskeletal and dermatological anomalies that could suggest a diagnosis of TS, such as Madelung's deformity (a rare congenital condition where the radius and ulna are misaligned), cubitus valgus, micrognathia, a high arched palate, nail hypoplasia, and the presence of many multi-pigmented nevi.

Roughly 95% of women with TS display reduced height and growth failure [1]. Issues with growth occur at various stages of development in TS, including in-utero growth restriction, linear growth failure during infancy and childhood, and impairment of the typical growth spurt seen in adolescence [2–4]. Without prompt diagnosis and treatment with growth hormone (GH), usually during the early elementary school years, a roughly 20 cm reduction in height from the female population mean is expected [3].

In TS, spontaneous puberty occurs between 14% and 33% of patients [5, 6]. Delayed puberty, delayed breast development, amenorrhea, and infertility are caused by primary hypogonadism due to impaired ovarian development. The classic description is of "streak gonads" in which germ cells are found to be replaced by connective tissue. The impairment of ovarian development itself is explained by various X chromosome anomalies, causing different degrees of monosomy of the X chromosome. The result is the hypergonadotropic hypogonadism often seen in TS, characterized by low levels of estrogen and androgen, and elevated follicle-stimulating hormone (FSH) and luteinizing hormone (LH) levels.

11.1.2 Epidemiology

The epidemiological analysis of TS is complicated by the fact that many individuals with mild phenotypes remain undiagnosed, making accurate estimation challenging [7]. Epidemiological studies of various populations estimate the prevalence of TS to be roughly 50 per 100,000 in female infants, with its incidence thought to range between 1-in-2,000 and 1-in-2,500 live female births [8–12]. However, when accounting for in-utero events, the loss of all or part of the X chromosome appears to happen much more frequently, with as many as 99% of such pregnancies ending in spontaneous miscarriages during the first trimester [8, 13, 14]. Estimates suggest that as many as 10% of miscarriages have chromosomal abnormalities consistent with TS [15, 16]. Overall, the incidence and prevalence of TS may now be lower than previous estimates, as the advent of prenatal ultrasound and associated genetic testing has resulted in some mothers choosing to electively terminate pregnancies thought to have a higher probability of TS [17, 18].

Turner syndrome is associated with a three-fold higher mortality rate than the general population, with an estimated 13-to-15-year reduction in lifespan [19, 20]. Excess mortality risk is present throughout the lifespan, though the highest excess risk occurs during adulthood. Notably, the risk is elevated for many of the major causes of death, though a significant amount of the excess mortality is caused by cardiovascular disease [20].

11.1.3 Genetic Mechanisms

Most cases of TS are not inherited, but rather arise from spontaneous meiotic or mitotic errors in cell division, which can occur before or after fertilization of the egg. *Monosomy X* (45, X) is the most common genotype and is found in 40–50% of TS cases [1]. It is caused by meiotic nondisjunction of the X chromosome, with errors most commonly occurring in paternal gametes.

Genetic mosaicism (45,X/46,XX) is the second most common abnormality and is responsible for 15–25% of cases [1]. It is caused by mitotic nondisjunction after fertilization, which causes only a subset of cell lines to lack an X chromosome. Mosaicism is thought to be associated with a milder phenotype, with lower risks of cardiovascular and lymphatic anomalies [1, 21, 22].

Rarer structural anomalies can also cause TS. *Isochromosome Xq*, which is characterized by an X chromosome with two copies of the long arm and none of the short arm, is perhaps the most common of these, representing 10–15% of cases [1]. Notably, Isochromosome Xq is associated with higher rates of autoimmune thyroiditis [23]. Less common structural anomalies include deletion of either the short or the long arm of an X chromosome (i.e., *Xp/Xq monosomy*). Another notable structural anomaly is *ring chromosome X*, which is caused by terminal breaks in the distal ends of Xp and Xq and their subsequent fusion. Ring chromosome X is particularly notable for its association with severe features such as developmental delay, syndactyly, and more pronounced growth restriction. These are attributed to the failure of X inactivation if the X-active specific transcript (XIS) locus is involved [24, 25].

Another important genetic subtype of TS is *Y-chromosome mosaicism* (45X/46XY), which should be considered in the presence of virilism, or if fluorescent in-situ-hybridization (FISH) testing finds evidence of a sex chromosome of unknown origin. Due to its association with an increased risk of gonadoblastoma, such results should be thoroughly investigated [26]. Roughly 10% of cases of TS may be attributed to Y-chromosome mosaicism [27]. Notably, 45X/46XY is associated with a number of phenotypes in addition to TS, and individuals may appear to be phenotypically male (often with issues of infertility) or present with ambiguous genitalia in the setting of mixed gonadal dysgenesis [27–29].

11.2 Assessment

11.2.1 Diagnosis of Turner Syndrome

While the mean age of diagnosis of TS is 15 years, due to the significant variation in phenotypic severity and presenting symptoms, the diagnosis is made across the lifespan, with peaks in infancy and adulthood [13]. With prenatal ultrasound, findings such as increased nuchal translucency, cystic hygroma, and cardiac anomalies like coarctation of the aorta should raise concern for TS [6, 30]. On prenatal quadruple marker screening, decreased alpha fetoprotein (AFP) and estriol with markedly increased human chorionic gonadotropin (hCG) and Inhibin A are also suggestive of TS. While these findings do raise suspicion for TS, karyotyping of fetal DNA obtained through amniocentesis or chorionic villous sampling is required to establish a prenatal diagnosis [6, 31]. Importantly, postnatal karyotyping is still required for diagnosis even if prenatal karyotyping indicates TS. This is because DNA obtained from amniocentesis or chorionic villi sampling is reflective of fibroblasts and may not be representative of postnatal genotype and the actual constitutional karyotype of the infant [1]. Notably, noninvasive forms of testing such as cell-free DNA analysis are unreliable screens for TS, and should not be used for prenatal diagnosis [32, 33].

Turner syndrome is not included in routine newborn screening tests, but should be pursued when female infants present with hallmark clinical findings such as webbed neck, cystic hygroma, or left-sided cardiac anomalies [6]. See Table 11.1 for recent practice guidelines that prompt chromosomal analysis for TS.

Karyotyping remains the gold standard for diagnosis. The American College of Medical Genetics recommends the standard 30-cell karyotype, which has been found to be able to detect mosaicism with high reliability [6, 34]. However, if the initial karyotyping yields negative results but clinical suspicion for TS remains high, it is reasonable to sample a second tissue (such as skin fibroblasts, buccal mucosa cells, or bladder epithelial cells) or to examine more metaphase spreads to exclude the possibility that the original testing missed the presence of mosaicism. Furthermore, Y-chromosome mosaicism may also be missed in karyotype analysis.

Table 11.1 Guidelines for chromosomal analysis in TS

A: At least one of the following clinical features is present
• Fetal cystic hygroma or hydrops fetalis
• Idiopathic short stature
• Obstructive left-sided congenital heart defect
• Unexplained delayed puberty or menarche
• Infertility
• Characteristic facial features
OR
B: At least two of the following clinical features are found to co-occur
• Renal anomaly
• Madelung deformity
• Neuropsychologic or psychiatric issues
• Multiple typical or melanocytic nevi
• Dysplastic or hyperconvex nails
• Other genital heart defects
• Hearing impairment <40 years of age together with short stature

Adapted from Gravholt et al. [1]

When this is suspected, FISH testing of buccal cells using sequences adjacent to the Y-centromere can be considered [6, 35]. Finally, it is worth mentioning that the practice of examining buccal smears for Barr bodies is outdated and no longer plays a role in the diagnosis of TS.

11.3 Signs and Symptoms of Common Psychiatric Comorbidities in TS Patients

11.3.1 Neurocognitive Disorders

As noted earlier, TS is associated with a range of developmental delays and psychiatric symptoms. Early identification and treatment of these conditions can improve outcomes and quality of life for patients.

Intellectual deficits are not the norm in TS, except in cases with ring chromosome X where patients may present with severe intellectual disability [25, 36]. Roughly 90% of women with TS will display average or above-average intelligence, while 10% will present with intellectual disability [1, 37]. This corresponds to a roughly eight-fold risk of intellectual disability in comparison to the general female population [38].

Even without formal intellectual disability, individuals with TS do tend to present with a characteristically uneven neurocognitive profile. Deficits occur in mathematical reasoning, visual-spatial skills, executive function, social communication, fine motor skills, and coordination [13, 38–41]. Difficulty with mathematics (dyscalculia) is estimated to occur in up to 50% of women with TS [42–44]. These deficits are usually identified in childhood but persist into adulthood [45]. Conversely, many women with TS will display advanced verbal skills [46]. As a result, it can be easy for a clinician with little experience with TS to miss deficits during a clinical interview [13]. If possible, women with TS should undergo neuropsychological testing to characterize their learning profile in more depth to ensure the provision of adequate educational and psychosocial supports.

Individuals with TS can also present with deficits in attention and executive functioning, for example with challenges in planning, multitasking, initiating tasks, and organizing [1]. If severe enough, this can lead to a diagnosis of attention-deficit/hyperactivity disorder (ADHD), which occurs in roughly 25% of cases [47–49]. This corresponds to an incidence rate of ADHD that is roughly 18 times higher than in the general female population [49].

Similarly, issues with social communication and cognition in TS may lead to diagnoses of social (pragmatic) communication disorder or autism spectrum disorder (ASD). Evidence suggests that TS women may have difficulty with face and emotion recognition, and perhaps impaired empathy [50–52]. A recent study found that as many as 83% of women with TS have significant difficulty with social communication, with roughly 23% of them meeting the full criteria for ASD [53]. The risk of ASD in TS was also recently estimated to be roughly four times higher than that of the general female population [38]. However, the true co-occurrence of ASD in TS remains controversial, as other authors argue that despite the impairments in social function observed in TS, the deficits may be different from those observed in ASD [54, 55].

Evidence also suggests that TS may increase the risk for other psychiatric comorbidities, such as mood disorders and anxiety. A common limitation of many of the studies that characterize the relationship between TS and comorbid psychiatric disorders are small sample sizes and selection bias [1]. As such, our understanding of psychopathology in TS remains limited. Nonetheless, it seems that as many as 50% of women with TS will struggle with clinically significant anxiety, including but not limited to generalized anxiety, social anxiety, phobias [56], or depression over the course of their lifespan [13, 57–59]. Both mood disorders and anxiety often arise in the context of psychosocial stressors such as difficulty with social pragmatics that compromises peer interactions, or frustration with academic subjects such as math that can lead to poor self-esteem, anxiety around tests, and depression [57].

A recent cross-sectional study undertaken in the UK noted that 34% of participants with TS met the criteria for at least one mental health disorder, which corresponded to a relative risk that was more than twice as high as that of typically developing girls [53]. Notably, 13% were diagnosed with anxiety, while only 1% had depression. Another recent retrospective cohort study in Sweden found that TS may increase the odds of schizophrenia and eating disorders [38]. To our knowledge, only one other study has found an association between TS and schizophrenia [59]. These studies, although inconclusive, highlight the importance of a thorough screening for psychiatric disorders in patients with TS as well as periodic monitoring across the lifespan.

11.3.2 Psychosocial Challenges

Psychosocial challenges for children with TS generally appear during the early school years. Furthermore, the issues with attention and executive function, as well as the cognitive phenotype described above can lead to educational challenges [42]. Between 40% and 70% of women with TS experience learning difficulties that complicate their education [53, 60, 61]. Despite this, most tend to achieve similar levels of educational attainment as the general population, with many completing 2- or 4-year college degrees and some pursuing graduate degrees [1, 62]. This corresponds to employment rates that are also similar to the general population [9, 61–63]. However, despite similar educational attainment, women with TS tend to report lower levels of occupational status than their peers [1, 64, 65].

Despite educational success and gainful employment, women with TS often remain dependent on their parents for longer than typically developing peers due to cognitive or emotional challenges that complicate independent living. Important skills such as health care autonomy and financial planning, which require complex cognitive skills, are often achieved later in life in TS [13, 60].

Psychosocial issues related to interpersonal relationships are also common in TS, and can impair friendships, romantic relationships, and sexual activity. Women with

TS have fewer close friendships and are less likely to marry [47, 62, 66]. Social difficulties often begin during childhood, where children with TS often spend less time with peers than would be expected in typical development, and often display difficulties forming and maintaining close friendships [60, 67]. Adolescents with TS are usually aware of their social interaction difficulties and may both welcome and benefit from social skills training [68]. Unfortunately, many women with TS will experience teasing related to atypical development, which can have lifelong negative impacts on self-esteem [69–72]. Interestingly, studies have failed to find a relationship between the presence of any specific hallmark physical feature of TS (e.g., webbed neck) and impairment of self-esteem or social function [73, 74].

Issues with psychosexual development begin in adolescence where, in the setting of delayed puberty and amenorrhea, many women with TS report later onset and reduced frequency of sexual intercourse [62]. Many also report impairment of self-esteem related to their perceived difficulties with sexual activity [75]. These issues extend into adulthood, where women with TS are less likely to be involved in a long-term active sexual partnership, and continue to display a reduced frequency of sexual activity [76].

11.4 Psychosocial Treatments

11.4.1 Neurocognitive and Psychiatric Assessment

Because of the neurocognitive and psychosocial issues discussed above, annual developmental and behavioral screenings through adulthood are a critical part of caring for girls with TS [1]. Formal neuropsychological testing is also recommended at major transitional stages, including preschool, school entry, and the start of high school [1, 6, 77]. Particularly relevant psychological tests are listed in Table 11.2.

11.4.2 Psychosocial Interventions

Targeted psychosocial interventions can help girls with TS to overcome issues related to academic and social impairment. Accommodations such as time extensions and tutoring are recommended to foster academic success, especially in the presence of dyscalculia [1]. Individualized educational plans and classroom interventions that seek to emphasize verbal strengths in the learning environment may also be beneficial. One way this can be done is to utilize verbal mnemonics or have lesson plans that incorporate spoken components [1]. Similarly, using oral testing may give young girls with TS the best ability to demonstrate their knowledge. Later in education, vocational counseling can be considered to help girls with TS navigate their way to careers in which they will thrive [1].

If psychiatric comorbidities such as ADHD or depression are present, referral to a psychiatrist or psychologist is recommended for evaluation and treatment planning [1]. Current guidelines for TS notably endorse the use of medications for both mood

Table 11.2 Common psychological tests used to assess neurocognitive skills

Psychological test	Utility
The Bayley Scales	Assesses cognitive, language, motor, social-emotional, and adaptive behavioral delays in infants [78]
Weschler Preschool and Primary Scale of Intelligence, Weschler Intelligence Scale for Children, Weschler Adult Intelligence Scale	Assesses verbal and nonverbal abilities across the lifespan [79]
The Developmental Neuropsychological Assessment	Assesses neurocognitive processes [60, 80, 81]
Social Skills Improvement System Rating Scale	To assess social and academic skills [82]
Kaufman Assessment Battery for Children	To assess presence of learning disabilities and developmental delay [83]
Achenbach System of Empirically Based Assessment	To assess depression, anxiety, and attention deficits [84]
The Child Behavior Checklist	To elicit information from the caregiver about day-to-day function of the child [60]

Adapted from Culen et al. [60]

disorders and ADHD [1]. These conditions are frequently managed with standard first-line treatments. Medication choice should be informed by the potential medical comorbidities of TS. As will be discussed in more detail later in this chapter, because of the potential for cardiovascular issues, an electrocardiogram (EKG) should be obtained before starting drugs that may prolong the QTc interval on an electrocardiogram. Cognitive behavioral therapy for mood and anxiety issues and group therapy to address social impairment may also be of benefit. Finally, referral to physical or occupational therapy may be considered if motor or visual-spatial impairments are present and impacting education or other activities of daily living such as driving.

The care of an individual with TS is complex, lifelong, and often requires a multidisciplinary team. The American Academy of Pediatrics Clinical Practice Guidelines recommend that transition planning for TS patients begin at age 14 years or earlier, and should include a multidisciplinary approach that addresses medical, educational, vocational, and psychosocial issues. Counseling should focus on building self-esteem, social skills, and independence, and should address issues such as sexuality, relationships, and family planning. In addition, counseling should address the potential for psychosocial challenges such as anxiety, depression, and social isolation, and should provide resources and support for addressing these challenges [1]. It is important for healthcare providers to work closely with patients and their families to develop individualized transition plans that address their unique needs and goals, and to provide ongoing support and guidance throughout the transition process.

Unfortunately, many patients with TS are lost to follow-up during the transition from pediatric to adult care [85]. While this transition is often challenging, it is exacerbated in TS by chronic issues of executive dysfunction and anxiety. For this reason, girls with TS often require a later and extended transition to adult care [13]. Current guidelines recommend that the pediatric endocrinologist, who is often a focal point of care for patients with TS, organize the transition as a staged process beginning in adolescence [1, 13]. Poor transitioning is associated not only with worse health outcomes but also with decreased quality of life secondary to reduced educational achievement and professional opportunities [13, 86]. As such, its importance cannot be overemphasized.

Finally, it is worth noting that some individuals with TS and intellectual disability may not be capable of achieving full independence from caregivers. In such a situation, patients should still be encouraged and allowed to aim for the maximal level of independence that is achievable within their limitations.

11.5 Biological Treatment

11.5.1 Growth

Recombinant Growth Hormone (GH) therapy is often used as a growth-promoting therapy in TS. The purpose of growth-promoting therapy is two-fold [1]. First, it minimizes physical limitations imposed on individuals with TS due to excessively short stature. Second, it allows for the initiation of estrogen replacement therapy in a timeframe such that puberty will occur along with their peers [87]. Evidence suggests that GH therapy results in the attainment of 5–8 cm of additional height on average, allowing girls with TS who receive GH to attain an adult height in the lower range of normal for adult females [88–90]. However, the efficacy is variable, and the attainment of taller adult heights is believed to be influenced by factors such as tall baseline height, tall parental height, early onset of GH therapy, increased duration of GH therapy, increased dose of GH, and longer length of GH therapy prior to puberty induction [1, 87, 91–93]. Current guidelines suggest beginning GH therapy between the ages of 4 and 6 years, with height measurements every 4–6 months to monitor treatment efficacy [1].

If initiation of GH therapy is significantly delayed or if the final adult height of the patient is predicted to be lower than preferred, guidelines recommend considering the addition of oxandrolone to GH therapy [1]. Oxandrolone is an anabolic steroid, which when added to GH therapy, may add an additional 2–5 cm to the final height [94–97]. However, patients must be counseled that this benefit comes with the risk of dose-dependent virilization and delayed breast development [1]. Patients must weigh the psychosocial impact of additional height against these potential negative side effects.

Growth hormone therapy in TS may be associated with a risk of slipped capital femoral epiphyses, intracranial hypertension, scoliosis, and pancreatitis [98, 99]. Authors of the recent treatment guidelines for TS note that while there is currently no evidence that GH therapy increases the risk of cardiovascular disease, metabolic disorders, bone mineralization, or hearing loss, most clinical trials have not been powered to be able to conclusively determine the rate of occurrence of these rare side effects [1]. They recommend monitoring insulin-like growth factor 1 (IGF-1) annually during GH therapy, and ensuring that IGF-1 levels do not exceed two standard deviations above the mean level for the patient's age because high levels of IGF-1 can result in gigantism in children and acromegaly in adults. Levels above three standard deviations should lead to a decrease in GH dose, while levels between two and three standard deviations are deferred to the clinical judgment of the clinician.

11.5.2 Puberty

As discussed earlier, patients with TS usually present with hypergonadotropic hypogonadism, and often require hormone replacement therapy (HRT) for the induction of puberty and to obtain female secondary sex characteristics. Hormone replacement therapy also assists with attaining optimal peak bone mass and uterine maturation. Current guidelines recommend starting to monitor FSH and LH levels to assess for hypergonadotropic hypogonadism around the age of 11 years, and to start low-dose transdermal 17-Beta estradiol therapy between 11 and 12 years of age if it is detected [1]. Progesterone should be added to the regimen either after breakthrough bleeding occurs or 2 years after the initiation of estrogen therapy, whichever occurs first. Evidence suggests that age-appropriate pubertal development due to HRT results in the improvement of health-related quality of life, and may also improve self-esteem, social functioning, and initiation of sexual activity in TS [62, 75, 100]. Treatment is often continued until the risks outweigh the benefits, which is often roughly the age of menopause in the general female population.

11.6 Common Medical Comorbidities

Individuals with TS are commonly diagnosed with cardiovascular, renal, and hepatic comorbidities. It is important to be aware of the potential for these comorbidities before prescribing psychotropic medications, and to ensure that patients have been appropriately screened for conditions that could impact the management of psychiatric illness such as ADHD, anxiety, and depression. Particularly relevant comorbidities and recommended screening guidelines are discussed briefly below, and the chapter concludes with suggested further reading for those readers requiring a more in-depth discussion.

11.6.1 Cardiovascular Comorbidities

Both congenital cardiovascular anomalies and acquired cardiovascular disease contribute significantly to morbidity and mortality in TS [101, 102]. The most widely appreciated cardiovascular issue in TS is congenital heart disease, which may occur in up to 50% of patients [20]. Congenital heart disease manifests broadly but is frequently left-sided, with notable examples including bicuspid aortic valve, aortic valve stenosis, aberrant right subclavian artery, hypoplastic left heart syndrome, atrial septal defects, ventricular septal defects, pulmonary valve stenosis, partial anomalous pulmonary venous drainage, coarctation of the aorta, aortic root dilation, and aortic dissection [1, 6]. Moreover, circulatory heart disease (including cerebrovascular disease, coronary artery disease, and systemic hypertension) accounts for 41% of the excess mortality observed in TS [20].

As such, a crucial part of care for women with TS is the appropriate screening and management of cardiovascular disease. Many girls with TS will require a referral to a cardiologist. Upon diagnosis of TS, it is appropriate to screen for congenital anomalies with a transthoracic echocardiogram (TTE) in infants [1]. Adults should receive both a TTE and cardiac magnetic resonance imaging (CMR) at the time of diagnosis. An EKG with QTc interval on an electrocardiogram corrected for heart rate measurement is recommended for all individuals at the time of diagnosis and before initiating any medications that may prolong the QTc interval, as the QTc interval is often found to be prolonged in women TS. Given the propensity for aortic dilation and dissection, it is important to continue to monitor the aortic root diameter in patients with TS. After the age of 16 years, or if the aortic size index is >2–2.3 cm/m^2, yearly TTE or CMR is recommended. It is also important to monitor blood pressure and lipids annually [1].

Careful screening and monitoring of cardiovascular risks in individuals with TS, particularly when considering the use of stimulant medications for ADHD, is important. Stimulants can increase heart rate and blood pressure, which may exacerbate cardiovascular risks in individuals with TS. Therefore, it is recommended that individuals with TS undergo a thorough cardiovascular evaluation, including echocardiography and electrocardiography, before initiating stimulant medications [31]. Additionally, updated guidelines in terms of cardiovascular screening before starting stimulant therapy for ADHD recommend regular monitoring of cardiovascular risk factors, such as blood pressure, lipid levels, and glucose tolerance throughout the lifespan of individuals with TS [1].

11.6.2 Metabolic Comorbidities

Obesity, diabetes, and glucose intolerance are commonly observed in TS. It is somewhat unclear if obesity occurs at a higher frequency in TS than in the general population, but some studies do suggest that elevated body mass index and reduced percentage of lean body mass occur in TS [1, 103, 104]. Evidence indicates an association between TS and both Type 1 and Type 2 diabetes, with estimates for the risk being as much as ten times higher than in age-matched controls [20, 105–107]. Moreover, many women with TS who do not meet the criteria for the diagnosis of diabetes still display issues with glucose homeostasis and intolerance concerning metabolic syndrome [108, 109]. Because of the association between these conditions and many of the cardiovascular diseases discussed above, it is critical that they are aggressively managed through both lifestyle modification and medication where appropriate. Current guidelines suggest counseling related to nutrition and physical activity beginning in childhood, as well as yearly hemoglobin A1c screening starting at age 10 years [1]. These issues are extremely important to keep in mind if the clinician is considering treatment with antipsychotic medication.

11.6.3 Autoimmune Comorbidities

Individuals with TS display an increased risk of developing a number of autoimmune disorders. Autoimmune disorders of the thyroid are the most frequent manifestation. Autoimmune thyroiditis is the most prevalent, but an association has also been observed with Grave's disease [110, 111]. Current guidelines suggest obtaining free T4 and TSH measurements annually to screen for thyroid dysfunction [1]. Other autoimmune conditions to be aware of in TS include Type 1 diabetes, celiac disease, uveitis, irritable bowel disease, and juvenile rheumatoid arthritis [107, 110]. Women with TS should be screened for celiac disease using transglutaminase antibodies every two years, starting at two years of age and continuing throughout childhood [1]. Symptomatic adults should also be screened.

11.6.4 Renal Comorbidities

Mortality due to renal disease in TS is estimated to be seven times higher than in the general population [20]. Renal anomalies occur in roughly 25–50% of cases of TS [112]. Ureteral and collecting duct anomalies can also occur, but are less frequent and only observed in 5–15% of cases. Classically, the association with horseshoe kidneys is emphasized, but duplication of the kidneys, absence of kidneys, multicystic kidneys, and ectopic kidneys are also seen [1]. Most patients with renal anomalies in TS do not progress to chronic renal failure, but many will develop frequent urinary tract infections (UTIs) secondary to obstructive issues [1]. It is important to have a high suspicion for UTIs and to promptly treat them to prevent renal scarring. Current guidelines suggest that patients with TS should be screened with renal ultrasound at the time of diagnosis [1]. Of course, any psychotropic medication that is renally excreted should only be initiated after evaluating the patient's renal function and adjusting the dose if indicated.

11.6.5 Hepatic Comorbidities

Though the mechanism is not currently understood, 20–80% of women with TS commonly present with asymptomatic abnormalities of aspartate aminotransferase, alanine transferase, and gamma-glutamyl transferase [113–117]. Most cases are of no clinical significance, but some may progress to cirrhosis, the risk of which is six times higher in TS than in the general population [105]. Doppler ultrasound of the liver is currently recommended as the initial step in the workup for individuals with liver enzyme abnormalities, and there is some evidence that estrogen replacement therapy significantly improves enzymatic elevation [1, 118, 119]. Current guidelines suggest starting estrogen replacement therapy between the ages of 11 and 12 years partially because of this benefit.

11.6.6 Otolaryngological Comorbidities

Early onset sensorineural hearing loss and conductive hearing loss secondary to middle ear effusion and otitis media are common features of TS. Hearing loss due to any cause is estimated to occur in roughly one-third of patients [120–122]. Chronic auditory dysfunction can lead to speech pathology, isolation, and depression, making its early identification and management a priority [1]. Given the social impairments faced by many women with TS, it is critical to ensure that hearing loss does not complicate an already difficult situation. Current guidelines recommend audiometric evaluation every 5 years starting at the time of diagnosis, and the aggressive treatment of both middle ear disease and otitis media with antibiotics or myringotomy, as deemed appropriate by an otolaryngologist [1].

References

1. Gravholt CH, Andersen NH, Conway GS, et al. Clinical practice guidelines for the care of girls and women with Turner syndrome: proceedings from the 2016 Cincinnati International Turner Syndrome Meeting. Eur J Endocrinol. 2017;177(3):G1–G70.
2. Davenport ML, Punyasavatsut N, Gunther D, Savendahl L, Stewart PW. Turner syndrome: a pattern of early growth failure. Acta Paediatr Suppl. 1999;88(433):118–21.
3. Brook CG, Murset G, Zachmann M, Prader A. Growth in children with 45,XO Turner's syndrome. Arch Dis Child. 1974;49(10):789–95.
4. Ranke MB, Pfluger H, Rosendahl W, et al. Turner syndrome: spontaneous growth in 150 cases and review of the literature. Eur J Pediatr. 1983;141(2):81–8.
5. Pasquino AM, Passeri F, Pucarelli I, Segni M, Municchi G. Spontaneous pubertal development in Turner's syndrome. Italian Study Group for Turner's Syndrome. J Clin Endocrinol Metab. 1997;82(6):1810–3.
6. Shankar RK, Backeljauw PF. Current best practice in the management of Turner syndrome. Ther Adv Endocrinol Metab. 2018;9(1):33–40.
7. Gunther DF, Eugster E, Zagar AJ, Bryant CG, Davenport ML, Quigley CA. Ascertainment bias in Turner syndrome: new insights from girls who were diagnosed incidentally in prenatal life. Pediatrics. 2004;114(3):640–4.
8. Gravholt CH, Juul S, Naeraa RW, Hansen J. Prenatal and postnatal prevalence of Turner's syndrome: registry study. BMJ. 1996;312(7022):16–21.
9. Stochholm K, Hjerrild B, Mortensen KH, Juul S, Frydenberg M, Gravholt CH. Socioeconomic parameters and mortality in Turner syndrome. Eur J Endocrinol. 2012;166(6):1013–9.
10. Nielsen J, Wohlert M. Sex chromosome abnormalities found among 34,910 newborn children: results from a 13-year incidence study in Arhus, Denmark. Birth Defects Orig Artic Ser. 1990;26(4):209–23.
11. Nielsen J, Wohlert M. Chromosome abnormalities found among 34,910 newborn children: results from a 13-year incidence study in Arhus, Denmark. Hum Genet. 1991;87(1):81–3.

12. Cockwell A, MacKenzie M, Youings S, Jacobs P. A cytogenetic and molecular study of a series of 45,X fetuses and their parents. J Med Genet. 1991;28(3):151–5.
13. Lin AE, Prakash SK, Andersen NH, et al. Recognition and management of adults with Turner syndrome: from the transition of adolescence through the senior years. Am J Med Genet A. 2019;179(10):1987–2033.
14. Hook EB, Warburton D. The distribution of chromosomal genotypes associated with Turner's syndrome: livebirth prevalence rates and evidence for diminished fetal mortality and severity in genotypes associated with structural X abnormalities or mosaicism. Hum Genet. 1983;64(1):24–7.
15. Levy B, Sigurjonsson S, Pettersen B, et al. Genomic imbalance in products of conception: single-nucleotide polymorphism chromosomal microarray analysis. Obstet Gynecol. 2014;124(2 Pt 1):202–9.
16. Romero ST, Geiersbach KB, Paxton CN, et al. Differentiation of genetic abnormalities in early pregnancy loss. Ultrasound Obstet Gynecol. 2015;45(1):89–94.
17. Iyer NP, Tucker DF, Roberts SH, Moselhi M, Morgan M, Matthes JW. Outcome of fetuses with Turner syndrome: a 10-year congenital anomaly register based study. J Matern Fetal Neonatal Med. 2012;25(1):68–73.
18. Baena N, De Vigan C, Cariati E, et al. Turner syndrome: evaluation of prenatal diagnosis in 19 European registries. Am J Med Genet A. 2004;129A(1):16–20.
19. Fuchs MM, Attenhofer Jost C, Babovic-Vuksanovic D, Connolly HM, Egbe A. Long-term outcomes in patients with Turner syndrome: a 68-year follow-up. J Am Heart Assoc. 2019;8(11):e011501.
20. Schoemaker MJ, Swerdlow AJ, Higgins CD, Wright AF, Jacobs PA, United Kingdom Clinical Cytogenetics Group. Mortality in women with Turner syndrome in Great Britain: a national cohort study. J Clin Endocrinol Metab. 2008;93(12):4735–42.
21. El-Mansoury M, Barrenas ML, Bryman I, et al. Chromosomal mosaicism mitigates stigmata and cardiovascular risk factors in Turner syndrome. Clin Endocrinol. 2007;66(5):744–51.
22. Denes AM, Landin-Wilhelmsen K, Wettergren Y, Bryman I, Hanson C. The proportion of diploid 46,XX cells increases with time in women with Turner syndrome--a 10-year follow-up study. Genet Test Mol Biomarkers. 2015;19(2):82–7.
23. Zinman B, Kabiawu SI, Moross T, et al. Endocrine, cytogenetic and psychometric features of patients with X-isochromosome 46, X, i(Xq) Turner's syndrome: a preliminary study in nine patients. Clin Invest Med. 1984;7(3):135–41.
24. Migeon BR, Luo S, Jani M, Jeppesen P. The severe phenotype of females with tiny ring X chromosomes is associated with inability of these chromosomes to undergo X inactivation. Am J Hum Genet. 1994;55(3):497–504.
25. Migeon BR, Luo S, Stasiowski BA, et al. Deficient transcription of XIST from tiny ring X chromosomes in females with severe phenotypes. Proc Natl Acad Sci USA. 1993;90(24):12025–9.
26. Schellhas HF. Malignant potential of the dysgenetic gonad. Part 1. Obstet Gynecol. 1974;44(2):298–309.
27. dos Santos AP, Andrade JG, Piveta CS, et al. Screening of Y chromosome microdeletions in 46,XY partial gonadal dysgenesis and in patients with a 45,X/46,XY karyotype or its variants. BMC Med Genet. 2013;14:115.
28. Lindhardt Johansen M, Hagen CP, Rajpert-De Meyts E, et al. 45,X/46,XY mosaicism: phenotypic characteristics, growth, and reproductive function--a retrospective longitudinal study. J Clin Endocrinol Metab. 2012;97(8):E1540–9.
29. Wu Q, Wang C, Shi H, Kong X, Ren S, Jiang M. The clinical manifestation and genetic evaluation in patients with 45,X/46,XY mosaicism. Sex Dev. 2017;11(2):64–9.
30. Bronshtein M, Zimmer EZ, Blazer S. A characteristic cluster of fetal sonographic markers that are predictive of fetal Turner syndrome in early pregnancy. Am J Obstet Gynecol. 2003;188(4):1016–20.
31. Bondy CA, Turner Syndrome Study Group. Care of girls and women with Turner syndrome: a guideline of the Turner Syndrome Study Group. J Clin Endocrinol Metab. 2007;92(1):10–25.

32. Gil MM, Quezada MS, Revello R, Akolekar R, Nicolaides KH. Analysis of cell-free DNA in maternal blood in screening for fetal aneuploidies: updated meta-analysis. Ultrasound Obstet Gynecol. 2015;45(3):249–66.
33. Meck JM, Kramer Dugan E, Matyakhina L, et al. Noninvasive prenatal screening for aneuploidy: positive predictive values based on cytogenetic findings. Am J Obstet Gynecol. 2015;213(2):214.e1–5.
34. Hook EB. Exclusion of chromosomal mosaicism: tables of 90%, 95% and 99% confidence limits and comments on use. Am J Hum Genet. 1977;29(1):94–7.
35. Freriks K, Timmers HJ, Netea-Maier RT, et al. Buccal cell FISH and blood PCR-Y detect high rates of X chromosomal mosaicism and Y chromosomal derivatives in patients with Turner syndrome. Eur J Med Genet. 2013;56(9):497–501.
36. Collins AL, Cockwell AE, Jacobs PA, Dennis NR. A comparison of the clinical and cytogenetic findings in nine patients with a ring (X) cell line and 16 45,X patients. J Med Genet. 1994;31(7):528–33.
37. Bender BG, Linden MG, Robinson A. Neurocognitive and psychosocial phenotypes associated with Turner syndrome. In: Atypical cognitive deficits in developmental disorders: implications for brain function. Lawrence Erlbaum Associates; 1994. p. 197–216.
38. Bjorlin Avdic H, Butwicka A, Nordenstrom A, et al. Neurodevelopmental and psychiatric disorders in females with Turner syndrome: a population-based study. J Neurodev Disord. 2021;13(1):51.
39. El-Mansoury M, Barrenas ML, Bryman I, Hanson C, Landin-Wilhelmsen K. Impaired body balance, fine motor function and hearing in women with Turner syndrome. Clin Endocrinol. 2009;71(2):273–8.
40. Knickmeyer RC, Hooper SR. The deep biology of cognition: moving toward a comprehensive neurodevelopmental model of Turner syndrome. Am J Med Genet C Semin Med Genet. 2019;181(1):91–9.
41. Temple CM, Carney RA. Intellectual functioning of children with Turner syndrome: a comparison of behavioural phenotypes. Dev Med Child Neurol. 1993;35(8):691–8.
42. Mazzocco MM. The cognitive phenotype of Turner syndrome: specific learning disabilities. Int Congr Ser. 2006;1298:83–92.
43. Rovet J, Holland J. Psychological aspects of the Canadian randomized controlled trial of human growth hormone and low-dose ethinyl oestradiol in children with Turner syndrome. The Canadian Growth Hormone Advisory Group. Horm Res. 1993;39(Suppl 2):60–4.
44. Murphy MM, Mazzocco MM, Gerner G, Henry AE. Mathematics learning disability in girls with Turner syndrome or fragile X syndrome. Brain Cogn. 2006;61(2):195–210.
45. Ross JL, Stefanatos GA, Kushner H, Zinn A, Bondy C, Roeltgen D. Persistent cognitive deficits in adult women with Turner syndrome. Neurology. 2002;58(2):218–25.
46. Temple CM, Shephard EE. Exceptional lexical skills but executive language deficits in school starters and young adults with Turners syndrome: implications for X chromosome effects on brain function. Brain Lang. 2012;120(3):345–59.
47. McCauley E, Feuillan P, Kushner H, Ross JL. Psychosocial development in adolescents with Turner syndrome. J Dev Behav Pediatr. 2001;22(6):360–5.
48. Green T, Naylor PE, Davies W. Attention deficit hyperactivity disorder (ADHD) in phenotypically similar neurogenetic conditions: Turner syndrome and the RASopathies. J Neurodev Disord. 2017;9:25.
49. Russell HF, Wallis D, Mazzocco MM, et al. Increased prevalence of ADHD in Turner syndrome with no evidence of imprinting effects. J Pediatr Psychol. 2006;31(9):945–55.
50. Burnett AC, Reutens DC, Wood AG. Social cognition in Turner's syndrome. J Clin Neurosci. 2010;17(3):283–6.
51. Hong DS, Bray S, Haas BW, Hoeft F, Reiss AL. Aberrant neurocognitive processing of fear in young girls with Turner syndrome. Soc Cogn Affect Neurosci. 2014;9(3):255–64.
52. Lawrence K, Campbell R, Swettenham J, et al. Interpreting gaze in Turner syndrome: impaired sensitivity to intention and emotion, but preservation of social cueing. Neuropsychologia. 2003;41(8):894–905.

53. Wolstencroft J, Mandy W, Skuse D. Mental health and neurodevelopment in children and adolescents with Turner syndrome. Womens Health. 2022;18:17455057221133635.
54. Hong DS, Dunkin B, Reiss AL. Psychosocial functioning and social cognitive processing in girls with Turner syndrome. J Dev Behav Pediatr. 2011;32(7):512–20.
55. Lepage JF, Lortie M, Deal CL, Theoret H. Empathy, autistic traits, and motor resonance in adults with Turner syndrome. Soc Neurosci. 2014;9(6):601–9.
56. Hutaff-Lee C, Bennett E, Howell S, Tartaglia N. Clinical developmental, neuropsychological, and social-emotional features of Turner syndrome. Am J Med Genet C Semin Med Genet. 2019;181(1):126–34. https://doi.org/10.1002/ajmg.c.31687.
57. Cardoso G, Daly R, Haq NA, et al. Current and lifetime psychiatric illness in women with Turner syndrome. Gynecol Endocrinol. 2004;19(6):313–9.
58. Schmidt PJ, Cardoso GM, Ross JL, Haq N, Rubinow DR, Bondy CA. Shyness, social anxiety, and impaired self-esteem in Turner syndrome and premature ovarian failure. JAMA. 2006;295(12):1374–6.
59. de Vries ALC, Roehle R, Marshall L, et al. Mental health of a large group of adults with disorders of sex development in six European countries. Psychosom Med. 2019;81(7):629–40.
60. Culen C, Ertl DA, Schubert K, Bartha-Doering L, Haeusler G. Care of girls and women with Turner syndrome: beyond growth and hormones. Endocr Connect. 2017;6(4):R39–51.
61. Sybert VP, McCauley E. Turner's syndrome. N Engl J Med. 2004;351(12):1227–38.
62. Naess EE, Bahr D, Gravholt CH. Health status in women with Turner syndrome: a questionnaire study on health status, education, work participation and aspects of sexual functioning. Clin Endocrinol. 2010;72(5):678–84.
63. Amundson E, Boman UW, Barrenas ML, Bryman I, Landin-Wilhelmsen K. Impact of growth hormone therapy on quality of life in adults with turner syndrome. J Clin Endocrinol Metab. 2010;95(3):1355–9.
64. Downey J, Elkin EJ, Ehrhardt AA, Meyer-Bahlburg HF, Bell JJ, Morishima A. Cognitive ability and everyday functioning in women with Turner syndrome. J Learn Disabil. 1991;24(1):32–9.
65. Fjermestad KW, Naess EE, Bahr D, Gravholt CH. A 6-year follow-up survey of health status in middle-aged women with Turner syndrome. Clin Endocrinol. 2016;85(3):423–9.
66. Gould HN, Bakalov VK, Tankersley C, Bondy CA. High levels of education and employment among women with Turner syndrome. J Womens Health (Larchmt). 2013;22(3):230–5.
67. Lepage JF, Dunkin B, Hong DS, Reiss AL. Impact of cognitive profile on social functioning in prepubescent females with Turner syndrome. Child Neuropsychol. 2013;19(2):161–72.
68. Wolstencroft J, Mandy W, Skuse D. Experiences of social interaction in young women with Turner syndrome: a qualitative study. Child Care Health Dev. 2020;46(1):46–55.
69. Boman UW, Bryman I, Halling K, Moller A. Women with Turner syndrome: psychological well-being, self-rated health and social life. J Psychosom Obstet Gynaecol. 2001;22(2):113–22.
70. Rickert VI, Hassed SJ, Hendon AE, Cunniff C. The effects of peer ridicule on depression and self-image among adolescent females with Turner syndrome. J Adolesc Health. 1996;19(1):34–8.
71. Sutton EJ, McInerney-Leo A, Bondy CA, Gollust SE, King D, Biesecker B. Turner syndrome: four challenges across the lifespan. Am J Med Genet A. 2005;139A(2):57–66.
72. Suzigan LZ, de Paiva e Silva RB, Guerra-Junior G, Marini SH, Maciel-Guerra AT. Social skills in women with Turner syndrome. Scand J Psychol. 2011;52(5):440–7.
73. McCauley E, Ross JL, Kushner H, Cutler G Jr. Self-esteem and behavior in girls with Turner syndrome. J Dev Behav Pediatr. 1995;16(2):82–8.
74. Boman UW, Bryman I, Moller A. Psychological well-being in women with Turner syndrome: somatic and social correlates. J Psychosom Obstet Gynaecol. 2004;25(3–4):211–9.
75. Carel JC, Elie C, Ecosse E, et al. Self-esteem and social adjustment in young women with Turner syndrome--influence of pubertal management and sexuality: population-based cohort study. J Clin Endocrinol Metab. 2006;91(8):2972–9.

76. Sheaffer AT, Lange E, Bondy CA. Sexual function in women with Turner syndrome. J Womens Health (Larchmt). 2008;17(1):27–33.
77. Heilbronner RL, Sweet JJ, Attix DK, Krull KR, Henry GK, Hart RP. Official position of the American Academy of Clinical Neuropsychology on serial neuropsychological assessments: the utility and challenges of repeat test administrations in clinical and forensic contexts. Clin Neuropsychol. 2010;24(8):1267–78.
78. Balasundaram P, Avulakunta ID. Bayley scales of infant and toddler development. Treasure Island (FL): StatPearls; 2023.
79. Hong DS, Reiss AL. Cognition and behavior in Turner syndrome: a brief review. Pediatr Endocrinol Rev. 2012;9 Suppl 2(0 2):710–2.
80. Ohmann S, Wurzer M, Popow C. Attention-deficit hyperactivity disorder and executive dysfunction in preschool children. A comparison of NEPSY and BRIEF-P assessments. Encéphale. 2022;48(3):232–40.
81. Ahmad SA, Warriner EM. Review of the NEPSY: a developmental neuropsychological assessment. Clin Neuropsychol. 2001;15(2):240–9.
82. DiPerna JC, Lei P, Bellinger J, Cheng W. Efficacy of the social skills improvement system class-wide intervention program (SSIS-CIP) primary version. Sch Psychol Q. 2015;30(1):123–41.
83. Kaufman AS, O'Neal MR, Avant AH, Long SW. Introduction to the Kaufman assessment battery for children (K-ABC) for pediatric neuroclinicians. J Child Neurol. 1987;2(1):3–16.
84. Rescorla LA. Assessment of young children using the Achenbach system of empirically based assessment (ASEBA). Ment Retard Dev Disabil Res Rev. 2005;11(3):226–37.
85. Rubin K. Transitioning the patient with Turner's syndrome from pediatric to adult care. J Pediatr Endocrinol Metab. 2003;16(Suppl 3):651–9.
86. Mahan JD, Betz CL, Okumura MJ, Ferris ME. Self-management and transition to adult health care in adolescents and young adults: a team process. Pediatr Rev. 2017;38(7):305–19.
87. Reiter EO, Blethen SL, Baptista J, Price L. Early initiation of growth hormone treatment allows age-appropriate estrogen use in Turner's syndrome. J Clin Endocrinol Metab. 2001;86(5):1936–41.
88. Pasquino AM, Pucarelli I, Segni M, Tarani L, Calcaterra V, Larizza D. Adult height in sixty girls with Turner syndrome treated with growth hormone matched with an untreated group. J Endocrinol Investig. 2005;28(4):350–6.
89. Chernausek SD, Attie KM, Cara JF, Rosenfeld RG, Frane J. Growth hormone therapy of Turner syndrome: the impact of age of estrogen replacement on final height. Genentech, Inc., Collaborative Study Group. J Clin Endocrinol Metab. 2000;85(7):2439–45.
90. Rosenfeld RG, Attie KM, Frane J, et al. Growth hormone therapy of Turner's syndrome: beneficial effect on adult height. J Pediatr. 1998;132(2):319–24.
91. van Pareren YK, de Muinck Keizer-Schrama SM, Stijnen T, et al. Final height in girls with turner syndrome after long-term growth hormone treatment in three dosages and low dose estrogens. J Clin Endocrinol Metab. 2003;88(3):1119–25.
92. Quigley CA, Crowe BJ, Anglin DG, Chipman JJ. Growth hormone and low dose estrogen in Turner syndrome: results of a United States multi-center trial to near-final height. J Clin Endocrinol Metab. 2002;87(5):2033–41.
93. Baxter L, Bryant J, Cave CB, Milne R. Recombinant growth hormone for children and adolescents with Turner syndrome. Cochrane Database Syst Rev. 2007;(1):CD003887.
94. Gault EJ, Perry RJ, Cole TJ, et al. Effect of oxandrolone and timing of pubertal induction on final height in Turner's syndrome: randomised, double blind, placebo controlled trial. BMJ. 2011;342:d1980.
95. Menke LA, Sas TC, de Muinck Keizer-Schrama SM, et al. Efficacy and safety of oxandrolone in growth hormone-treated girls with turner syndrome. J Clin Endocrinol Metab. 2010;95(3):1151–60.
96. Zeger MP, Shah K, Kowal K, Cutler GB Jr, Kushner H, Ross JL. Prospective study confirms oxandrolone-associated improvement in height in growth hormone-treated adolescent girls with Turner syndrome. Horm Res Paediatr. 2011;75(1):38–46.

97. Sas TC, Gault EJ, Bardsley MZ, et al. Safety and efficacy of oxandrolone in growth hormone-treated girls with Turner syndrome: evidence from recent studies and recommendations for use. Horm Res Paediatr. 2014;81(5):289–97.
98. Darendeliler F, Karagiannis G, Wilton P. Headache, idiopathic intracranial hypertension and slipped capital femoral epiphysis during growth hormone treatment: a safety update from the KIGS database. Horm Res. 2007;68(Suppl 5):41–7.
99. Bell J, Parker KL, Swinford RD, Hoffman AR, Maneatis T, Lippe B. Long-term safety of recombinant human growth hormone in children. J Clin Endocrinol Metab. 2010;95(1):167–77.
100. Bannink EM, Raat H, Mulder PG, de Muinck Keizer-Schrama SM. Quality of life after growth hormone therapy and induced puberty in women with Turner syndrome. J Pediatr. 2006;148(1):95–101.
101. Silberbach M, Roos-Hesselink JW, Andersen NH, et al. Cardiovascular health in Turner syndrome: a scientific statement from the American Heart Association. Circ Genom Precis Med. 2018;11(10):e000048.
102. Stochholm K, Juul S, Juel K, Naeraa RW, Gravholt CH. Prevalence, incidence, diagnostic delay, and mortality in Turner syndrome. J Clin Endocrinol Metab. 2006;91(10):3897–902.
103. Ostberg JE, Thomas EL, Hamilton G, Attar MJ, Bell JD, Conway GS. Excess visceral and hepatic adipose tissue in Turner syndrome determined by magnetic resonance imaging: estrogen deficiency associated with hepatic adipose content. J Clin Endocrinol Metab. 2005;90(5):2631–5.
104. Elsheikh M, Conway GS. The impact of obesity on cardiovascular risk factors in Turner's syndrome. Clin Endocrinol. 1998;49(4):447–50.
105. Bakalov VK, Cooley MM, Troendle J, Bondy CA. The prevalence of diabetes mellitus in the parents of women with Turner's syndrome. Clin Endocrinol. 2004;60(2):272.
106. Gravholt CH, Juul S, Naeraa RW, Hansen J. Morbidity in Turner syndrome. J Clin Epidemiol. 1998;51(2):147–58.
107. Jorgensen KT, Rostgaard K, Bache I, et al. Autoimmune diseases in women with Turner's syndrome. Arthritis Rheum. 2010;62(3):658–66.
108. Bakalov VK, Cooley MM, Quon MJ, et al. Impaired insulin secretion in the Turner metabolic syndrome. J Clin Endocrinol Metab. 2004;89(7):3516–20.
109. Caprio S, Boulware S, Diamond M, et al. Insulin resistance: an early metabolic defect of Turner's syndrome. J Clin Endocrinol Metab. 1991;72(4):832–6.
110. Mortensen KH, Cleemann L, Hjerrild BE, et al. Increased prevalence of autoimmunity in Turner syndrome--influence of age. Clin Exp Immunol. 2009;156(2):205–10.
111. Aversa T, Lombardo F, Valenzise M, et al. Peculiarities of autoimmune thyroid diseases in children with Turner or Down syndrome: an overview. Ital J Pediatr. 2015;41:39.
112. Sagi L, Zuckerman-Levin N, Gawlik A, et al. Clinical significance of the parental origin of the X chromosome in turner syndrome. J Clin Endocrinol Metab. 2007;92(3):846–52.
113. Salerno M, Di Maio S, Gasparini N, Rizzo M, Ferri P, Vajro P. Liver abnormalities in Turner syndrome. Eur J Pediatr. 1999;158(8):618–23.
114. Albareda MM, Gallego A, Enriquez J, Rodriguez JL, Webb SM. Biochemical liver abnormalities in Turner's syndrome. Eur J Gastroenterol Hepatol. 1999;11(9):1037–9.
115. Wojcik M, Ruszala A, Janus D, Starzyk JB. Liver biochemical abnormalities in adolescent patients with Turner syndrome. J Clin Res Pediatr Endocrinol. 2019;11(4):395–9.
116. Calanchini M, Moolla A, Tomlinson JW, et al. Liver biochemical abnormalities in Turner syndrome: a comprehensive characterization of an adult population. Clin Endocrinol. 2018;89(5):667–76.
117. Koulouri O, Ostberg J, Conway GS. Liver dysfunction in Turner's syndrome: prevalence, natural history and effect of exogenous oestrogen. Clin Endocrinol. 2008;69(2):306–10.
118. Fedor I, Zold E, Barta Z. Liver abnormalities in Turner syndrome: the importance of estrogen replacement. J Endocr Soc. 2022;6(10):bvac124.
119. Gravholt CH, Poulsen HE, Ott P, Christiansen JS, Vilstrup H. Quantitative liver functions in Turner syndrome with and without hormone replacement therapy. Eur J Endocrinol. 2007;156(6):679–86.

120. King KA, Makishima T, Zalewski CK, et al. Analysis of auditory phenotype and karyotype in 200 females with Turner syndrome. Ear Hear. 2007;28(6):831–41.
121. Hederstierna C, Hultcrantz M, Rosenhall U. Estrogen and hearing from a clinical point of view; characteristics of auditory function in women with Turner syndrome. Hear Res. 2009;252(1–2):3–8.
122. Dhooge IJ, De Vel E, Verhoye C, Lemmerling M, Vinck B. Otologic disease in Turner syndrome. Otol Neurotol. 2005;26(2):145–50.

Further Reading

Culen C, Ertl DA, Schubert K, Bartha-Doering L, Haeusler G. Care of girls and women with turner syndrome: beyond growth and hormones. Endocr Connect. 2017;6(4):R39–51.

Gravholt CH, Andersen NH, Conway GS, et al. Clinical practice guidelines for the care of girls and women with turner syndrome: proceedings from the 2016 Cincinnati international turner syndrome meeting. Eur J Endocrinol. 2017;177(3):G1–G70.

Lin AE, Prakash SK, Andersen NH, et al. Recognition and management of adults with turner syndrome: from the transition of adolescence through the senior years. Am J Med Genet A. 2019;179(10):1987–2033.

Shankar RK, Backeljauw PF. Current best practice in the management of turner syndrome. Ther Adv Endocrinol Metab. 2018;9(1):33–40.

Rett Syndrome

12

Susanna B. Mierau

12.1 Overview of Neurodevelopmental Disorders Associated with MeCP2 Dysfunction

12.1.1 MeCP2 Role in Neurodevelopmental and Neurological Dysfunction

In 1999, loss-of-function mutations in *MECP2,* a gene on the X chromosome that codes for the MeCP2 protein, were identified as the cause of most cases of Rett syndrome, a rare neurodevelopmental disorder primarily affecting females [1]. This discovery inspired further basic and translational neuroscience research into the function of MeCP2 in the brain revealing that MeCP2 acts both as a gene regulator and chromatin remodeler [2–4]. Further investigations of different *MECP2* mutations in clinical populations, and in mouse and human in vitro models of Rett syndrome, have revealed critical functions for MeCP2, both in early brain development and in the maintenance of brain cell function in adulthood [5]. Importantly, MeCp2-deficient mice that were genetically engineered to reexpress Mecp2 in adulthood showed rescue of multiple neurological and behavioral deficits [6], providing hope that targeted therapies could restore neurological function in children and adults with Rett syndrome.

At the time *MECP2* mutations were identified in Rett syndrome, few genes were known, and few clinical screens were available for identifying genetic causes of intellectual disability (ID). Thus, *MECP2* mutations were screened for in both

S. B. Mierau (✉)
Lurie Center for Autism, Massachusetts General Hospital, Lexington, MA, USA

Division of Cognitive and Behavioral Neurology, Brigham and Women's Hospital, Boston, MA, USA

Harvard Medical School, Boston, MA, USA
e-mail: smierau@mgh.harvard.edu

R. P. Thom, C. J. McDougle (eds.), *Neuropsychiatric Care for Genetic Syndromes and Other Neurodevelopmental Disorders*,
https://doi.org/10.1007/978-3-031-76269-7_12

female and male children with developmental delay and/or ID, including those who did not have the clinical features that define Rett syndrome. The increase in the number of children receiving genetic testing revealed that, while too little functional MeCP2 led to Rett syndrome, overexpression of MeCP2 also impaired neurodevelopment. *MECP2* duplication syndrome was first identified in a girl with atypical Rett syndrome and in multiple boys with severe developmental delay and ID [7–9]. As genetic technologies improved, a wider range of *MECP2*-related disorders were identified, in which partial loss of function can lead to mild intellectual impairment and/or other neuropsychiatric phenotypes [10].

Although *MECP2* mutations were identified over 20 years ago, there have been many challenges in developing preventative and disease-modifying treatments. Due to X-inactivation, females with Rett syndrome show mosaicism. Instead of each cell expressing half of the amount of MeCP2, on average 50% of the cells show normal MeCP2 expression and the other 50% show no MeCP2 expression. Thus, strategies such as gene therapy would need to increase MeCP2 expression selectively in the MeCP2-deficient cells without increasing gene expression in the cells with normal MeCP2 expression [11]. Mouse models of Rett syndrome have also revealed cell-type specific effects of loss of Mecp2 that alter the timing of brain cell maturation in excitatory and inhibitory cells [12, 13]. Thus, cell-type specific targeted therapies may be necessary early in life to support brain development. Fortunately, it appears that downstream targets for supporting neuronal function may improve function. The first Food and Drug Administration (FDA) approval for a Rett syndrome-specific medication, trofinetide, occurred in March 2023 [14].

12.1.2 Epidemiology of Neurodevelopmental Disorders Caused by MeCP2 Dysfunction

Rett syndrome occurs in one in 10,000–15,000 live female births. It is one of the leading causes of profound ID in females. While the same *MECP2* mutations in rare familial cases led to Rett syndrome in females and lethal neonatal encephalopathy in males, there are males surviving with Rett syndrome [15]. Rather than male lethality, the female predominance in Rett syndrome may be, at least in part, due to a higher incidence of de novo mutations arising from the paternal X chromosome in sperm, which only female offspring inherit [16, 17]. Over 300 people with *MECP2* duplication syndrome have been reported in the literature [18]. The incidence is unknown, but it has been estimated to be 1% of males with moderate-to-severe ID, or 1 in 100,000 live male births [19]. *MECP2* mutations, distinct from those that cause Rett syndrome, have been identified in males and females with ID and/or autism spectrum disorder (ASD) who do not meet the criteria for Rett syndrome. These are termed *MECP2*-related disorders, and the clinical phenotype varies depending on the specific *MECP2* mutation.

12.1.3 Common Clinical Features

12.1.3.1 Rett Syndrome

Rett syndrome is a severe neurological disorder in which children, primarily girls, have a devastating loss of language, social, and motor function [11]. Although Rett syndrome is typically diagnosed after 6–18 months of age, a review of home videos reveals behavioral differences that are already apparent at birth (Einspieler et al. 2016). The clinical criteria for Rett syndrome include the partial or complete loss of purposeful hand skills and spoken language, gait abnormalities, and stereotyped hand movements such as hand wringing [20]. Other symptoms may include seizures, autistic features, gastrointestinal problems, breathing disturbances, teeth grinding, impaired sleep patterns, abnormal muscle tone, peripheral vasomotor disturbances, skeletal abnormalities (i.e., scoliosis, kyphosis), slow growth, and small, cold hands or feet. Ninety-five to 97% of children meeting the clinical criteria for classic (typical) Rett syndrome have mutations in *MECP2* [21]. Out of the over 200 different *MECP2* mutations identified in typical Rett syndrome, the eight most common mutations are found in 58–60% of patients [16, 21]. Mutations in *MECP2* or other genes (e.g., *CDKL5*, *FOXG1*) can be found in atypical or other variants of Rett syndrome, in which affected individuals do not meet all of the clinical criteria for classic Rett syndrome. Four stages have been characterized in the developmental progression of Rett syndrome. In Stage 1, developmental maturation slows or stalls between 6 and 18 months. In Stage 2 (typically ages 18 months to 4 years), there is regression with loss of previously acquired skills including purposeful hand movements and expressive language. Hand stereotypies and gait difficulties also appear in Stage 2. Stage 3 typically begins after 2 years of age and is marked by a plateau period. In this stage, seizures and other medical comorbidities may become the dominant concern. In Stage 4 (typically after age 10 years old into adulthood), there is decreased mobility and motor deterioration. In some affected individuals, there may be Parkinsonian features as well [16, 21]. Survival has improved with advances in medical care. Over 70% of classic Rett syndrome patients live past 50 years of age [22].

12.1.3.2 *MECP2* Duplication Syndrome

Males with *MECP2* duplication syndrome described in the medical literature typically have ID and developmental delay (100% of males, most moderate-to-severe), hypotonia in infancy (95%), feeding difficulties (60%), and delayed or absent speech (60%). The hypotonia in early infancy typically leads to gross motor delays in sitting and crawling. Spasticity may also develop in early childhood. Only 55% learn to walk, either independently or with support. Epilepsy is also common, affecting ~50% of patients. Recurrent respiratory infections occur in ~75% of patients and may lead to early death, with 25% mortality reported by age 25 years [11] (Van Esch 1993).

Females with *MECP2* duplication combined with extreme or complete skewing of X-inactivation have been identified as asymptomatic carriers in mothers of affected sons. Interestingly, a closer study has revealed anxiety, depression, and/or autistic features that began prior to motherhood, which may be related to the *MECP2* duplication [23, 24]. Symptomatic females with the *MECP2* duplication syndrome have also been identified and typically have a less severe clinical presentation than males [23].

12.1.3.3 Other *MECP2*-Related Disorders

Loss-of-function or partial loss-of-function *MECP2* mutations have also been identified in males and females with ASD, ID, or specific learning disorders who do not have the full clinical features of Rett syndrome [10]. These *MECP2*-related disorders are typically caused by a set of mutations distinct from those that cause Rett syndrome. The most common identified so far is the A140V mutation (estimated to be 0.6% of all *MECP2* mutations). Symptoms may include mild-to-severe ID, speech difficulties, social impairment, small stature and head size, and later development of spasticity, tremor, dystonia, and/or other Parkinsonian features in adolescence to adulthood [25]. There have also been reports of childhood- or adolescent-onset psychosis and cognitive decline as the presenting symptoms.

12.2 Signs and Symptoms of Common Psychiatric Comorbidities

Recognizing the signs and symptoms of common psychiatric comorbidities such as anxiety or depression in children and adults with Rett syndrome or other *MECP2*-related disorders can be particularly challenging because of the co-occurrence of intellectual and expressive language impairments. In many cases, the diagnosis and appropriate management of psychiatric comorbidities depends on a collaboration between caregivers and clinicians. A recent caregiver survey from a cohort of 925 patients with Rett syndrome (641 patients with classic, 84 with atypical), *MECP2* duplication syndrome (74), CDKL5 deficiency disorder (67), or FOXG1 syndrome (59) showed communication as the top caregiver concern. Behavioral symptoms were also the top concern for a small percentage of patients including screaming episodes (3%), anxiety (2%), self-abusive behaviors (1%), and aggressiveness (1%) [26].

12.2.1 Anxiety

Symptoms suggestive of generalized anxiety disorder in Rett syndrome may include worsening of hyperventilation or breath holding, panic attacks, difficulty relaxing, inconsolable crying, appearing nervous, tense, or trembling in the absence of frightening stimuli, or screaming episodes [27]. A small observational study of five females with Rett syndrome (ages 4–47 years) compared anxiety-related behaviors in stressful (e.g., a household chore the patient cannot complete without help) and non-stressful (free play) conditions [28]. They found that distressed vocalizations, facial grimacing, and trembling were associated with the stress-inducing condition.

However, the frequency of hand stereotypies (e.g., hand clasping)—which was previously thought to be a sign of stress or anxiety—did not change. Signs of social anxiety may also be apparent in behaviors such as avoiding eye contact and social interaction. The U.S. Rett Natural History Study, which included 861 females with Rett syndrome (ages 3–66 years), found that internalizing behaviors such as crying, acting upset, or being nervous were present at a mild-to-moderate severity in almost all of the participants [27]. Anxiety behaviors were more likely to be recognized in patients with milder Rett syndrome phenotypes, likely due to better motor skills for nonverbal communication. In the second U.S. Rett Natural History Study, 77.5% of the 662 people with Rett syndrome were reportedly anxious or nervous at least occasionally, indicating that many parents or caregivers are aware of the signs. 24.1% of affected individuals appeared anxious frequently or very often suggesting that anxiety is likely common in Rett syndrome [29]. The authors estimated that the frequency of anxiety or anxiety-like behaviors in Rett syndrome at ~15%, compared to ~6.5% in the general pediatric population and ~25% in ASD [29]. However, the prevalence of anxiety may be higher than these estimates, considering the language, motor, and social interaction impairments prominent in Rett syndrome. Indeed, a recent systematic review of anxiety in genetic syndromes with ID estimated the prevalence of anxiety in Rett syndrome to be much higher, at 73% [30].

12.2.2 Mood Disorders

Symptoms or signs of mood disorders in children or adults with Rett syndrome may include abrupt changes in mood, spells of inconsolable crying or screaming for no apparent reason, periods of time when they function worse than other times, vocalizing for no apparent reason, and grimacing [31]. These symptoms were identified in a study of 143 girls with Rett syndrome from caregiver reports. However, these symptoms were also observed in adults with Rett syndrome along with social withdrawal and lethargy. In this study, 8 of 56 adults with Rett syndrome (14.3%) met the criteria for depression based on the Psychiatric Assessment Schedule for Adults with Developmental Disabilities (PAS-ADD) Checklist completed by their caregivers [32]. In the second U.S. Rett Natural History Study, caregivers reported on whether the individual with Rett syndrome was receiving treatment for appearing sad, miserable, or uncomfortable (12.2% of participants), rapid changes in mood (9%), irritability (8.2%), screaming episodes (6.6%), self-injurious behavior (4.1%), or aggressive behavior (3.4%). These signs, along with loss of appetite, loss of interest in prior interests, and alteration in sleep can also be observed in children and adults with Rett syndrome and other *MECP2*-related disorders with depression. Of note, mood symptoms may be more often recognized in individuals who are less severely affected by Rett syndrome and have better communication skills.

12.2.3 Psychosis

Childhood- or adolescent-onset psychosis has been identified in males and females with *MECP2*-related disorders [33–35]. The A140V *MECP2* mutation is the most common cause of MeCP2-related disorders identified so far and comprises 0.6% of all *MECP2* mutations in some geographic regions [36]. A case report of a 15-year-old woman, for example, in Canada documented a 3-year history of behavioral changes including social withdrawal, low mood, decreased appetite, socially inappropriate phone calls and social media posts, decreased sleep, and new-onset obsessive-compulsive behaviors [36]. Based on these reports, another study screened for *MECP2* mutations in a population of 404 patients with schizophrenia (171 females and 233 males) and 390 control subjects without psychosis [37]. Interestingly, six rare missense mutations (five previously identified in *MECP2*-related disorders and one novel double-missense mutation) were identified, suggesting that psychotic features may appear in multiple *MECP2*-related disorders. Other studies have suggested that specific *MECP2* mutations that are more likely to include childhood-onset cognitive decline and schizophrenia may affect the intervening domain of the MeCP2 protein in contrast to the most common mutations that cause Rett syndrome that affect the methyl-CpG-binding or transcription repression domains [35]. Interestingly, mutations in the intervening domain may affect binding to the brain-derived neurotrophic factor (*BDNF*) promoter region [35]. Thus, it will be exciting to see whether the first FDA-approved drug for Rett syndrome, trofinetide (a small molecule analog of insulin-like growth factor-1 (IGF-1) which supports neuronal survival and synaptic maturation through the same pathways as BDNF in the brain [38, 39]), may also have efficacy for psychotic and other cognitive symptoms in this group of *MECP2*-related disorders.

12.3 Assessment

Knowledge of the specific *MECP2* mutation can be particularly informative when assessing changes in behavior and potential psychiatric comorbidities. For Rett syndrome, specific mutations in *MECP2* may have a higher incidence of anxiety or other medical comorbidities likely to lead to anxiety, screaming episodes, or self-abusive behaviors [26, 40]. Specific *MECP2* mutations also confer different risks for epilepsy, which should be considered in the setting of behavioral changes, particularly in nonverbal individuals [41]. Seizures are less common before the age of five years and typically peak between ages 16 and 20 years [41, 42]. Specific mutations in *MECP2*-related disorders (e.g., A140V) have been associated with adolescent-onset psychosis with or without anxiety and depression. Sleep disturbances are common in Rett syndrome and can also contribute to changes in behavior and other psychiatric signs or symptoms. Particularly, in limited verbal and nonverbal individuals, evaluating for a new or worsening medical problem as an underlying cause of behavior change (with or without signs of anxiety or depression) should be considered to avoid inappropriately treating common ailments (e.g., constipation, broken molar from excessive teeth grinding) with psychiatric medications. Identifying underlying causes of low mood, anxiety, or irritability in adults with Rett syndrome can be particularly important, as many have reduced access to routine medical and/or dental care [43].

There is no specific clinical scale for anxiety, depression, or other psychiatric comorbidities validated for Rett syndrome. Clinical scales such as the Rett Syndrome Behavior Questionnaire (RSBQ) or the Mental Health/Well-being (MH) scale from the Child Health Questionnaire-Parent Form 50 (CHQ-PF50) have been used to assess internalizing behaviors such as anxiety [29, 31, 44]. This includes questions regarding whether the individual is observed to be "feeling lonely or like crying" or "acting upset or nervous." Higher scores from parental reports were seen for patients with more mild *MECP2* variants (e.g., R133C) versus more moderate or severe forms of Rett syndrome [27] in the first U.S. Rett Natural History Study; however, this correlation was not reproduced in the second natural history study [29]. A smaller study of 74 children (ages 2–11 years) combined the RSBQ with the Anxiety, Depression, and Mood Scale (ADAMS) and the Aberrant Behavior Checklist-Community (ABC-C) to assess anxiety [40]. The latter two scales have been previously used in people with ID, ASD, and/or Fragile X syndrome. The Psychiatric Assessment Schedule for Adults with Developmental Disabilities (PAS-ADD Checklist) was also used to identify depression in women with Rett syndrome (ages 18–65 years) in a small study by interviewing their caregivers [32]. A Rett syndrome-specific scale to screen for anxiety and mood disorders is needed.

12.4 Psychosocial Treatments

Caregiver education is essential for both identifying symptoms and signs of psychiatric comorbidities along with monitoring the response to treatment. Due to the significant impairments in language and social communication, common therapies employed in Rett syndrome include physical therapy, occupational therapy, and speech therapy. A study in Polish children with Rett syndrome ($n = 23$ children, ages 2–12 years) showed higher quality of life scores for those receiving at least 10 hours of therapy per week than those receiving only 5–10 hours per week [45]. The U.S. Rett Natural History Study revealed other common interventions in Rett syndrome, including therapeutic horseback riding (15.9% of study participants), music therapy (16.1%), and swimming therapy (16.3%), that have all been utilized in females with Rett syndrome [27, 46]. It is not yet established whether these therapies are efficacious in Rett syndrome for addressing psychiatric symptoms, particularly anxiety and depressed mood. However, meta-analyses and natural history studies have found a correlation between improved quality of life and more mobility [47]. Mobility in Rett syndrome is also correlated with longer survival.

12.5 Biological Treatments

The first FDA-approved drug for Rett syndrome, trofinetide (brand name Daybue), was approved in March 2023 [14, 48]. This novel analog of IGF-1 resulted in mild improvement in parent/caregiver-reported behavioral assessments of female patients ages 5–20 years who were treated for 12 weeks [38]. This included social communication, fine motor skills, and breathing. However, common side effects included diarrhea (80% in the trofinetide versus 2% in the placebo group) and vomiting (26.9% in the trofinetide versus 9.6% in the placebo group). As of March 2023, there are currently three other drugs in clinical trials for Rett syndrome, including two Phase I trials for gene therapy (TSHA-120 and NGN-401). A Phase 3 trial for blarcamesine (brand name Anavex 2–73) has reportedly shown improvement in emotional-behavioral symptoms in 52.9% of women with Rett syndrome treated with blarcamesine, versus 8.3% in the placebo group, based on parent/caregiver-reported behavioral assessments [49]. Blarcamesine activates sigma-1 receptors in the endoplasmic reticulum (ER), which may reduce the ER stress response [50], and was previously in clinical trials for the treatment of Alzheimer's dementia [51]. Common side effects reported were headache and dizziness, likely related to the effect on muscarinic acetylcholine receptors.

In the absence of studies specifically comparing efficacy in Rett syndrome, the pharmacologic treatment of psychiatric conditions including anxiety and depression is similar to that in children or adults without Rett syndrome [52]. In the U.S. Rett National History Study, 15.6% of the 687 females with Rett syndrome (age 3–66 years) had been treated with selective serotonin reuptake inhibitors (SSRIs). Up to 17.3% had received a medication for anxiety and 11.9% were on an SSRI for anxiety during the time of the three-year observational portion of the study [27]. Interestingly, pharmacologic treatment for anxiety appears to be effective in Rett syndrome. Anxiety treated with any medication, anxiety treated with an SSRI, and any SSRI use were all associated with lower parent-reported internalizing behaviors based on the MH scale from the CHQ-PF50 [27]. Studies will be necessary to determine whether the treatment of psychosis for *MECP2*-related disorders differs from current treatments for other causes of psychosis.

12.6 Common Medical Comorbidities

Rett syndrome is a multisystem disorder and MeCP2 function is important for many cell-types in the body outside of the nervous system. Clinicians considering pharmacotherapy for psychiatric comorbidities should be aware of the following medical problems common in Rett syndrome that may affect prescribing:

- Epilepsy (estimated prevalence 90% across the lifespan in Rett syndrome)
- Autonomic dysfunction including abnormal breathing patterns (~100%)
- Sleep dysfunction (80–93%)

- Gastrointestinal: constipation (80%), acid reflux (40%), and gallbladder dysfunction (4%)
- Cardiac: prolonged QTc interval (10–18%)
- Endocrine: low bone density (59%), premature or delayed puberty (19–28%), and thyroid dysfunction (18%)
- Orthopedic problems: scoliosis (80%), hip displacement (50%), and fractures (28–32%)

The estimated prevalences were made in a meta-analysis of 104 studies of Rett syndrome patients worldwide [53]. Psychiatric medications that can lower the seizure threshold (e.g., bupropion), cause hypotension (e.g., propranolol, clonidine), or worsen constipation (e.g., multiple SSRI and antipsychotic medications) should be avoided or used with caution. For example, a case report on the use of propranolol 10 mg in a child with Rett syndrome noted a paradoxical increase in heart rate and distress, necessitating discontinuation [54]. Impaired swallowing and even choking or gagging on food and liquids are also common in Rett syndrome. This can limit treatments to medications with formulations that can be crushed, given via a G-tube, and/or administered as a liquid or patch.

Key Points to Remember

- Rett syndrome primarily affects females but can also affect males.
- Mutations in *MECP2* on the X chromosome cause 95–97% of cases of Rett syndrome. However, distinct mutations from those that cause Rett syndrome cause *MECP2* duplication syndrome or other *MECP2*-related disorders.
- Caregiver report suggests that anxiety and mood disturbances are common in Rett syndrome and other *MECP2* disorders; however, they may be underrecognized by clinicians due to the language and social interaction difficulties in Rett syndrome.
- Two large natural history studies in the U.S. show improvement in behavioral scores with medical treatment of anxiety with SSRIs or other anxiety medications.
- Rett syndrome is a multisystem disorder. New or worsening medical causes for anxiety and/or changes in behavior should be investigated.
- Medication selection for treating psychiatric symptoms should consider many possible medical comorbidities and risks, especially the risk of seizures, prolonged QTc interval, and worsening constipation or sleep.

References

1. Amir RE, Van den Veyver IB, Wan M, Tran CQ, Francke U, Zoghbi HY. Rett syndrome is caused by mutations in X-linked MECP2, encoding methyl-CpG-binding protein 2. Nat Genet. 1999;23(2):185–8.

2. Cohen S, Gabel HW, Hemberg M, et al. Genome-wide activity-dependent MeCP2 phosphorylation regulates nervous system development and function. Neuron. 2011;72(1):72–85.
3. Ebert DH, Gabel HW, Robinson ND, et al. Activity-dependent phosphorylation of MeCP2 threonine 308 regulates interaction with NCoR. Nature. 2013;499(7458):341–5.
4. Lewis JD, Meehan RR, Henzel WJ, et al. Purification, sequence, and cellular localization of a novel chromosomal protein that binds to methylated DNA. Cell. 1992;69(6):905–14.
5. McGraw CM, Samaco RC, Zoghbi HY. Adult neural function requires MeCP2. Science. 2011;333(6039):186.
6. Guy J, Gan J, Selfridge J, Cobb S, Bird A. Reversal of neurological defects in a mouse model of Rett syndrome. Science. 2007;315(5815):1143–7.
7. Ariani F, Mari F, Pescucci C, et al. Real-time quantitative PCR as a routine method for screening large rearrangements in Rett syndrome: report of one case of MECP2 deletion and one case of MECP2 duplication. Hum Mutat. 2004;24(2):172–7.
8. Van Esch H, Bauters M, Ignatius J, et al. Duplication of the MECP2 region is a frequent cause of severe mental retardation and progressive neurological symptoms in males. Am J Hum Genet. 2005;77(3):442–53.
9. Meins Á, Lehmann J, Gerresheim F, et al. Submicroscopic duplication in Xq28 causes increased expression of the MECP2 gene in a boy with severe mental retardation and features of Rett syndrome. Journal of Medical Genetics. 2005;42(2):e12.
10. Pascual-Alonso A, Martínez-Monseny AF, Xiol C, Armstrong J. *MECP2*-related disorders in males. Int J Mol Sci. 2021;22(17):9610.
11. Sandweiss AJ, Brandt VL, Zoghbi HY. Advances in understanding of Rett syndrome and MECP2 duplication syndrome: prospects for future therapies. Lancet Neurol. 2020;19(8):689–98.
12. Durand S, Patrizi A, Quast KB, et al. NMDA receptor regulation prevents regression of visual cortical function in the absence of Mecp2. Neuron. 2012;76(6):1078–90.
13. Mierau SB, Patrizi A, Hensch TK, Fagiolini M. Cell-specific regulation of N-methyl-D-aspartate receptor maturation by Mecp2 in cortical circuits. Biol Psychiatry. 2016;79(9):746–54.
14. Harris E. Trofinetide receives FDA approval as first drug for Rett syndrome. JAMA. 2023;329(14):1142.
15. Villard L. MECP2 mutations in males. J Med Genet. 2007;44(7):417–23.
16. Collins BE, Neul JL. Rett syndrome and MECP2 duplication syndrome: disorders of mecp2 dosage. Neuropsychiatr Dis Treat. 2022;18:2813–35.
17. Wen Y, Wang J, Zhang Q, Yang X, Wei L, Bao X. MECP2 germline mosaicism plays an important part in the inheritance of Rett syndrome: a study of MECP2 germline mosaicism in males. BMC Med. 2023;21(1):155.
18. Van Esch H. MECP2 duplication syndrome. In: Pagon RA, Adam MP, Ardinger HH, et al., editors. GeneReviews(®). Seattle (WA): University of Washington; 2008 Jan 18 [updated 2020 May 21]. Available from: https://www.ncbi.nlm.nih.gov/books/NBK1284/
19. Giudice-Nairn P, Downs J, Wong K, et al. The incidence, prevalence and clinical features of MECP2 duplication syndrome in Australian children. J Paediatr Child Health. 2019;55(11):1315–22.
20. Neul JL, Kaufmann WE, Glaze DG, et al. Rett syndrome: revised diagnostic criteria and nomenclature. Ann Neurol. 2010;68(6):944–50.
21. Cuddapah VA, Pillai RB, Shekar KV, Lane JB, Motil KJ, Skinner SA, et al. Methyl-CpG-binding protein 2 (MECP2) mutation type is associated with disease severity in Rett syndrome. J Med Genet. 2014;51(3):152–8.
22. Tarquinio DC, Hou W, Neul JL, et al. The changing face of survival in Rett syndrome and MECP2-related disorders. Pediatr Neurol. 2015;53(5):402–11.
23. El Chehadeh S, Touraine R, Prieur F, et al. Xq28 duplication including MECP2 in six unreported affected females: what can we learn for diagnosis and genetic counselling? Clin Genet. 2017;91(4):576–88.
24. Ramocki MB, Peters SU, Tavyev YJ, et al. Autism and other neuropsychiatric symptoms are prevalent in individuals with MeCP2 duplication syndrome. Ann Neurol. 2009;66(6):771–82.

25. Lambert S, Maystadt I, Boulanger S, et al. Expanding phenotype of p.Ala140Val mutation in MECP2 in a 4 generation family with X-linked intellectual disability and spasticity. Eur J Med Genet. 2016;59(10):522–5.
26. Neul JL, Benke TA, Marsh ED, et al. Top caregiver concerns in Rett syndrome and related disorders: data from the US Natural History Study. J Neurodev Disord. 2023a;15(1):33.
27. Buchanan CB, Stallworth JL, Scott AE, et al. Behavioral profiles in Rett syndrome: data from the natural history study. Brain and Development. 2019;41(2):123–34.
28. Quest KM, Byiers BJ, Payen A, Symons FJ. Rett syndrome: a preliminary analysis of stereotypy, stress, and negative affect. Res Dev Disabil. 2014;35(5):1191–7.
29. Buchanan CB, Stallworth JL, Joy AE, et al. Anxiety-like behavior and anxiolytic treatment in the Rett syndrome natural history study. J Neurodev Disord. 2022;14(1):31.
30. Edwards G, Jones C, Pearson E, et al. Prevalence of anxiety symptomatology and diagnosis in syndromic intellectual disability: a systematic review and meta-analysis. Neurosci Biobehav Rev. 2022;138:104719.
31. Mount RH, Charman T, Hastings RP, Reilly S, Cass H. The Rett syndrome behaviour questionnaire (RSBQ): refining the behavioural phenotype of Rett syndrome. J Child Psychol Psychiatry. 2002;43(8):1099–110.
32. Hryniewiecka-Jaworska A, Foden E, Kerr M, Felce D, Clarke A. Prevalence and associated features of depression in women with Rett syndrome. J Intellect Disabil Res. 2016;60(6):564–70.
33. Curie A, Lesca G, Bussy G, et al. Asperger syndrome and early-onset schizophrenia associated with a novel MECP2 deleterious missense variant. Psychiatr Genet. 2017;27(3):105–9.
34. Klauck SM, Lindsay S, Beyer KS, Splitt M, Burn J, Poustka A. A mutation hot spot for nonspecific X-linked mental retardation in the MECP2 gene causes the PPM-X syndrome. Am J Hum Genet. 2002;70(4):1034–7.
35. Sheikh TI, Harripaul R, Ayub M, Vincent JB. MeCP2 AT-Hook1 mutations in patients with intellectual disability and/or schizophrenia disrupt DNA binding and chromatin compaction in vitro. Hum Mutat. 2018;39(5):717–28.
36. Venkateswaran S, McMillan HJ, Doja A, Humphreys P. Adolescent onset cognitive regression and neuropsychiatric symptoms associated with the A140V MECP2 mutation. Dev Med Child Neurol. 2014;56(1):91–4.
37. Chen C-H, Cheng M-C, Huang A, Hu T-M, Ping L-Y, Chang Y-S. Detection of rare methyl-CpG binding protein 2 gene missense mutations in patients with schizophrenia. Front Genet. 2020;11:476.
38. Neul JL, Percy AK, Benke TA, et al. Trofinetide for the treatment of Rett syndrome: a randomized phase 3 study. Nat Med. 2023b;29(6):1468–75.
39. Tropea D, Giacometti E, Wilson NR, et al. Partial reversal of Rett syndrome-like symptoms in MeCP2 mutant mice. Proc Natl Acad Sci USA. 2009;106(6):2029–34.
40. Barnes KV, Coughlin FR, O'Leary HM, et al. Anxiety-like behavior in Rett syndrome: characteristics and assessment by anxiety scales. J Neurodev Disord. 2015;7(1):30.
41. Glaze DG, Percy AK, Skinner S, et al. Epilepsy and the natural history of Rett syndrome. Neurology. 2010;74(11):909–12.
42. Tarquinio DC, Hou W, Berg A, et al. Longitudinal course of epilepsy in Rett syndrome and related disorders. Brain. 2017;140(2):306–18.
43. Lai YYL, Downs JA, Wong K, Zafar S, Walsh LJ, Leonard HM. Enablers and barriers in dental attendance in Rett syndrome: an international observational study. Spec Care Dentist. 2022;42(6):565–74.
44. Oberman LM, Leonard H, Downs J, et al. Rett syndrome behaviour questionnaire in children and adults with Rett syndrome: psychometric characterization and revised factor structure. Am J Intellect Dev Disabil. 2023;128(3):237–53.
45. Rozensztrauch A, Sebzda A, Śmigiel R. Clinical presentation of Rett syndrome in relation to quality of life and family functioning. J Int Med Res. 2021;49(4):3000605211007714.
46. Chou M-Y, Chang N-W, Chen C, et al. The effectiveness of music therapy for individuals with Rett syndrome and their families. J Formos Med Assoc. 2019;118(12):1633–43.

47. Corchón S, Carrillo-López I, Cauli O. Quality of life related to clinical features in patients with Rett syndrome and their parents: a systematic review. Metab Brain Dis. 2018;33(6):1801–10.
48. FDA Website. FDA approves first treatment for Rett syndrome. [cited 2023 Mar 4]. Available from: https://www.fda.gov/drugs/news-events-human-drugs/fda-approves-first-treatment-rett-syndrome
49. Anavex Website. Blarcamesine phase 3 trial met primary and secondary efficacy endpoints. [cited 2023 Mar 4]. Available from: https://www.anavex.com/post/anavex-2-73-blarcamesine-avatar-phase-3-trial-met-primary-and-secondary-efficacy-endpoints
50. Hayashi T, Su TP. Sigma-1 receptor chaperones at the ER-mitochondrion interface regulate Ca(2+) signaling and cell survival. Cell. 2007;131(3):596–610.
51. Su TP, Su TC, Nakamura Y, Tsai SY. The sigma-1 receptor as a pluripotent modulator in living systems. Trends Pharmacol Sci. 2016;37(4):262–78.
52. Persico AM, Ricciardello A, Cucinotta F. The psychopharmacology of autism spectrum disorder and Rett syndrome. Handb Clin Neurol. 2019;165:391–414.
53. Fu C, Armstrong D, Marsh E, et al. Multisystem comorbidities in classic Rett syndrome: a scoping review. BMJ Paediatr Open. 2020;4(1):e000731.
54. Santosh PJ, Bell L, Lievesley K, Singh J, Fiori F. Paradoxical physiological responses to propranolol in a Rett syndrome patient: a case report. BMC Pediatr. 2016;16(1):194.

Further Reading

Persico AM, Ricciardello A, Cucinotta F. The psychopharmacology of autism spectrum disorder and Rett syndrome. Handb Clin Neurol. 2019;165:391–414. https://doi.org/10.1016/B978-0-444-64012-3.00024-1.

Sandweiss AJ, Brandt VL, Zoghbi HY. Advances in understanding of Rett syndrome and MECP2 duplication syndrome: prospects for future therapies. Lancet Neurol. 2020;19(8):689–98.

Phelan–McDermid Syndrome

13

Paige Hickey Townsend, Heli Patel,
and Ann M. Neumeyer

13.1 Overview of the Neurodevelopmental Disorder

13.1.1 Epidemiology

Phelan–McDermid syndrome (PMS) is a rare genetic syndrome caused by a change in the end of the long arm of chromosome 22 or a change (pathogenic variant) in the *SHANK3* gene. There is no cure for PMS currently. While the true incidence and prevalence of PMS remain undetermined, more than 1,200 individuals were identified with the condition globally in 2015 and 3,100 individuals in 2023 [1, 2]. Additionally, PMS has been detected in 0.5% of individuals diagnosed with autism [3]. However, these numbers are likely an underestimate, as adults with milder phenotypic presentations (i.e., without intellectual disability (ID), regression, or presence of physical or medical comorbidities) may be less likely to be diagnosed.

13.1.2 Underlying Genetic/Neurobiological Mechanisms

PMS is a genetic condition that arises from the haploinsufficiency of *SHANK3*, a gene located on chromosome 22q13.3. In PMS, a loss of function of *SHANK3* can occur in a few different ways. The most common cause is a deletion (either interstitial or terminal; see Fig. 13.1) of chromosome 22q13.3, which occurs in 65% of cases of PMS [4]. Terminal deletions may be indicative of ring chromosome 22 or inherited unbalanced translocations, which may impact *SHANK3* functioning. Although there have been some cases of interstitial deletions to 22q13.3 that do not

P. H. Townsend · H. Patel · A. M. Neumeyer (✉)
Lurie Center for Autism, Massachusetts General Hospital, Lexington, MA, USA
e-mail: ptownsend2@mgh.harvard.edu; Heli.patel12@umassmed.edu;
Aneumeyer@mgh.harvard.edu

R. P. Thom, C. J. McDougle (eds.), *Neuropsychiatric Care for Genetic Syndromes and Other Neurodevelopmental Disorders*,
https://doi.org/10.1007/978-3-031-76269-7_13

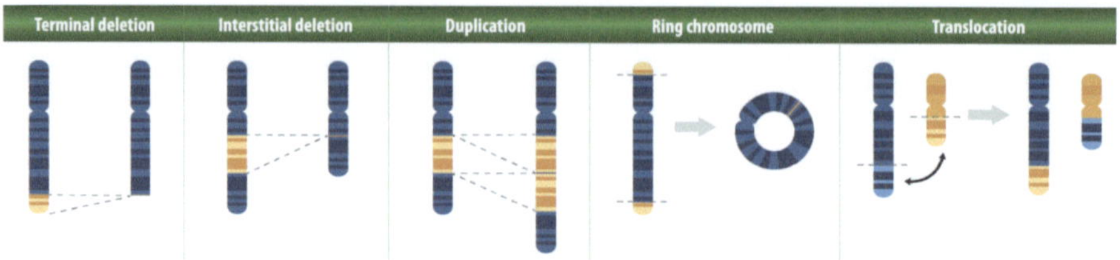

Fig. 13.1 Types of genetic mutations that can be observed on chromosome 22 in patients with PMS. This figure was originally published on the Phelan–McDermid Syndrome Foundation (PMSF) website (https://pmsf.org/diagnosis/) [2] and is being used with their permission

affect *SHANK3*, the majority of deletions include *SHANK3* [5]. Sequence variants of *SHANK3* also account for 18% of PMS cases [4].

SHANK3 is expressed throughout the body [1], which is why individuals with PMS can present with a range of different behavioral and medical phenotypic characteristics. In the brain, it is found in the cortex, thalamus, striatum, hippocampus, dentate gyrus, and cerebellum [6]. In addition to the brain, *SHANK3* is expressed in the intestine, skeletal muscle, liver, kidney, spleen, and thymus [7].

SHANK3 plays a crucial role in shaping and organizing the synapse of glutamatergic neurons. *SHANK3* codes for proteins that contribute to scaffolding the postsynaptic membrane of glutamatergic neurons [6, 8–10]. In mouse models, knocking out *SHANK3* leads to a decrease in the amount of these proteins present in the postsynaptic terminal [11, 12]. *SHANK3* knockout mice also have fewer α-amino-3-hydroxy-5-methyl-4-isoxazolepropionic acid (AMPA) and N-methyl-D-aspartate (NMDA) receptors, suggesting that *SHANK3* may also influence receptor density on the postsynaptic membrane [6, 11–13]. Disrupting *SHANK3* can lead to reduced input resistance (excitability) and impair the communication between and the functioning of AMPA and NMDA receptors, suggesting that SHANK3 might also impact the functioning of excitatory neurons [8, 10–12, 14–18]. Furthermore, *SHANK3* is believed to be important for synaptogenesis and the formation of dendritic spikes [13, 16, 19]. In knockout mouse models of *SHANK3*, there are fewer and shorter dendritic spines compared to wild-type mice [12, 13, 15, 19].

The inhibitory functioning of parvalbumin interneurons can also be affected by deletions to *SHANK3*. *SHANK3* knockout mice have a reduced number of parvalbumin neurons and decreased expression of parvalbumin in the striatum compared to wild-type mice [20, 21]. Gogolla et al. also found that *SHANK3* deletions compromised perineuronal nets in the insular cortex [21]. Since perineuronal nets surround parvalbumin interneurons in the cortex, disruptions to perineuronal nets can also impact inhibitory signaling from parvalbumin neurons [6]. Taken together, disruptions to *SHANK3* may alter inhibitory functioning, supporting the idea of an excitatory-inhibitory imbalance in PMS [6].

Finally, *SHANK3* is also involved in regulating sleep and circadian cycles [18]. One study by Ingiosi et al. found that *SHANK3* regulates circadian transcription factors that maintain circadian rhythms in both mice and humans [22]. This work suggests that *SHANK3* may be closely tied to disruptions to sleep and circadian cycles in patients with PMS.

13.1.3 Common Clinical Features

Common clinical features associated with PMS can be categorized into three broad categories: physical, medical, and behavioral/developmental features as shown in Table 13.1.

The phenotypic presentation of individuals with PMS is variable and can be partially attributed to genetics. For example, larger deletions to chromosome 22q13.3

Table 13.1 Clinical characteristics

	Clinical characteristics
Physical/ Dysmorphology	• Distinct facial characteristics – Dolichocephaly (long skull), wide brow, flat midface, wide nasal bridge, bulbous nose, deep-set eyes, ptosis (drooping upper eyelid), long eyelashes, full/puffy eyelids, full/puffy cheeks, poorly formed and large ears, pointed chin, sacral dimple, long philtrum, high-arched palate, malocclusion/wide-spaced teeth • Large, fleshy hands • Dysplastic toenails • Neonatal hypotonia • Syndactyly of toes 2–3
Medical	Neurological • Hypotonia • Decreased pain perception • Heat intolerance • Decreased perspiration • Seizure disorders • Arachnoid cysts Endocrine • Hypothyroidism • Precocious or delayed puberty Cardiovascular • Lymphedema • Cardiac defects Renal • Renal cysts • Hypoplasia • Vesicoureteral reflux • Urinary tract infections Gastrointestinal • Gastroesophageal reflux • Constipation • Feeding challenges Vision/hearing • Strabismus • Hearing loss (Eustachian tube dysfunction)

(continued)

Table 13.1 (continued)

	Clinical characteristics
Behavioral/ developmental/ psychiatric	• Absent to severely delayed speech • Mild-to-global developmental delay • Autism spectrum disorder (ASD) • Mouthing and chewing behaviors • Regressions • Catatonia • Attention-deficit/hyperactivity disorder (ADHD) • Learning and intellectual disabilities

This table is modified from Phelan et al. (2012) [23]

are associated with more severe ID and language impairment [24–27], more significant medical [25] and dysmorphic features [28, 29], and a higher risk of epilepsy [27, 28, 30]. Alternatively, psychiatric symptoms [25, 31, 32] and regressions [25] appear to be more common in patients with smaller deletions or *SHANK3* sequence variants. Involvement of other genes [24] may also contribute to specific phenotypes in PMS. For example, deletion of *CELSR1*, a gene affected in terminal deletions >4.3 Mb, has been associated with the development of lymphedema [33]. More work is needed to fully understand the genetic contributions of PMS.

13.2 Signs and Symptoms of Common Psychiatric Comorbidities

In the following section, we will discuss the signs and symptoms of common psychiatric comorbidities that are associated with PMS.

13.2.1 Autism Spectrum Disorder (ASD)

Phelan–McDermid syndrome is one of the most common genetic causes of ASD [17, 34]. Many patients with PMS have either a diagnosis of ASD or symptoms consistent with ASD. However, the presentation of ASD symptoms may be very different in individuals with PMS compared to other autistic individuals. For example, those with PMS often exhibit fewer and less severe restrictive, repetitive behaviors; less social withdrawal; and more mood-related symptoms [31]. Due to this unique presentation, identifying ASD symptoms may be challenging in this patient population.

13.2.2 Sleep Disorders

Sleep disturbances occur frequently in individuals with PMS, often begin early in life, and affect up to 90% of individuals [18]. Commonly reported sleep problems include nighttime incontinence, bruxism, restlessness during sleep, frequent night awakenings, and difficulty falling asleep during childhood [18]. While many of these conditions improve with age, certain problems such as delayed sleep onset, sleep anxiety, parasomnias, and difficulty falling and remaining asleep persist into adulthood. Additionally, there is increased evidence of parasomnias with age. The identification and treatment of sleep disorders within this population is crucial, as sleep impairment can have major impacts on overall health, behavior, functioning, and development.

13.2.3 Hyperactive and Agitated Behaviors

Hyperactive and agitated behaviors have commonly been reported in individuals with PMS [31]. Such behaviors mostly consist of motoric restlessness, impulsivity, and distractibility. Hyperactivity, in particular, was reported in around 29% of patients with PMS with a 22q13 deletion [27, 35, 36]. The prevalence of hyperactivity was much higher (~72%) in patients with PMS with *SHANK3* variants [36, 37].

13.2.4 Bipolar Disorder

Diagnoses of bipolar disorder have repeatedly been reported in individuals with PMS, particularly post-adolescence [31, 38]. Specific symptoms include behavioral instability, irritability, aggression, screaming, mood cycling, distractibility, hypersexuality, and sleep disturbances [38]. There is some variability in the presentation of episodes. A recent study focused on 38 individuals with PMS enriched for those with a history of psychiatric symptoms reported a combination of manic episodes, depressive episodes, mixed mood and anxiety symptoms, and possibly brief psychotic episodes [32]. Following these acute episodes, there was persistence of anxiety and irritability along with regression. While the connection between bipolar disorder and PMS remains understudied, it is important to closely monitor and assess mood symptoms to facilitate rapid treatment.

13.2.5 Catatonia

Catatonia is a psychomotor syndrome that often co-occurs with various psychiatric disorders that are highly prevalent within the PMS population, such as ASD and bipolar disorder. Clinical symptoms of catatonia include motor and behavioral disturbances [39]. Motor symptoms may include stereotyped postures and movements such as bending limbs, a stooped posture, constant restlessness, or a complete lack of movement [31]. Other symptoms include mutism, oppositional behavior, or motoric slowing [31]. The age of onset of catatonic symptoms is variable, but it may be as early as 16 years [32]. Considering the high mortality and morbidity associated with catatonia, timely treatment is crucial [32].

13.2.6 Anxiety

While anxiety has historically been difficult to detect in patients with profound ID or limited verbal capabilities, there are many observable symptoms of anxiety in patients with PMS [32]. These include heightened irritability and agitation, disruptive behavior (shouting, self-injury, etc.), avoidance and withdrawal, increased repetitive behaviors, increased echolalia, and sleep disturbances [40].

13.2.7 Schizophrenia Spectrum and Other Psychotic Disorders

While the prevalence of psychotic disorders in the PMS population remains undetermined, cases of psychotic illness have been reported in the literature [40, 41]. Common behaviors that may warrant further assessment for a primary psychotic disorder include aggressive outbursts, apathy, mood disturbances, loss of initiative, loss of skills, flat affect, and mood dysregulation [31, 40].

13.2.8 Regressions

Patients with *SHANK3* variants are at an increased risk for regression (loss of previously acquired skills) and this is a highly common feature of PMS. This risk of behavioral and cognitive regression increases with age and recovery is often minimal, if at all [40]. In individuals with idiopathic ASD, regression typically occurs during earlier childhood and primarily impacts social skills and language capabilities [30]. In contrast, regressions in PMS may occur during mid-childhood, disrupting both developmental and self-help skills [30]. Neuropsychiatric disorders such as bipolar disorder, catatonia, and psychosis may also present following regression of skills [40]. The medical assessment for regression is detailed below.

13.3 Assessments

When PMS is suspected, several steps should be taken. An initial behavioral assessment and family history should be obtained. Children presenting with autistic symptoms, ID, delayed speech development, physical characteristics consistent with PMS; hypotonia without a known cause; or regressions in development should be considered for genetic testing. Genetic testing for PMS includes assessing for both 22q13.3 deletions and *SHANK3* sequence variants that are present throughout the genome [42, 43]. This comprehensive evaluation is essential for confirming the diagnosis as well as guiding further interventions and support for individuals suspected to have PMS.

13.3.1 Diagnostic Genetic Testing

Genetic testing for 22q13.3 deletions is commonly performed using chromosomal microarray (CMA), which is designed to detect copy number variants or changes in the amount of DNA present in a chromosome. CMA provides a higher resolution compared to traditional karyotyping and can identify interstitial and terminal chromosomal deletions or duplications but does not reveal the structural aspects of the chromosome, such as translocations or ring chromosomes (Fig. 13.1). Translocations and ring chromosome 22 are more prevalent in individuals with terminal 22q13.3 deletions, rather than interstitial deletions. Therefore, individuals with terminal deletions may require further genetic testing [42].

SHANK3 sequence variants are typically identified using next-generation sequencing (NGS) methods such as whole exome sequencing (WES) or whole genome sequencing (WGS) [42]. Whole exome sequencing assesses the exome, which consists of the protein-coding regions of genes that play crucial roles in cellular functions. Alternatively, WGS sequences every gene in the genome. These technologies enable a detailed analysis of the genome, providing comprehensive information about the genes and their variations.

Based on the results of the initial CMA and NGS testing, individuals with PMS can be categorized based on the size of their deletion and involvement of *SHANK3*. Small 22q13.3 deletions that only affect *SHANK3* or *SHANK3* and neighboring genes, and *SHANK3* sequence variants that occur outside of chromosome 22 are typically categorized as Class I deletions. Alternatively, longer 22q13.3 deletions are categorized as Class II deletions. The majority of individuals with PMS experience loss of *SHANK3* as part of either a Class I or Class II deletion [25, 44]. However, a small subset of patients with PMS experience interstitial deletions that do not affect *SHANK3* [44]. Language distinguishing the involvement of *SHANK3* (PMS-SHANK3 related versus PMS-SHANK3 unrelated) has recently been adopted [43, 45].

Additional genetic testing is often conducted to further characterize the mutation, particularly in individuals with 22q13.3 terminal deletions [42, 43]. One commonly used method is karyotyping, which involves examining the chromosomes to identify larger structural abnormalities, such as the presence of a ring chromosome 22. Ring chromosomes can be formed when the distal long arm and distal short arm of the chromosome break and reconnect, resulting in a circular structure. A ring chromosome 22 is present in 10–20% of individuals with PMS [4, 46–48]. Individuals with ring chromosome 22 have an increased risk of developing neurofibromatosis type 2 (NF2), highlighting the importance of screening for this abnormality [46]. In some cases, individuals with PMS may present with an unbalanced translocation. The presence of a terminal 22q13.3 deletion and duplication of other genetic information may point to an unbalanced translocation, which can be confirmed using fluorescence in situ hybridization (FISH), a technique that can identify the location of a gene on the chromosome.

Genetic testing should also evaluate whether mutations were inherited or occurred spontaneously (de novo). Some mutations associated with PMS, such as ring chromosome 22 or balanced translocations, are more likely to be inherited, whereas others (i.e., *SHANK3* sequence variants) are more commonly de novo [42]. FISH is recommended for affected individuals and their parents to determine whether mutations present in an individual with PMS are inherited versus attained de novo [49]. FISH has the capability to detect various types of mutations, including mosaic or non-mosaic deletions, translocations, or other balanced rearrangements. Parents who exhibit mosaic or non-mosaic mutations should be offered further testing to determine the risk of PMS in future children [43, 46].

Screening for autosomal recessive single-gene disorders is also essential [40]. For example, the *ARSA* gene is deleted in 77% of PMS patients [24]. Defects in this gene can cause metachromatic leukodystrophy (MLD), an autosomal recessively inherited disorder characterized by progressive neurological deterioration. While cases of MLD have been observed in patients with PMS, the carrier frequency of MLD is low (estimated in 1:100–1:200), making MLD rare in this population [50–52]. Early detection of MLD is critical because individuals who are presymptomatic or in the early stages may elect to undergo experimental treatments such as hematopoietic stem cell transplantation or gene therapy [43]. Metachromatic leukodystrophy can be identified using genetic testing or analysis of sulfatides present in the urine. Screening for megalencephalic leukoencephalopathy with subcortical cysts (*MLC1* defect), deletions in *CHKB* and *ALG12*, which cause congenital muscular dystrophy and congenital disorder of glycosylation (CGC), respectively, and *TCF20*, which is associated with seizures, should also be considered. A comprehensive description of potential single-gene disorders in PMS is also described by Vitrac et al. [24].

13.3.2 Medical Assessments

In addition to genetic testing, individuals diagnosed with PMS should be referred to a series of medical specialists and psychologists to assess baseline functioning and monitor progress over time. Medical and behavioral assessments that may be useful in individuals with PMS are described below [43, 53].

13.3.2.1 Primary Care

Primary care providers play an important role in identifying individuals with PMS. Since PMS is a rare genetic disorder, it can be difficult to detect. However, screening for the physical and medical features described at the beginning of the chapter during annual visits can help identify individuals with PMS. After receiving a diagnosis of PMS, it is important for primary care physicians to ensure that the child undergoes ophthalmology and audiology evaluations [43, 54]. Challenges with vision, such as strabismus and ptosis, are known to impact individuals with PMS [28, 34]. Many individuals with PMS also demonstrate decreased responses to auditory stimuli [23, 55, 56]. For individuals with ring chromosome 22, additional screening measures should be implemented for NF2 [46, 57]. These include: (1) annual hearing tests for vestibular schwannomas [58] and (2) regular dermatology evaluations to screen for skin tumors and other dermatologic signs of NF2 [43, 58]. Patients with PMS can also have challenges with body temperature regulation, so primary care doctors should discuss protective strategies [43]. Primary care providers also sometimes become the initial coordinating physician responsible for assembling an interdisciplinary care team for the patient [59].

13.3.2.2 Neurology

Neurologists also serve an important role in caring for individuals with PMS. A baseline neurological examination is recommended for all patients after a PMS diagnosis has been established [43]. Considering the high prevalence of hypotonia in PMS, this examination should focus on gross motor skills, gait, fine motor coordination, speech and language skills, sensory reactivity, reflexes, and other behaviors (i.e., visual tracking, eye contact, attention, impulsivity, or aggressiveness) [53, 60]. The neurological examination should also assess head circumference, as 17% of individuals with PMS have macrocephaly and 16% have microcephaly [44].

In addition, neurologists are encouraged to obtain a baseline magnetic resonance imaging (MRI) of the brain and spinal column after initial diagnosis [53]. Structural brain abnormalities are more common in individuals with PMS compared with typically developing peers [53, 60]. White matter hyperintensities, periventricular leukomalacia, enlarged ventricles, arachnoid cysts, atrophy of the cortical gray matter in the cerebellum and corpus callosum, and the presence of subdural hematomas are some of the most frequent MRI abnormalities that have been observed in patients with PMS [53, 60–63]. Individuals with MRI abnormalities should continue to be monitored over time. Repeated MRIs might also be recommended to others with PMS. Given the increased risk of NF2-related acoustic neuromas, vestibular schwannomas, and spinal tumors, individuals with ring chromosome 22 should receive brain and spinal MRIs with gadolinium contrast every 1–2 years in accordance with the NF2 guidelines [64]. Individuals with microcephaly and macrocephaly may also benefit from periodic MRI scans. The presence of seizures, electroencephalogram (EEG) abnormalities, or behavioral regressions may also warrant an MRI.

Epilepsy and seizures are significant concerns for individuals with PMS and should be continuously monitored by neurologists. The prevalence rate of epilepsy in PMS is highly variable across studies (15–70%) and may reflect differences in sample and inclusionary criteria [28, 43, 65, 66]. However, Sarasua and colleagues [28] found that over 60% of individuals with PMS had at least one seizure during their lifetime, and that the presence of seizures increased with age [28]. Even individuals without a formal epilepsy diagnosis can exhibit epileptiform activity on EEG recordings, highlighting the importance of monitoring seizures in PMS [65]. Neurologists are recommended to order an initial EEG recording that includes periods of sleep for PMS patients suspected of having seizures or diagnosed with epilepsy. If the initial EEG does not provide conclusive evidence but there is a strong clinical suspicion of seizures, a follow-up EEG should be performed [43, 66]. Additionally, if new symptoms suggestive of seizures arise or there is unexplained developmental regression, particularly in language or motor abilities, an EEG should be performed [43, 66].

13.3.2.3 Psychiatry and Psychology

The mental health of individuals with PMS requires ongoing evaluation and monitoring. Individuals with PMS are at risk of developing a number of different behavioral and psychiatric conditions, including hyperactivity, anxiety, bipolar disorder, catatonia, and psychosis [32, 40]. After the diagnosis of PMS has been established, it is important to complete an initial evaluation of the patient's baseline mental status and intellectual ability [29, 53]. Monitoring the cognitive, linguistic, and motor development of individuals with PMS is also encouraged. Many children with PMS qualify for a diagnosis of ID, have limited language abilities, and have fewer adaptive skills [23, 26, 31, 54, 67, 68]. Conducting an initial neuropsychological assessment provides valuable insights into the child's current level of functioning, which can be leveraged to help children access appropriate services that are tailored to their specific needs. Since neuropsychological assessments are standardized to the general population, it may be necessary to use raw scores, mental age, or ratio IQs instead of standard scores to accurately evaluate the child's relative strengths and weaknesses [29]. Cognitive, language, and motor skills should be monitored over time as well, given the prevalence of behavioral regressions involving loss of speech and motor skills in PMS [30–32, 40, 54].

If a change in mental state or developmental or language skills is noticed, it is crucial to rule out underlying medical conditions or psychosocial stressors that may explain changes in behavior. If medical causes are ruled out, it may be necessary to refer patients for a comprehensive psychiatric assessment to provide appropriate pharmacologic care and support [31].

13.3.2.4 Cardiology

As part of the comprehensive evaluation for individuals with PMS, a standard cardiac assessment should be conducted by a cardiologist including physical examination with echocardiography and electrocardiography. Most, if not all, cardiac defects associated with PMS are congenital, so further support from a cardiologist may only be necessary if congenital heart defects are present [23, 43].

13.3.2.5 Gastroenterology

Patients with PMS can present with a wide range of gastrointestinal conditions (see Common Clinical Features). The care team should ensure they are monitoring for warning signs of these conditions. Symptoms such as lack of appetite, teeth grinding, and vomiting may be indicative of gastroesophageal reflux disease (GERD). If GERD is suspected, a gastroenterologist may need to conduct a gastrointestinal tract examination, gastroscopy with biopsies, screening for drug toxicity, and impedance testing [69]. For children with constipation, questionnaires and x-rays might be needed to better characterize the problem [69]. Zinc, B12, and copper deficiencies have been reported in PMS [43, 70]. Ongoing measurement of zinc concentrations in the plasma, nails, or urine may also be useful for identifying individuals with PMS with zinc deficiencies.

13.3.2.6 Nephrology/Urology

Structural renal abnormalities and genitourinary problems are reported in as many as 38% of patients with PMS [28, 34]. An initial evaluation should include a physical examination, blood pressure measurement, and blood tests for urea, creatinine, and electrolyte levels [43]. Renal and bladder sonography is also recommended for individuals with larger, Class II deletions. If any abnormalities are found during the diagnostic screening tests, referral to a pediatric nephrologist and/or urologist for further monitoring or treatment is advised.

13.3.2.7 Endocrinology

Hypothyroidism is observed in 3–6% of individuals with PMS and can have detrimental effects on brain function and behavior [28, 34, 71]. Fortunately, hypothyroidism is treatable with thyroid hormone replacement therapy [72]. Thyroid function tests should be conducted after the initial diagnosis of PMS and monitored regularly in teens and young adults to promptly detect hypothyroidism and initiate treatment if needed.

13.4 Psychosocial Treatments

In the following section, we will discuss the recommendations for psychosocial interventions that can be used to treat PMS. While there is currently no known cure for PMS, various interventions targeting cognitive, language, and motor skills, as well as improving sleep quality and addressing challenging behaviors, may benefit individuals with PMS. Due to the complex phenotypic presentation of individuals with PMS, a combination of psychosocial treatments should be considered.

13.4.1 Applied Behavioral Analysis Therapy

Applied Behavioral Analysis (ABA) therapy is one intervention that can be utilized in PMS [73]. Applied Behavioral Analysis therapy is widely utilized in the treatment of ASD and other neurodevelopmental disorders due to its effectiveness in addressing a wide range of developmental areas. For example, it has been shown to enhance language and communication skills, improve attention and focus, promote the development of the social skills necessary for building relationships and participating in social activities, facilitate academic progress, and reduce problem behaviors that may hinder daily functioning [74, 75]. There is a close association between ASD and PMS. Phelan–McDermid syndrome is one of the most prevalent genetic forms of ASD, making up 0.5% of ASD cases [1]. Previous studies characterizing the PMS phenotype have also reported that between 57 and 79% of individuals with PMS meet the criteria for ASD [44]. Thus, ABA therapy should be considered in individuals with PMS and ASD.

ABA therapy may also be beneficial for individuals with PMS who do not meet full diagnostic criteria for ASD. Individuals with PMS (with and without ASD) can also present with sensory processing deficits, such as mouthing or chewing, or experiencing tactile hyperreactivity [44]. Techniques used in ABA therapy may be useful to help children disengage from mouthing or chewing behaviors, and to become more tolerant of sensory input. Techniques from ABA may also help alleviate challenging behaviors, such as aggression or self-injury. In cases of comorbid mood cycling or bipolar disorder with or without psychotic symptoms, a more intensive behavioral program based on the principles of ABA, in addition to treatment with psychiatric medications, may be necessary.

13.4.2 Gross and Fine Motor Skills

Motor dysfunction is a common trait among individuals with PMS. Gross motor deficits, such as hypotonia, are observed in >75% of cases of PMS and can have a negative impact on gait and feeding [60]. Gross motor skills can also be stunted by physical features associated with PMS, such as genu valgus, pes planovalgus, joint hypermobility, and leg length discrepancy. In some cases, gross motor skills are severely affected, resulting in the inability to walk independently. Fine motor skills can also be affected. For example, in a study by Frank et al., researchers found that all of the 51 participants in the study had challenges with fine motor coordination and visuomotor integration [60]. A prolonged loss of both gross and fine motor skills can also occur during regressive episodes in PMS later in childhood. Motor skills are critical for many activities of daily living, such as oral hygiene, dressing, and feeding, highlighting the importance of treatments that address motor functioning in individuals with PMS.

Physical therapy (PT) may be warranted to help improve gross motor skills in PMS [23, 53]. Physical therapists help children acquire new movement skills, improve stamina and coordination, and develop daily routines that can be used in the home and in the classroom. It is recommended to choose a physical therapist who is specialized in pediatrics or has experience working with individuals with developmental disabilities. Other therapeutics, such as aqua therapy, hippotherapy, and adaptive tricycles, can also be utilized in addition to PT to improve gross motor capabilities [43]. Some individuals may also benefit from using orthoses for their wrists, arms, legs, or feet to support or realign the outer extremities. When considering the use of orthoses, it is also important to take into account sensory sensitivities present in the individual. Many people with PMS report hyperreactivity to tactile stimuli, so orthoses that are too rigid or too tight may be challenging to implement.

Occupational therapy (OT) may also be useful in developing fine motor and daily living skills that may be lost or impaired in PMS [23, 53]. For example, occupational therapists can focus on improving wrist and hand alignment in PMS and create goals to promote toilet training, dressing, and eating independently. Occupational therapists can also offer strategies for responding to sensory information in the environment. Like with PT, it is important to identify an occupational therapist with expertise working with individuals with neurodevelopmental disorders. For individuals with PMS presenting with failure to thrive or other challenges surrounding eating, we recommend consulting with a feeding specialist [23]. Feeding therapy can target a range of different skills that are necessary for eating independently that can be impacted in PMS, including learning how to use and coordinate the muscles used for sucking or swallowing and learning to tolerate different food textures.

13.4.3 Interventions to Improve Communication

Deficits in verbal and nonverbal communication skills are another core characteristic of PMS [23, 31, 54, 67, 68]. Receptive and expressive language skills are significantly reduced, and less integrated into social interactions in individuals with PMS [76]. Expressive language skills appear to be more severely impacted and can be lost during some episodes of regression in PMS [30, 54]. Because limited language skills may be associated with the presence of challenging behaviors such as self-injury and aggression, we recommend that individuals with PMS seek treatments that promote functional communication.

One potential intervention to address communication deficits in PMS is speech therapy [53, 54]. Speech therapists frequently work with children with developmental delays and ASD to help encourage the use of both verbal and nonverbal communication strategies in social settings or when making requests. Importantly, children with PMS appear to have relative strengths in functional, symbolic, and pretend play skills, and intact social intent that can be leveraged in speech therapy. For individuals who are nonverbal or minimally verbal, the use of augmentative and alternative communication (AAC) may also be beneficial [23, 77]. There are many types of AAC systems, including American Sign Language (ASL), Picture Exchange Communication Systems (PECS), iPad applications, or speech-generating devices. Using AAC has been shown to have positive effects on communication in minimally verbal children (<10 words) with developmental delays, suggesting that AAC devices may be beneficial for developing speech production abilities [78, 79].

13.4.4 Educational Services

Educational services should be sought for children with PMS. Children under 3 years old (in the United States) who are diagnosed with PMS are eligible for Early Intervention (EI) services, which include access to ABA therapy, PT, OT, and speech therapy, as well as playgroups to address social skills. Before receiving EI services, children undergo a neuropsychological evaluation to capture their baseline skills.

Goals are also communicated to families to promote the use of the skills learned during EI at home.

Older children may also be eligible for individualized education programs (IEPs) that provide additional services in the school setting. Some individuals with PMS, particularly those with limited language or ID, may require placement in special education or substantially separate classrooms that are taught by teachers and aides trained to work with children with developmental disabilities. Individualized education programs might also offer 1:1 aides to accompany children with PMS in the classroom to address difficulties with attention, set academic goals, or mitigate challenging behaviors. Like with EI, the goals and services provided by the IEP will be determined based on the child's skills.

13.4.5 Sleep

Individuals with PMS report a high rate of sleep disturbances, such as having difficulty falling asleep or waking up frequently throughout the night, which results in reduced total sleep time [18, 26, 80–82]. These types of sleep disturbances emerge early in childhood and have been observed in children as young as 4–5 months of age and become more prevalent through adulthood [81, 82]. Sleep is important for learning, memory, attention, emotional regulation, and sleep disruptions can exacerbate ASD-related symptoms and challenging behaviors [83–85]. Engaging in good sleep hygiene is encouraged to help improve sleep quality [83]. Sleep hygiene can be improved by setting and maintaining consistent bedtime routines, eliminating or reducing light and noise in the bedroom, and minimizing stimulating activities before bedtime [23].

13.5 Biological Treatments

As PMS is quite rare, few treatment studies have been completed. Studies have largely sought to increase or improve synaptic function. Insulin-like growth factor-1 (IGF-1) has been shown to reverse social and motor deficits in mouse models [86] of PMS as well as in pilot human studies [87–89]. In one placebo-controlled, double-blind crossover pilot study of IGF-1 [87], nine children were administered three months of treatment and three months of placebo. There were no serious adverse events, suggesting that IGF-1 can be tolerated by children with PMS. Importantly, some clinical improvement in social withdrawal, hyperactivity, sensory symptoms, and repetitive behaviors was observed during the treatment phase. Improvements in sensory symptoms, repetitive behaviors, and hyperactivity were also observed in an extension of this clinical trial that included ten children with PMS [89]. Others have investigated recombinant human growth hormone (rhGH) as a potential alternative to IGF-1 in patients with PMS. One study found that after three months of treatment in a double-blind crossover study of six children, there were significant improvements in behavior without serious adverse events [90]. Specifically, children had higher scores on the Gesell Development

Scale (GDS), which measures motor and language development, adaptive skills, and social behavior, post-treatment. Compared to placebo, rhGH also resulted in reductions in the Simplified Chinese Aberrant Behavior Checklist (SC-ABC). These pilot studies suggest that IGF-1 and rhGH may be viable interventions for PMS in the future. However, further investigation of IGF-1 and rhGH in larger clinical trials is required before these potential interventions can be utilized clinically.

13.5.1 Pharmacological Management of Psychiatric Comorbidities

Psychopharmacology may also help with the management of psychiatric comorbidities present in PMS. The most common psychiatric comorbidities and the medications used for treatment are described in Table 13.2. However, it is important to note that while typical pharmacological interventions may be effective, they may not always be tolerated by individuals with PMS. Considerations and recommendations for pharmacological treatment are also included in Table 13.2.

Table 13.2 Common psychiatric comorbidities

Comorbidity	Potential medications	Considerations
ADHD	• Alpha agonists (guanfacine, clonidine) [43]. • Methylphenidate [41, 43], amphetamine salts. • Atomoxetine [91, 92].	Atomoxetine may be less effective or carry more side effects in patients with variants of *CYP2D6*, a gene located on chromosome 22q13.2 [91, 92]. Methylphenidate is poorly tolerated in some patients with PMS [36, 67, 69], causing increased insomnia and aggression [93]. **Recommendation**: Alpha agonists should be used as the first-line treatment for ADHD in patients with PMS [43].
Anxiety	• Buspirone [43]. • SSRIs [32, 43]. • *N*-acetylcysteine [43]. • Gabapentin [43].	Patients with PMS have a higher likelihood of experiencing side effects, such as mania or aggression, from SSRIs [32, 43]. **Recommendation**: Patients with PMS who are prescribed SSRIs should be started on low doses and monitored. If SSRIs are poorly tolerated, alternative medications, such as buspirone, gabapentin, or *N*-acetylcysteine, may be effective [43].
Bipolar disorder	• Anticonvulsants (divalproex sodium, lamotrigine) [40, 41]. • Lithium [40–42, 93, 94]. • Second-generation antipsychotics [35, 38, 40, 93].	Lithium may also be used to treat catatonia and regression [40, 42, 43, 93]. Antipsychotics should be used with caution and at low doses, as they can induce catatonia or neuroleptic malignant syndrome[a] in some patients with PMS [43]. **Recommendations**: Lithium, divalproex sodium, or lamotrigine should be the first line of treatment for bipolar disorder [40, 43, 95]. Lithium should be used if the patient also presents with catatonia or regression [42].

(continued)

Table 13.2 (continued)

Comorbidity	Potential medications	Considerations
Catatonia	• Lorazepam [41–43]. • Lithium [40–43, 93].	**Recommendations**: Lorazepam is generally effective in treating catatonia in PMS [43]. Patients with co-occurring mood disorders or regression may also benefit from lithium [42]. Electroconvulsive therapy may also be useful in treating catatonia in PMS [32]. Antipsychotics are typically not recommended [43, 95].
Psychosis	• Antipsychotics [40, 41].	Antipsychotics are usually ineffective and poorly tolerated in PMS [43, 91, 95]. Antipsychotics have induced catatonia or neuroleptic malignant syndrome[a] in some PMS patients [43], and can increase aggression [32, 95]. **Recommendation**: Patients with PMS who are using antipsychotics should be monitored closely for signs of catatonia.

ADHD attention-deficit hyperactivity disorder, *CYP2D6* cytochrome P450 family 2 subfamily D member 6, *SSRIs* selective serotonin reuptake inhibitors

[a]Neuroleptic malignant syndrome is a life-threatening adverse reaction to neuroleptic or antipsychotic drugs which induces high-fever, sweating, and unstable blood pressure

13.6 Common Medical Comorbidities

The presence of other medical comorbidities makes prescribing safe and effective pharmacologic treatments for patients with PMS more complex. Table 13.3 identifies some of the most common medical comorbidities present in PMS and medications that are used to address those comorbidities.

Key Points to Remember

- Phelan–McDermid syndrome is a rare genetic condition caused by deletions to 22q13.3 or sequence variants of SHANK3.
- Individuals with PMS have a broad range of complex medical and behavioral phenotypes that might reflect variation in the underlying genetic change.
- Primary care physicians should be aware of, and screen for the physical, medical, and behavioral characteristics present in patients with PMS.
- A cross-disciplinary team of providers, involving primary care physicians, geneticists, neurologists, psychiatrists, psychologists, gastroenterologists, and therapists should be organized by the coordinating physician to care for patients with PMS.

Table 13.3 Common medical comorbidities

Comorbidity	Potential medications	Considerations
Congenital heart defects	None-treated with surgery	
Epilepsy	Carbamazepine; clorazepate; ethosuximide; felbamate; lacosamide; lamotrigine; levetiracetam; lorazepam; methsuximide; oxcarbazepine; perampanel; phenobarbital; phenytoin; rufinamide; topiramate; valproate; zonisamide [63, 65, 66]	A combination of two or more medications may be required for individuals with multiple types of seizures [65]. **Recommendation**: Treatment of epilepsy in PMS should be in accordance with local guidelines [66].
GI disorders		
Constipation/ diarrhea	Oral laxatives; zinc supplements [69]	Changes in sleep and behavior can sometimes be attributed to GI disorders in PMS [43].
Cyclic vomiting	Miralax	
GERD	Cyproheptadine; amitriptyline [96] Proton pump inhibitors [69]	
Hypothyroidism	Levothyroxine [72]	
Hypotonia	None-treated with physical therapy	**Recommendation**: Route of drug administration should be considered for patients with swallowing difficulties
Lymphedema	None-treated with compression bandages [23] and physical therapy	
Renal defects	None	
Sleep disturbance	Melatonin; clonidine or guanfacine; trazodone; amitriptyline; antihistamines; 5-hydroxytryptophan; gabapentin; melatonin orexin antagonist [18, 41]	**Recommendation**: A combination of medication and behavioral interventions (i.e., sleep hygiene) should be used to treat sleep disturbances

GERD gastroesophageal reflux disease, *GI* gastrointestinal, *SJS* Stevens-Johnson syndrome

Photographs of Individuals with the Syndrome

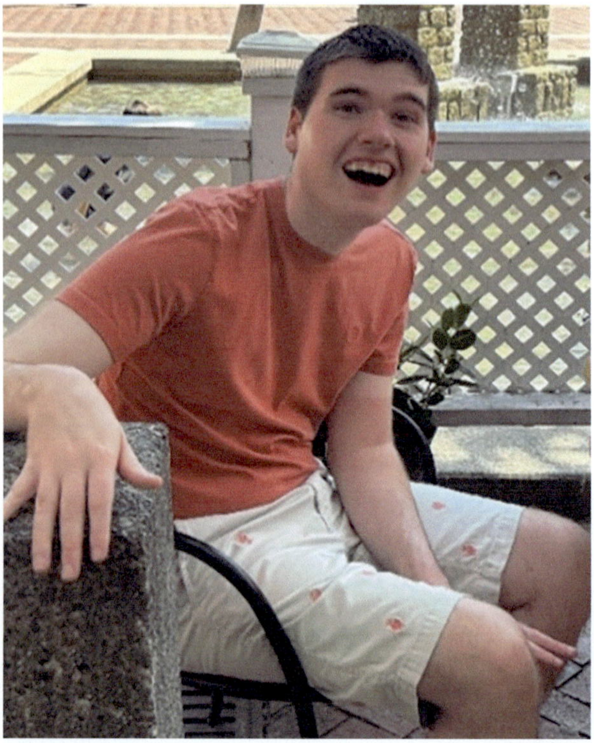

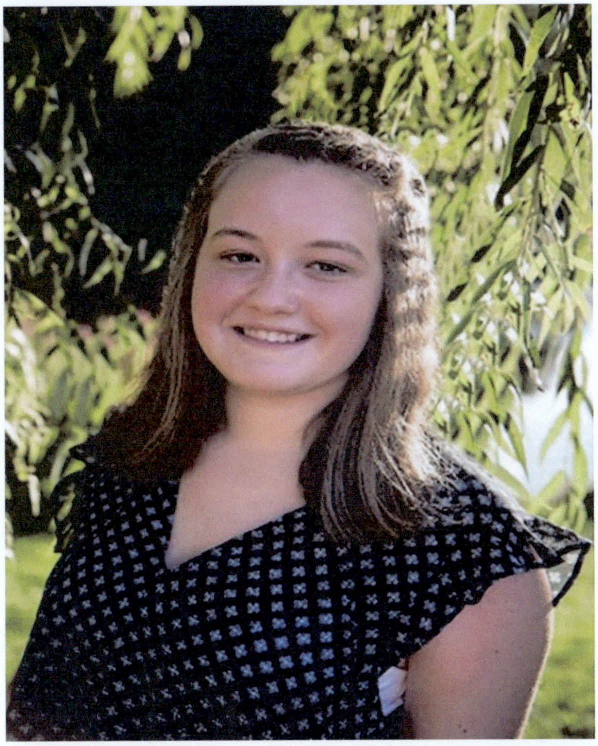

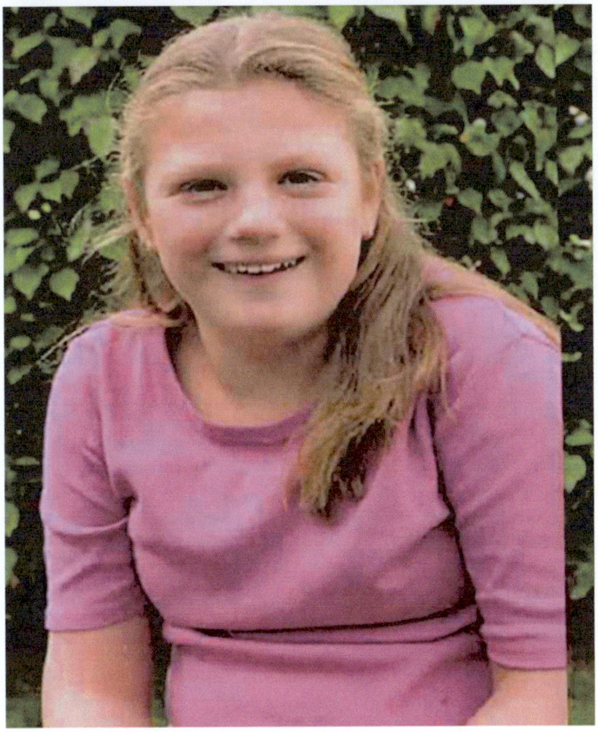

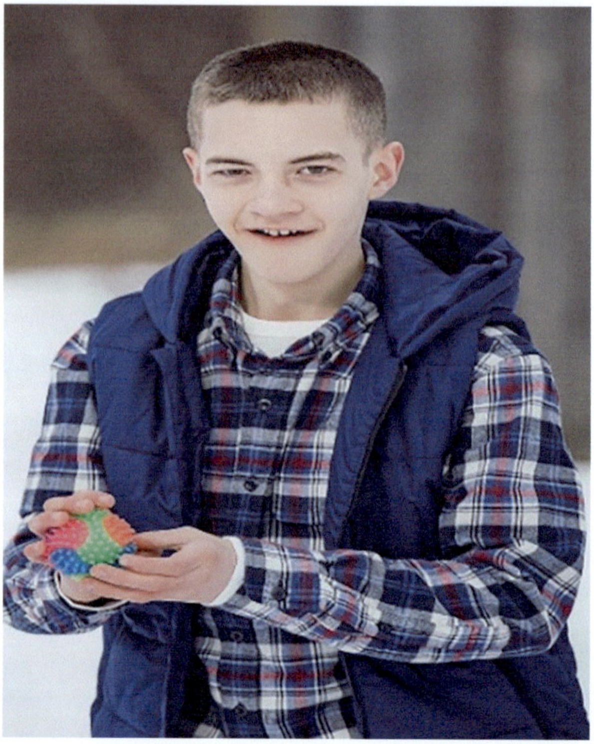

References

1. Costales JL, Kolevzon A. Phelan-McDermid Syndrome and SHANK3: implications for treatment. Neurotherapeutics. 2015;12(3):620–30. https://doi.org/10.1007/s13311-015-0352-z.
2. Home - Phelan-McDermid Syndrome Foundation - An international alliance of science and support [Internet]. Phelan-McDermid Syndrome Foundation. [cited 2023 Jun 28]. Available from: https://pmsf.org/
3. Betancur C, Buxbaum JD. SHANK3 haploinsufficiency: a "common" but underdiagnosed highly penetrant monogenic cause of autism spectrum disorders. Mol Autism. 2013;4(1):17. https://doi.org/10.1186/2040-2392-4-17.
4. Landlust AM, Koza SA, Carbin M, et al. Parental perspectives on Phelan-McDermid syndrome: results of a worldwide survey. Eur J Med Genet. 2023;66(7):104771. https://doi.org/10.1016/j.ejmg.2023.104771.
5. Disciglio V, Lo Rizzo C, Mencarelli MA, et al. Interstitial 22q13 deletions not involving SHANK3 gene: a new contiguous gene syndrome. Am J Med Genet. 2014;164A(7):1666–76. https://doi.org/10.1002/ajmg.a.36513.
6. Monteiro P, Feng G. SHANK proteins: roles at the synapse and in autism spectrum disorder. Nat Rev Neurosci. 2017;18(3):147–57. https://doi.org/10.1038/nrn.2016.183.
7. Harony-Nicolas H, De Rubeis S, Kolevzon A, Buxbaum JD. Phelan McDermid Syndrome: from genetic discoveries to animal models and treatment. J Child Neurol. 2015;30(14):1861–70. https://doi.org/10.1177/0883073815600872.

8. Sheng M, Kim E. The Shank family of scaffold proteins. J Cell Sci. 2000;113(11):1851–6. https://doi.org/10.1242/jcs.113.11.1851.
9. Sala C, Vicidomini C, Bigi I, Mossa A, Verpelli C. Shank synaptic scaffold proteins: keys to understanding the pathogenesis of autism and other synaptic disorders. J Neurochem. 2015;135(5):849–58. https://doi.org/10.1111/jnc.13232.
10. Yi F, Danko T, Botelho SC, et al. Autism-associated SHANK3 haploinsufficiency causes Ih channelopathy in human neurons. Science. 2016;352(6286):aaf2669. https://doi.org/10.1126/science.aaf2669.
11. Peça J, Feliciano C, Ting JT, et al. Shank3 mutant mice display autistic-like behaviors and striatal dysfunction. Nature. 2011;472(7344):437–42. https://doi.org/10.1038/nature09965.
12. Mei Y, Monteiro P, Zhou Y, et al. Adult restoration of Shank3 expression rescues selective autistic-like phenotypes. Nature. 2016;530:481–4.
13. Roussignol G, Ango F, Romorini S, et al. Shank expression is sufficient to induce functional dendritic spine synapses in aspiny neurons. J Neurosci. 2005;25(14):3560–70. https://doi.org/10.1523/JNEUROSCI.4354-04.2005.
14. Wang X, Bey A, Katz B, et al. Altered mGluR5-Homer scaffolds and corticostriatal connectivity in a Shank3 complete knockout model of autism. Nat Commun. 2017;7:11459. https://doi.org/10.1038/ncomms11459.
15. Zhao Y, Kaiser T, Monteiro P, et al. Mice with Shank3 mutations associated with ASD and Schizophrenia display both shared and distinct defects. Neuron. 2016;89(1):147–62. https://doi.org/10.1016/j.neuron.2015.11.023.
16. Arons MH, Thynne CJ, Grabrucker AM, et al. Autism-associated mutations in ProSAP2/Shank3 impair synaptic transmission and neurexin-neuroligin-mediated transsynaptic signaling. J Neurosci. 2012;32(43):14966–78. https://doi.org/10.1523/JNEUROSCI.2215-12.2012.
17. Sakai Y, Okuzono S, Schaaf CP, et al. Translational pediatrics: clinical perspective for Phelan–McDermid syndrome and autism research. Pediatr Res. 2022;92:373–7. https://doi.org/10.1038/s41390-021-01806-x.
18. San José Cáceres A, Landlust AM, Carbin JM, European Phelan-McDermid Syndrome consortium, Loth E. Consensus recommendations on sleeping problems in Phelan-McDermid syndrome. Eur J Med Genet. 2023;66(6):104750. https://doi.org/10.1016/j.ejmg.2023.104750.
19. Sala C, Piëch V, Wilson NR, Passafaro M, Liu G, Sheng M. Regulation of dendritic spine morphology and synaptic function by Shank and Homer. Neuron. 2001;31(1):115–30. https://doi.org/10.1016/S0896-6273(01)00339-7.
20. Filice F, Vörckel KJ, Sungur AO, Wöhr M, Schwaller B. Reduction in parvalbumin expression not loss of the parvalbumin-expressing GABA interneuron subpopulation in genetic parvalbumin and shank mouse models of autism. Mol Brain. 2016;9:10. https://doi.org/10.1186/s13041-016-0192-8.
21. Gogolla N, Takesian AE, Feng G, Fagiolini M, Hensch TK. Sensory integration in mouse insular cortex reflects GABA circuit maturation. Neuron. 2014;83(4):894–905. https://doi.org/10.1016/j.neuron.2014.06.033.
22. Ingiosi AM, Schoch H, Wintler T, et al. Shank3 modulates sleep and expression of circadian transcription factors. eLife. 2019;8:e42819.
23. Phelan K, McDermid HE. The 22q13.3 deletion syndrome (Phelan-McDermid Syndrome). Mol Syndromol. 2012;2(3–5):186–201. https://doi.org/10.1159/000334260.
24. Vitrac A, Leblond CS, Rolland T, et al. Dissecting the 22q13 region to explore the genetic and phenotypic diversity of patients with Phelan-McDermid syndrome. Eur J Hum Genet. 2023;66(5):104732. https://doi.org/10.1016/j.ejmg.2023.104732.
25. Levy HC, O'Bryan EM, Tolin DF. A meta-analysis of relapse rates in cognitive-behavioral therapy for anxiety disorders. J Anxiety Disord. 2021;81:102407. https://doi.org/10.1016/j.janxdis.2021.102407.
26. Nevado J, García-Miñaúr S, Palomares-Bralo M, et al. Variability in Phelan-McDermid syndrome in a cohort of 210 individuals. Front Genet. 2022;13:652454. https://doi.org/10.3389/fgene.2022.652454.

27. Tabet AC, Rolland T, Ducloy M, et al. A framework to identify contributing genes in patients with Phelan-McDermid syndrome. NPJ Genom Med. 2017;2:32. https://doi.org/10.1038/s41525-017-0035-2.
28. Sarasua SM, Boccuto L, Sharp JL, et al. Clinical and genomic evaluation of 201 patients with Phelan-McDermid syndrome. Hum Genet. 2014;133(7):847–59. https://doi.org/10.1007/s00439-014-1423-7.
29. Soorya L, Leon J, Trelles MP, Thurm A. Framework for assessing individuals with rare genetic disorders associated with profound intellectual and multiple disabilities (PIMD): the example of Phelan McDermid Syndrome. Clin Neuropsychol. 2018;32(7):1226–55. https://doi.org/10.1080/13854046.2017.1413211.
30. Reierson G, Bernstein J, Froehlich-Santino W, et al. Characterizing regression in Phelan McDermid Syndrome (22q13 deletion syndrome). J Psychiatr Res. 2017;91:139–44. https://doi.org/10.1016/j.jpsychires.2017.03.010.
31. van Balkom IDC, Burdeus-Olavarrieta M, Cooke J, et al. Consensus recommendations on mental health issues in Phelan-McDermid syndrome. Eur J Hum Genet. 2023;66(6):104770. https://doi.org/10.1016/j.ejmg.2023.104770.
32. Kohlenberg TM, Trelles MP, McLarney B, Betancur C, Thurm A, Kolevzon A. Psychiatric illness and regression in individuals with Phelan-McDermid syndrome. J Neurodev Disord. 2020;12(1):7. https://doi.org/10.1186/s11689-020-9309-6.
33. Smith MS, Sarasua SM, Rogers C, Phelan K, Boccuto L. Lymphedema is associated with CELSR1 in Phelan-McDermid syndrome. Clin Genet. 2023;104:472–8. https://doi.org/10.1111/cge.14364.
34. Soorya L, Kolevzon A, Zweifach J, et al. Prospective investigation of autism and genotype-phenotype correlations in 22q13 deletion syndrome and SHANK3 deficiency. Mol Autism. 2013;4(1):18. https://doi.org/10.1186/2040-2392-4-18.
35. Denayer A, Van Esch H, de Ravel T, et al. Neuropsychopathology in 7 patients with the 22q13 deletion syndrome: presence of bipolar disorder and progressive loss of skills. Mol Syndromol. 2012;3(1):14–20. https://doi.org/10.1159/000339119.
36. Xu N, Lv H, Yang T, et al. A 29 Mainland Chinese cohort of patients with Phelan-McDermid syndrome: genotype-phenotype correlations and the role of SHANK3 haploinsufficiency in the important phenotypes. Orphanet J Rare Dis. 2020;15(1):335. https://doi.org/10.1186/s13023-020-01592-5.
37. De Rubeis S, Siper PM, Durkin A, et al. Delineation of the genetic and clinical spectrum of Phelan-McDermid syndrome caused by SHANK3 point mutations. Mol Autism. 2018;9:31. https://doi.org/10.1186/s13229-018-0205-9.
38. Egger JI, Zwanenburg RJ, van Ravenswaaij-Arts CM, Kleefstra T, Verhoeven WM. Neuropsychological phenotype and psychopathology in seven adult patients with Phelan-McDermid syndrome: implications for treatment strategy. Genes Brain Behav. 2016;15(4):395–404. https://doi.org/10.1111/gbb.12285.
39. Walther S, Strik W. Catatonia. CNS Spectr. 2016;21(4):341–8. https://doi.org/10.1017/S1092852916000274.
40. Kolevzon A, Delaby E, Berry-Kravis E, Buxbaum JD, Betancur C. Neuropsychiatric decompensation in adolescents and adults with Phelan-McDermid syndrome: a systematic review of the literature. Mol Autism. 2019;10:50. https://doi.org/10.1186/s13229-019-0291-3.
41. Verhoeven WMA, Egger JIM, de Leeuw N. A longitudinal perspective on the pharmacotherapy of 24 adult patients with Phelan McDermid syndrome. Eur J Med Genet. 2020;63(3):103751. https://doi.org/10.1016/j.ejmg.2019.103751.
42. Phelan K, Rogers RC, Boccuto L. Phelan-McDermid syndrome. In: Adam MP, Mirzaa GM, Pagon RA, et al., editors. GeneReviews. Seattle (WA): University of Washington; 2005 May 11 [updated 2018 Jun 7]. Available from: https://www.ncbi.nlm.nih.gov/books/NBK1198/
43. Srivastava S, Sahin M, Buxbaum JD, et al. Updated consensus guidelines on the management of Phelan-McDermid syndrome. Am J Med Genet. 2023;191:2015–44. https://doi.org/10.1002/ajmg.a.63312.

44. Schön M, Lapunzina P, Nevado J, et al. Definition and clinical variability of SHANK3-related Phelan-McDermid syndrome. Eur J Hum Genet. 2023;66(7):104754. https://doi.org/10.1016/j.ejmg.2023.104754.
45. Phelan K, Boccuto L, Powell CM, et al. Phelan-McDermid syndrome: a classification system after 30 years of experience. Orphanet J Rare Dis. 2022;17(1):27. https://doi.org/10.1186/s13023-022-02180-5.
46. Koza SA, Tabet AC, Bonaglia MC, et al. Consensus recommendations on counseling in Phelan-McDermid syndrome, with special attention to recurrence risk and to ring chromosome 22. Eur J Hum Genet. 2023;66(7):104773. https://doi.org/10.1016/j.ejmg.2023.104773.
47. Bonaglia MC, Giorda R, Beri S, et al. Molecular mechanisms generating and stabilizing terminal 22q13 deletions in 44 subjects with Phelan/McDermid syndrome. PLoS Genet. 2011;7(7):e1002173. https://doi.org/10.1371/journal.pgen.1002173.
48. Levy T, Foss-Feig JH, Betancur C, et al. Strong evidence for genotype-phenotype correlations in Phelan-McDermid syndrome: results from the developmental synaptopathies consortium. Hum Mol Genet. 2022;31(4):625–37. https://doi.org/10.1093/hmg/ddab280.
49. Richards S, Aziz N, Bale S, et al. Standards and guidelines for the interpretation of sequence variants: a joint consensus recommendation of the American College of Medical Genetics and Genomics and the Association for Molecular Pathology. Genet Med. 2015;17(5):405–24. https://doi.org/10.1038/gim.2015.3.
50. Bisgaard AM, Kirchhoff M, Nielsen JE, et al. Chromosomal deletion unmasking a recessive disease: 22q13 deletion syndrome and metachromatic leukodystrophy. Clin Genet. 2009;75(2):175–9. https://doi.org/10.1111/j.1399-0004.2008.01113.x.
51. Ahn H, Seo GH, Keum C, et al. Diagnosis of metachromatic leukodystrophy in a patient with regression and Phelan-McDermid syndrome. Brain and Development. 2020;42(5):414–7. https://doi.org/10.1016/j.braindev.2020.02.003.
52. Mingbunjerdsuk D, Wong M, Bozarth X, Sun A. Co-occurrence of metachromatic leukodystrophy in Phelan-McDermid syndrome. J Child Neurol. 2021;36(2):148–51. https://doi.org/10.1177/0883073820960308.
53. Kolevzon A, Angarita B, Bush L, et al. Phelan-McDermid syndrome: a review of the literature and practice parameters for medical assessment and monitoring. J Neurodev Disord. 2014;6(1):39. https://doi.org/10.1186/1866-1955-6-39.
54. Burdeus-Olavarrieta M, Nevado J, van Weering-Scholten S, Parker S, European Phelan-McDermid syndrome consortium, Swillen A. Consensus recommendations on communication, language and speech in Phelan-McDermid syndrome. Eur J Hum Genet. 2023;66(5):104745. https://doi.org/10.1016/j.ejmg.2023.104745.
55. Isenstein EL, Grosman HE, Guillory SB, et al. Neural markers of auditory response and habituation in Phelan-McDermid Syndrome. Front Neurosci. 2022;16:815933. https://doi.org/10.3389/fnins.2022.815933.
56. Engineer CT, Rahebi KC, Borland MS, et al. Shank3-deficient rats exhibit degraded cortical responses to sound. Autism Res. 2018;11(1):59–68. https://doi.org/10.1002/aur.1883.
57. Ziats MN, Ahmad A, Bernat JA, et al. Genotype-phenotype analysis of 523 patients by genetics evaluation and clinical exome sequencing. Pediatr Res. 2020;87(4):735–9. https://doi.org/10.1038/s41390-019-0611-5.
58. Ardern-Holmes S, Fisher G, North K. Neurofibromatosis type 2: presentation, major complications, and management, with a focus on the pediatric age group. J Child Neurol. 2017;32(1):9–22. https://doi.org/10.1177/0883073816666736.
59. van Eeghen AM, Stemkens D, Fernández-Fructuoso JR, et al. Consensus recommendations on organization of care for individuals with Phelan-McDermid syndrome. Eur J Hum Genet. 2023;66(7):104747. Available from: https://www.sciencedirect.com/science/article/pii/S1769721223000538?via%3Dihub
60. Frank Y. A prospective study of neurological abnormalities in Phelan-Mcdermid Syndrome. Orphanet J Rare Dis. 2017;5(1):1–13.
61. Omansky GL, Abdulhayoglu E, Zhurbilo B. Phelan-McDermid syndrome. Neonatal Netw. 2017;36(2):98–100. https://doi.org/10.1891/0730-0832.36.2.98.

62. Aldinger KA, Kogan J, Kimonis V, et al. Cerebellar and posterior fossa malformations in patients with autism-associated chromosome 22q13 terminal deletion. Am J Med Genet. 2013;161A(1):131–6. https://doi.org/10.1002/ajmg.a.35700.
63. Figura M, Gaweł M, Kolasa A, Janik P. Cerebellar ataxia with neuropathy and vestibular areflexia syndrome (CANVAS) - a case report and review of literature. Neurol Neurochir Pol. 2014;48(5):368–72. https://doi.org/10.1016/j.pjnns.2014.08.003.
64. Halliday D, Emmanouil B, Evans DGR. Updated protocol for genetic testing, screening and clinical management of individuals at risk of NF2-related schwannomatosis. Clin Genet. 2023;103(5):540–52. https://doi.org/10.1111/cge.14310.
65. Holder JL, Quach MM. The spectrum of epilepsy and electroencephalographic abnormalities due to SHANK3 loss-of-function mutations. Epilepsia. 2016;57(10):1651–9. https://doi.org/10.1111/epi.13506.
66. de Coo IFM, Jesse S, Le TL, Sala C, European Phelan-McDermid syndrome consortium. Consensus recommendations on dpilepsy in Phelan-McDermid syndrome. Eur J Med Genet. 2023;66(6):104746. https://doi.org/10.1016/j.ejmg.2023.104746.
67. Phelan MC, Rogers RC, Saul RA, et al. 22q13 deletion syndrome. Am J Med Genet. 2001;101(2):91–9. https://doi.org/10.1002/1096-8628(20010615)101:2<91::aid-ajmg1340>3.0.co;2-c.
68. Burdeus-Olavarrieta M, San José-Cáceres A, García-Alcón A, González-Peñas J, Hernández-Jusdado P, Parellada-Redondo M. Characterisation of the clinical phenotype in Phelan-McDermid syndrome. J Neurodev Disord. 2021;13(1):26. https://doi.org/10.1186/s11689-021-09370-5.
69. Matuleviciene A, Siauryte K, Kuiper E, Grabrucker AM, European Phelan-McDermid syndrome guideline consortium. Consensus recommendations on chewing, swallowing and gastrointestinal problems in Phelan-McDermid syndrome. Eur J Med Genet. 2023;66(6):104763. https://doi.org/10.1016/j.ejmg.2023.104763.
70. Pfaender S, Sauer AK, Hagmeyer S, et al. Zinc deficiency and low enterocyte zinc transporter expression in human patients with autism related mutations in SHANK3. Sci Rep. 2017;7:45190. https://doi.org/10.1038/srep45190.
71. Eslami-Amirabadi M, Sajjadi SA. The relation between thyroid dysregulation and impaired cognition/behaviour: an integrative review. J Neuroendocrinol. 2021;33(3):e12948. https://doi.org/10.1111/jne.12948.
72. Chaker L, Razvi S, Bensenor IM, et al. Publisher correction: hypothyroidism. Nat Rev Dis Primers. 2022;8:39. https://doi.org/10.1038/s41572-022-00373-7.
73. Schroeder KA, Witts BN, Traub MR. Opportunities for ABA intervention in Phelan-McDermid syndrome. Int J Dev Disabil. 2021;68(6):984–9. https://doi.org/10.1080/20473869.2021.1895698.
74. Yu Q, Li E, Li L, Liang W. Efficacy of interventions based on applied behavior analysis for autism spectrum disorder: a meta-analysis. Psychiatry Investig. 2020;17(5):432–43. https://doi.org/10.30773/pi.2019.0229.
75. Peters-Scheffer N, Didden R, Korzilius H, Sturmey P. A meta-analytic study on the effectiveness of comprehensive ABA-based early intervention programs for children with autism spectrum disorders. Res Autism Spectr Disord. 2011;5(1):60–9. https://doi.org/10.1016/j.rasd.2010.03.011.
76. Brignell A, Krahe M, Downes M, Kefalianos E, Reilly S, Morgan A. Interventions for children and adolescents who stutter: a systematic review, meta-analysis, and evidence map. J Fluen Disord. 2021;70:105843. https://doi.org/10.1016/j.jfludis.2021.105843.
77. Marrus N, Hall L. Intellectual disability and language disorder. Child Adolesc Psychiatr Clin N Am. 2017;26(3):539–54. https://doi.org/10.1016/j.chc.2017.03.001.
78. Romski M, Sevcik RA, Adamson LB, et al. Randomized comparison of augmented and nonaugmented language interventions for toddlers with developmental delays and their parents. J Speech Lang Hear Res. 2010;53(2):350–64. https://doi.org/10.1044/1092-4388(2009/08-0156).

79. Chavers TN, Morris M, Schlosser RW, Koul R. Effects of a systematic augmentative and alternative communication intervention using a speech-generating device on multistep requesting and generic small talk for children with severe autism spectrum disorder. Am J Speech Lang Pathol. 2021;30(6):2476–91. https://doi.org/10.1044/2021_AJSLP-20-00353.
80. Smith-Hicks C, Wright D, Kenny A, et al. Sleep abnormalities in the synaptopathies-SYNGAP1-related intellectual disability and Phelan-McDermid Syndrome. Brain Sci. 2021;11(9):1229. https://doi.org/10.3390/brainsci11091229.
81. Bro D, O'Hara R, Primeau M, Hanson-Kahn A, Hallmayer J, Bernstein JA. Sleep disturbances in individuals with Phelan-McDermid syndrome: correlation with caregivers' sleep quality and daytime functioning. Sleep. 2017;40(2) https://doi.org/10.1093/sleep/zsw062.
82. Moffitt BA, Sarasua SM, Ward L, et al. Sleep and Phelan-McDermid Syndrome: lessons from the international registry and the scientific literature. Mol Genet Genomic Med. 2022;10(10):e2035. https://doi.org/10.1002/mgg3.2035.
83. Veatch OJ, Maxwell-Horn AC, Malow BA. Sleep in autism spectrum disorders. Curr Sleep Med Rep. 2015;1:131–40. https://doi.org/10.1007/s40675-015-0012-1.
84. Malow BA, Marzec ML, McGrew SG, Wang L, Henderson LM, Stone WL. Characterizing sleep in children with autism spectrum disorders: a multidimensional approach. Sleep. 2006;29(12):1563–71. https://doi.org/10.1093/sleep/29.12.1563.
85. Goldman SE, Surdyka K, Cuevas R, Adkins K, Wang L, Malow BA. Defining the sleep phenotype in children with autism. Dev Neuropsychol. 2009;34(5):560–73. https://doi.org/10.1080/87565640903133509.
86. Bozdagi O, Tavassoli T, Buxbaum JD. Insulin-like growth factor-1 rescues synaptic and motor deficits in a mouse model of autism and developmental delay. Mol Autism. 2013;4:9. https://doi.org/10.1186/2040-2392-4-9.
87. Kolevzon A, Bush L, Wang AT, et al. A pilot controlled trial of insulin-like growth factor-1 in children with Phelan-McDermid syndrome. Mol Autism. 2014;5:54. https://doi.org/10.1186/2040-2392-5-54.
88. Shcheglovitov A, Shcheglovitova O, Yazawa M, et al. SHANK3 and IGF1 restore synaptic deficits in neurons from 22q13 deletion syndrome patients. Nature. 2013;503:267–71. https://doi.org/10.1038/nature12618.
89. KolevzonA BMS, Siper PM, Halpern D, et al. Clinical trial of insulin-like growth factor-1 in Phelan-McDermid syndrome. Mol Autism. 2022;13:17. https://doi.org/10.1186/s13229-022-00493-7.
90. Li T, Xie R, Zhao J, et al. Effectiveness of recombinant human growth hormone therapy for children with Phelan-McDermid syndrome: an open-label, cross-over, preliminary study. Front Psych. 2022;13:763565. https://doi.org/10.3389/fpsyt.2022.763565.
91. Brown JT, Bishop JR, Sangkuhl K, et al. Clinical pharmacogenetics implementation consortium guideline for cytochrome P450 (CYP) 2D6 genotype and atomoxetine therapy. Clin Pharmacol Ther. 2019;106:94–102.
92. Dyar B, Meaddough E, Sarasua SM, Rogers C, Phelan K, Boccuto L. Genetic findings as the potential basis of personalized pharmacotherapy in Phelan-McDermid Syndrome. Genes. 2021;12(8):1192. https://doi.org/10.3390/genes12081192.
93. Serret S, Thümmler S, Dor E, Vesperini S, Santos A, Askenazy F. Lithium as a rescue therapy for regression and catatonia features in two SHANK3 patients with autism spectrum disorder: case reports. BMC Psychiatry. 2015;15:107. https://doi.org/10.1186/s12888-015-0490-1.
94. Egger JIM, Verhoeven WMA, Groenendijk-Reijenga R, Kant SG. Phelan-McDermid syndrome due to a SHANK3 mutation in an intellectually disabled adult male: successful treatment with lithium. BMJ Case Rep. 2017;2017:bcr-2017-220778.
95. Frank Y. The neurological manifestations of Phelan-McDermid Syndrome. Pediatr Neurol. 2021;122:59–64. https://doi.org/10.1016/j.pediatrneurol.2021.06.002.
96. Romano C, Dipasquale V, Rybak A, Comito D, Borrelli O. An overview of the clinical management of cyclic vomiting syndrome in childhood. Curr Med Res Opin. 2018;34(10):1785–91. https://doi.org/10.1080/03007995.2018.1445983.

Further Reading

Recommendations from the European Consensus Guideline in Phelan–McDermid syndrome:

van Ravenswaaij-Arts CMA, van Balkom IDC, Jesse S, Bonaglia MC. Editorial: towards a European consensus guideline for Phelan-McDermid syndrome. Eur J Med Genet. 2023;66(5):104736. https://doi.org/10.1016/j.ejmg.2023.104736.

PMS family foundations:

Phelan-McDermid Syndrome Foundation: https://pmsf.org/
Phelan-McDermid Asociacion Sindome: https://22q13.org.es

More information about past and previous clinical trials for PMS can be found by visiting:

https://www.clinicaltrials.gov/search?cond=Phelan-McDermid%20Syndrome

Smith–Lemli–Opitz Syndrome 14

Kelly K. Noah and Elaine Tierney

14.1 Overview of the Neurodevelopmental Disorder

Smith–Lemli–Opitz syndrome (SLOS, OMIM 270400) is an autosomal recessive disorder due to an inborn error of post-squalene cholesterol biosynthesis [1], caused by mutations in *DHCR7* (OMIM 602858) located on chromosome 11q12–13 [2–4]. The enzyme, 7-dehydrocholesterol reductase (DHCR7; EC 1.3.1.21; 3β-hydroxysterol Δ^7-reductase), reduces the Δ^7-double bond in 7-dehydrocholesterol (7DHC; cholesta-5,7-dien-3β-ol), the precursor molecule to cholesterol, via the Kandutsch-Russell pathway [5, 6]. A deficiency of DHCR7 activity experienced by individuals with SLOS often results in decreased levels of cholesterol and increased levels of 7DHC and its isomer, 8-dehydrocholesterol (8DHC; cholesta-5,8(9)-dien-3β-ol), in plasma and tissues [1, 7, 8] (Fig. 14.1).

The incidence of SLOS ranges from 1/20,000 [9, 10] to 1/60,000 [11, 12], varying among populations. Current SLOS carrier frequency estimates rank individuals of Ashkenazi Jewish descent (1 in 43) and Northern European descent (1 in 54) highest, while individuals of African or Asian descent are rarely identified. Prenatal demise may be a relatively common outcome, occurring in approximately 42% to 88% of affected conceptuses [13]. Smith–Lemli–Opitz syndrome is characterized by a wide and variable spectrum of phenotypic abnormalities, including intellectual disability and multiple congenital malformations. Physical clinical features of

K. K. Noah
Smith-Lemli-Opitz Foundation, Fargo, ND, USA
e-mail: knoah@smithlemliopitz.org

E. Tierney (✉)
Kennedy Krieger Institute, Baltimore, MD, USA

Department of Psychiatry and Behavioral Sciences, Johns Hopkins University School of Medicine, Baltimore, MD, USA
e-mail: tierney@kennedykrieger.org

R. P. Thom, C. J. McDougle (eds.), *Neuropsychiatric Care for Genetic Syndromes and Other Neurodevelopmental Disorders*,
https://doi.org/10.1007/978-3-031-76269-7_14

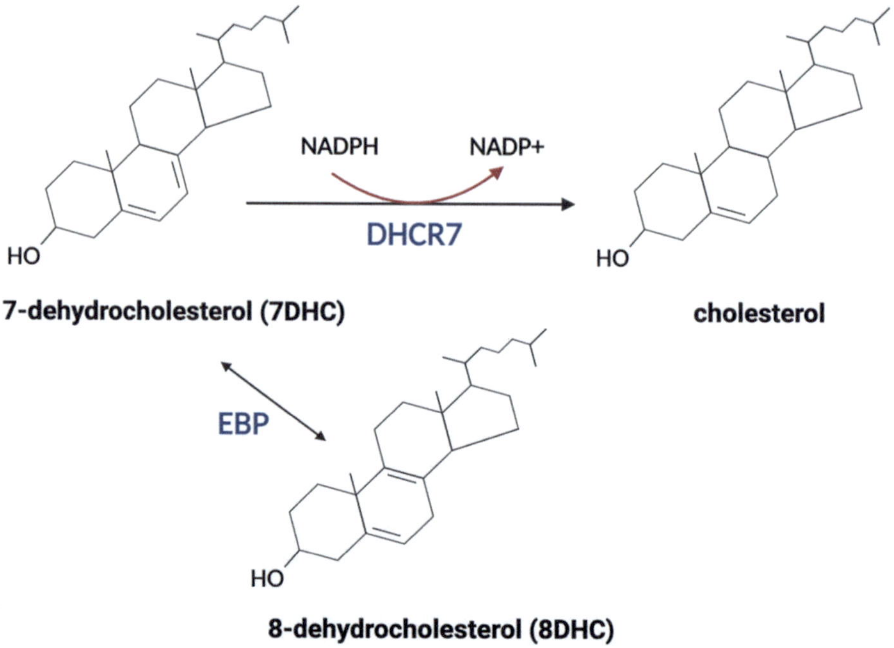

Fig. 14.1 Function of 7-dehydrocholesterol reductase (DHCR7). DHCR7 (EC 1.3.1.21; 3β-hydroxysterol Δ^7-reductase) catalyzes the final step in cholesterol biosynthesis by reducing 7-dehydrocholesterol (7DHC; cholesta-5,7-dien-3β-ol) to cholesterol. 7DHC isomerization to 8-dehydrocholesterol (8DHC; cholesta-5,8(9)-dien-3β-ol) occurs due to the functioning of emopamil-binding protein (EBP; EC 5.3.3.5; 3β-hydroxysterol-Δ^8,Δ^7-isomerase)

SLOS include distinct facial features (narrow forehead, epicanthal folds, ptosis, short nose, anteverted nares, and low-set and small ears); oral malformations (high-arched cleft palate, bifid uvula, and short mandible with preservation of jaw width); microcephaly, growth restriction, and limb anomalies (short, proximally placed thumbs, single palmar creases, postaxial polydactyly, clinodactyly, and 2–3 toe syndactyly); cardiovascular, pulmonary, renal, skeletal, and gastrointestinal anomalies; underdeveloped external genitalia in males; photosensitivity, and a variety of other structural defects. Individuals with SLOS may also experience impacts on the central nervous system, presenting with conditions including holoprosencephaly, agenesis or partial agenesis of the corpus callosum, and hypotonia [14, 15]. While syndactyly of the second and third toes is a normal variant, its presence in individuals in conjunction with other physical and behavioral features of SLOS (Table 14.1) should prompt consideration of a SLOS diagnosis [15].

Table 14.1 Clinical features of Smith–Lemli–Opitz syndrome

Physical features	Behavioral features
• Distinct facial features (narrow forehead, epicanthal folds, ptosis, short nose, anteverted nares, low-set and small ears) • Oral malformations (high-arched cleft palate or bifid uvula, and short mandible with preservation of jaw width) • Microcephaly • Growth restriction • Limb anomalies (short, proximally placed thumbs, single palmar creases, clinodactyly, postaxial polydactyly, and 2nd/3rd toe syndactyly) • Cardiovascular, pulmonary, renal, skeletal, and gastrointestinal anomalies • Underdeveloped external genitalia in males • Photosensitivity • Central nervous system anomalies (holoprosencephaly, agenesis or partial agenesis of the corpus callosum, and hypotonia)	• Autism spectrum disorder • Social impairment • Communication disorder • Intellectual disability • Repetitive and ritualistic behaviors • Self-injury • Opisthokinesis • Severe sleep disturbance • Attention-deficit/hyperactivity disorder • Sensory hyperreactivity • Anxiety

14.2 Signs and Symptoms of Common Psychiatric Comorbidities

Autism spectrum disorder (ASD) is frequently observed in SLOS and is associated with approximately 50–86% of cases [16–18]. In some instances, the rate of ASD clinical diagnosis appears to be artificially increased due to lower levels of cognitive function observed in many individuals with SLOS. The degree of gross neurologic pathology in SLOS is inversely correlated with cholesterol levels measured at birth. The ratio of 7DHC + 8DHC to cholesterol in both plasma and cerebrospinal fluid (CSF) was also significantly correlated with the SLOS anatomical severity score [16, 19]. The cognitive abilities of individuals with SLOS vary from no intellectual disability to profound intellectual disability [20–22]. Plasma cholesterol was positively correlated with IQ and Vineland Adaptive Behavior Scales-II (Vineland-II scores), while CSF cholesterol was not significantly correlated with the IQ or Vineland-II scores. In both plasma and CSF, 7DHC + 8DHC was significantly related to all IQ and Vineland-II scores [16].

Clinical features of behavior that are common in SLOS include intellectual disability, cognitive delay, sensory hyperreactivity, irritability, sleep difficulties, syndrome-specific motor movements, ASD, and self-injurious behavior. Individuals with SLOS can also experience significant language impairment [8, 23], with better receptive than expressive language abilities [24]. In a cohort of 49 subjects (age range 0.8–32.4 years; mean age of 8.2 ± 7.8 years) whose language functioning was captured on the MacArthur Communicative Development Inventory, 21 (43%) had an expressive language age below 8 months and 38 (78%) had an expressive language age of 30 months or less, with the individual showing substantially greater receptive than expressive abilities [17]. New social situations and changes in routine may be distressing to some individuals [25].

Overactivity [26, 27] and attention-deficit/hyperactivity disorder (ADHD) [28, 29] have been diagnosed in individuals with SLOS, with biochemically mild individuals having more severe overactivity and ADHD symptoms. Attention-deficit/hyperactivity disorder can present in the same manner as is observed in the typically developing population, with the degree of hyperactivity and inattention varying greatly from one individual to another. Males tend to have a higher activity level than females and extreme levels of activity have been observed (Tierney, unpublished clinical observation). Of 85 clinical electroencephalographs (EEGs) in 23 individuals with SLOS, 43 (51%) were abnormal, largely due to interictal epileptiform discharges (IEDs). While epileptiform discharges are common in SLOS, there is a relatively low prevalence of epilepsy and seizures. Fluctuations in the presence of IEDs may be associated with the variability in ADHD symptoms [30].

Self-injury and aggression can also commonly occur in SLOS. Self-biting occurs frequently and is most often at the wrists and thenar eminence. Tissue damage can be severe and occurs by biting through the skin, bruising, and breaking of the skin on the forehead due to self-injury. Ryan and colleagues reported that 8 (35%) of the study population ($n = 23$) displayed self-injurious behavior and 12 (52%) displayed aggressive behavior [12]. In another SLOS cohort ($n = 56$), 50 (89%) had a history of repeated self-injury, with 30 (54%) biting themselves (primarily on the wrist and thenar eminence of the thumb), 27 (48%) banging their heads on objects, and 30 (54%) exhibiting a syndrome-specific quick motor activity of backward-thrusting arching motion of the head and trunk ("opisthokinesis") that was most commonly observed in infancy and lessened with age. Sometimes this motion would result in self-injury [12, 17].

Affect dysregulation has also been noted in SLOS [23, 24] with individuals, starting in infancy, making a high-pitch cry that can last between hours to overnight for weeks at a time per parental reports [31]. The individuals have been described as being inconsolable [27] and hypersensitive to stimulation [32], although this primarily occurs during infancy and toddlerhood. Irritability is expressed at later stages with a sad affect, impatience, low frustration tolerance, inappropriate screaming, anxiety, and quick mood changes [33]. These behavioral aspects appear to be secondary to temperament that is present with most individuals with SLOS, rather than depressive or cyclical mood disorders.

Tactile [12, 23] and auditory hypersensitivity [23] have been reported in individuals with SLOS. Tierney and colleagues compared the sensory profile of 35 SLOS subjects (age range 3.2–32.4 years) to datasets from typical subjects. The SLOS subjects had greater auditory, oral, visual, and tactile processing difficulties that were greater than two standard deviations from the mean observed with a group of typical subjects. A group of 30 SLOS subjects demonstrated statistically greater difficulties with these behaviors compared to typical subjects, subjects with ADHD, Asperger's disorder, idiopathic ASD, and other developmental disorders [17]. These individuals tend to avoid walking on grass or sand barefoot [25].

Severe sleep cycle disturbances have been reported in individuals with SLOS [23]. Ryan and colleagues surveyed the parents of 23 individuals with SLOS and found that 70% reported abnormal sleeping patterns, including difficulties settling down or awakening during the night. Sedatives were ineffective in most reports [12]. Zarowski and colleagues had the parents of 18 individuals with SLOS (age range 2–31 years) complete questionnaires on sleep. The individuals with SLOS had symptoms of sleep-disordered breathing, including snoring (50%) and mouth breathing (67%). These are postulated to be exacerbated by the characteristic facial anomalies associated with SLOS [12, 15, 34]. Individuals with SLOS were also observed to suffer from problems with sleep onset, including difficulty falling asleep (61%) and sleep onset time >30 minutes (62%). Sleep maintenance issues such as waking up screaming (61%), waking up more than twice (44%), having trouble falling back to sleep (67%), waking up early in the morning (61%), and restless sleep (50%), were also reported. Sleep-time associated rituals [needing parents in the room to fall asleep (50%), watch TV or listen to music to fall asleep (44%), and bed sharing (33%)], sleep-anxiety, and symptoms of excessive daytime sleepiness [unrefreshed in the morning (39%), daytime sleepiness (44%), and daytime naps (56%)] were frequently reported [35]. Biochemical severity of SLOS was associated with decreased sleep duration and increased latency to sleep onset [36].

14.3 Assessment

Smith–Lemli–Opitz syndrome should be suspected in individuals with any of the clinical features mentioned previously (Table 14.1) [14, 15, 29]. Because specific testing and partial treatment with cholesterol supplementation for SLOS are available, the threshold should be low for obtaining a sterol analysis for SLOS in an individual with ASD and one physical or behavioral feature [29]. The distinct facial malformations of many individuals with SLOS can be viewed on the Smith–Lemli–Opitz Syndrome Foundation website https://www.smithlemliopitz.org/ [37]. The characteristic biochemical indicator of SLOS is an increase in 7DHC levels observed in plasma or tissues. This is confirmed by plasma sterol analysis, typically done utilizing gas-chromatography-mass spectroscopy (GC-MS) [19]. Ultraviolet (UV) spectroscopy, gas chromatography, time-of-flight mass spectrometry, particle-beam LC/MS, electrospray tandem MS, colorimetric assays, or UV absorbance are other analytical methods that can be utilized in the detection of 7DHC in plasma, amniotic fluid, or chorionic villus samples [15, 38]. Midgestational maternal urine testing to examine the concentrations of steroid markers can also be utilized in the prenatal diagnosis of SLOS [39]. Low cholesterol levels are not required for SLOS diagnosis, as approximately 10% of individuals with SLOS have been observed to have normal plasma cholesterol levels [40]. Additionally, the standard laboratory cholesterol test does not distinguish between cholesterol and 7DHC, potentially resulting in a normal "cholesterol" value due to the presence of dehydrocholesterol (DHC) in the sample. While elevations in 7DHC levels are relatively specific to SLOS, mild elevations can be observed in individuals treated with some psychiatric drugs, as well as conditions of upregulation of cholesterol biosynthesis such as cerebrotendinous xanthomatosis [15]. In these cases, 7DHC reductase enzymatic assay or sterol biosynthesis analysis in cultured cells can aid in diagnosis. *DHCR7* mutational analysis can also be utilized to confirm a diagnosis of SLOS or in equivocal biochemical cases [19, 41, 42]. A staged approach can be utilized to reduce the cost of mutational analysis, as the sequencing of exons 6–9 identifies approximately 85% of *DHCR7* mutations [15].

Behavioral assessments include checking for the presence of self-injury, aggression, and disruptive behavior, determining the amount of impairment and the safety risk of those behaviors, will be further discussed below in the psychosocial treatments section. Ideally, a referral should be made to a speech and language pathologist with a specialty in augmentative communication techniques if the individual has difficulty with functional communication. Speech pathologists with such expertise can work with behavioral psychologists to implement functional communication as part of the behavioral treatment. There should also ideally be an assessment for co-occurring psychiatric disorders and referral for further assessment and treatment as necessary. This treatment might include behavioral programming, cognitive behavioral therapy, and/or medication use.

14.4 Psychosocial Treatments

There should be an assessment of psychosocial stressors including physical and sexual abuse, bullying, parental stress, classroom or program structure, and family characteristics.

Challenging behaviors in individuals with SLOS include self-injurious behavior and major disruptive behavior. Due to their severity of intensity, frequency, and duration, these behaviors often result in tissue injury and family disruption. Treatments can be selected based upon the availability of services in the region as well as the nature of the behaviors.

Behavioral treatment approaches are often used in combination with psychiatric assessment and the use of psychotropic medications [43]. Applied behavioral analysis-based assessment is an approach to identify factors that are precipitating and maintaining behaviors (known as environmental contingencies). Sometimes these variables can be identified based upon careful interview and observation of the individual. However, others require a "functional analysis" during which there is a process of manipulating the environment to better understand antecedent and consequent events. Then a treatment for these behaviors is created by manipulating these environmental contingencies to bring about a desired behavioral change with positive reinforcement and/or behavioral extinction. Parent or caregiver training on how to implement behavioral treatment is key to the success of behavioral treatment. Social skills training can also be helpful, as well as exercise and relaxation techniques [44].

The inability of individuals with SLOS to express themselves verbally due to mixed receptive-expressive language disorder is often accompanied by behavioral difficulties that improve when additional means of communication are taught. The different forms of augmentative communication that can be used include sign or modified sign techniques, and physical tools such as picture boards and electronic devices that have picture icons for communication (either photos or drawings). Ideally, a behavioral specialist will work with the speech pathologist who has experience with augmentative communication techniques in order to identify which icons the patient will understand, and these can be incorporated into the behavioral program.

14.5 Biological Treatments

The treatment of SLOS has focused on enhancing cholesterol production and decreasing the accumulation of 7DHC and 8DHC precursor molecules, as both likely contribute to the pathogenesis of SLOS. Clinical goals include improving feeding, sleep, growth, development, and behaviors [45]. Primary therapeutic treatments have concentrated on dietary or other forms of cholesterol supplementation in individuals with SLOS. Providing cholesterol supplementation through either egg yolk or cholesterol suspension began in 1993 after the discovery of the metabolic etiology of the disorder [1, 8]. Cholesterol supplementation has been observed to increase plasma cholesterol levels [46–48] and lowers 7DHC and 8DHC levels in some individuals with SLOS [48, 49]. While the biochemical goals of increasing cholesterol and decreasing 7DHC and 8DHC are rational, two studies found no significant improvement in developmental progress after cholesterol supplementation was initiated [12, 50]. However, parents have reported decreased irritability [23, 26], happier affect [1, 23, 27, 51], decreased hyperactivity, improved attention [26], decreased self-injury [1, 12], and decreased aggression [12, 23], accompanied by decreases in temper outbursts, trichotillomania and tactile defensiveness [23]. With supplementation, individuals with SLOS have also been reported to be calmer [51] and more sociable [23]. Other improvements noted after cholesterol supplementation were increases in alertness and activity in subjects who were abnormally passive [1, 12], and improved sleep patterns [12]. From parental reports of 51 SLOS subjects on cholesterol supplementation, 38 (75%) parents reported that they felt their children's behavior and adjustment were better after beginning cholesterol supplementation [17]. Irons and colleagues demonstrated that antenatal supplementation of cholesterol by fetal intravenous and intraperitoneal transfusions of fresh frozen plasma increased levels of fetal cholesterol measured in cordocentesis samples. An increase in fetal erythrocyte cell mean corpuscular volume was also identified, indicating some urgency to the early detection of SLOS [52].

Statins have also been suggested for the treatment of SLOS. Simvastatin is a 3-hydroxy-3-methylglutaryl coenzyme A (HMG-CoA) reductase inhibitor that inhibits the cholesterol biosynthesis pathway prior to the enzymatic deficiency observed in SLOS, with a goal of decreasing levels of the potentially harmful precursors, 7DHC and 8DHC [53]. A double-blind placebo-controlled study of simvastatin in individuals with SLOS who were being treated with cholesterol supplementation compared outcomes to 7DHC levels and Aberrant Behavior Checklist-Community scale (ABC-C) irritability subscale scores [54]. The study showed that the individuals who received simvastatin had significantly lower plasma

7DHC levels and trended toward having a significant decrease in 7DHC CSF levels. The individuals treated with simvastatin also had a significant decrease in their irritability, as measured by the ABC-C. However, the potential benefit of treatment with simvastatin is outweighed by the potential adverse effects of the medication, as one of the individuals in the trial developed cataracts after the trial ended. The development of cataracts in SLOS is rare after infancy [55].

7DHC and its related oxysterols may contribute to SLOS pathogenesis, as they have been observed to exert cytotoxicity, reduce cell proliferation, and induce cell differentiation and gene transcript changes [56, 57]. In an animal model of SLOS, treatment with antioxidant supplementation led to dramatic protection from light-induced deleterious change [58]. In fibroblasts from individuals with SLOS, treatment with antioxidant supplements led to decreased levels of 7DHC-derived oxysterols [59]. In an unblinded clinical trial, supplementation with vitamin E (a strong antioxidant), corrected low-normal plasma levels and resulted in reduced aggression, self-injury, irritability, hyperactivity, inattention, repetitive behaviors, sleep disturbance, and skin photosensitivity or eczema in half of the subjects [60]. A clinical trial using cholesterol supplementation plus a mixture of vitamins and other compounds with antioxidant properties is currently ongoing. Outcome measures of the trial include electroretinograms, brainstem audiometry measurements, serum oxysterol levels, and clinical findings [61].

Bile acids are essential for the absorption and digestion of lipids and lipid-soluble compounds in the small intestine, as well as to regulate cholesterol homeostasis [62, 63]. Individuals with SLOS can exhibit reduced production of bile acids [64, 65], in turn, preventing dietary cholesterol from being absorbed properly. More mildly affected individuals have been observed to have normal bile acid synthesis [66]. Supplementation with cholic acid, a major bile acid made in the body that improves fat absorption, is currently under investigation for its potential beneficial effects on individuals with SLOS [67]. There is evidence that tauroursodeoxycholic acid (TUDCA), a taurine-conjugated bile acid with antioxidant, antiapoptotic and neuroprotective properties crosses the blood–brain barrier [68].

Gene therapy has been investigated in a mouse model of SLOS [69] as another potential treatment option, and surgical intervention may be necessary to correct some of the physical abnormalities associated with the disorder [70]. Micrognathia, palatal anomalies, and prominent incisors can cause difficulties in airway management, causing an increased risk for complications during anesthesia and perioperatively. Suctioning of gastric contents and the use of strict fasting guidelines can minimize postoperative risks of aspiration from gastroesophageal reflux, as it is commonly observed in individuals with SLOS [45].

14.6 Psychiatric Medication Treatment Strategy

Psychopharmacological intervention should be considered for individuals who have impairment in functioning in the home or school/residential setting and the clinician can choose a medication in the manner that one would if treating a child with typical development or another developmental disability. When addressing ADHD symptoms, a trial of one or more stimulants may be performed. Individuals with SLOS will have a higher chance of having side effects or not responding positively to stimulant medications, as is also seen in individuals with ASD. Also, many individuals with SLOS have difficulty with appetite and might not be able to tolerate any further decrease in appetite that can occur with stimulants. The alpha-adrenergic agonist medications, guanfacine and clonidine, tend to be well tolerated in individuals with SLOS and can improve sleep (which is usually impaired) as well as decrease ADHD symptoms, as will be further detailed below.

Individuals who have aggression or self-injury could be demonstrating these behaviors for a communicative function or to obtain attention independent of communication needs. However, due to the severity of the behaviors, pharmacologic intervention will often need to be used to keep the individual safe until additional services can be provided (if such services can even be located for the individual). Problem behaviors often include striking the head, which can result in cataract formation and retinal detachment, and aggression. Therefore, antipsychotic medication may need to be prescribed to maintain the safety of the individual with SLOS and/or the safety of family members and school/residential center staff. Individuals with SLOS tend to respond well to the use of risperidone (Tierney, unpublished clinical observation), which has US Food and Drug Administration (FDA) approval for the treatment of irritability in individuals with ASD [60]. Usually, the risperidone treatment side effect of increased appetite is helpful to individuals with SLOS.

However, when choosing which medication to use, the clinician should be aware that in the typical population and control cell lines, commonly used psychiatric medications have been shown to inhibit sterol biosynthesis by inhibiting DHCR7. Thus, the use of these medications increases 7DHC levels, which will give rise to a variety of oxysterol products, some of which are toxic, and therefore should be avoided, if possible, in individuals with SLOS. However, the benefit of the medication may outweigh the effects that result from the increase in 7DHC levels. These medications are listed below in approximate decreasing order of the tendency to increase 7DHC levels in control animals, control cells, or individuals without SLOS [71–74]. Importantly, the effect of many other psychotropic medications on 7DHC levels has not been tested:

- Antipsychotics: haloperidol, cariprazine, aripiprazole, and to lesser extents, brexpiprazole and risperidone (aripiprazole had a 30 times greater effect of increasing 7DHC levels than risperidone, while risperidone, clozapine, and olanzapine did not affect circulating 7DHC levels in a study of humans [73]).
- Antidepressants: nefazadone, trazodone, buspirone, bupropion, sertraline, nortriptyline, clomipramine, maprotiline, amitriptyline, desipramine, amoxapine, imipramine, mosapride, doxepin, and to a lesser extent fluoxetine (escitalopram and citalopram had no effect on circulating 7DHC levels in humans [73]).
- Beta-blockers: propranolol, metoprolol, nebivolol, and atenolol.

Animal model studies with some of these medications show decreased cholesterol biosynthesis and increased levels of 7DHC in the brain [56]. The antipsychotics clozapine and chlorpromazine have also been found to modulate the enzyme that is affected in SLOS [75] and maternal cariprazine exposure inhibited embryonic and postnatal brain cholesterol biosynthesis in the SLOS mouse model [76]. In addition, haloperidol, risperidone, and ziprasidone inhibited the production of cholesterol [77]. Lamotrigine had no effect on circulating 7DHC levels in humans [73]. Hydroxyzine, an antihistamine, decreased 7DHC levels in SLOS fibroblasts for unknown reasons (Korade, personal communication, 2023).

Individuals with SLOS have photosensitivity independent of psychotropic medications [78]. Photosensitivity with psychotropic medications can occur through phototoxicity and photoallergy [79]. 7DHC has been implicated in phototoxicity [80], so any psychotropic medication that has been reported to result in photosensitivity might be through the mechanism of increased 7DHC levels in the tissues. The following medications are additional compounds known to cause clinical photosensitivity in individuals who do not have SLOS:

- Antipsychotics: chlorpromazine, fluphenazine, perphenazine, thioridazine, chlorproethazine, flupenthixol, olanzapine, clozapine
- Antidepressants: imipramine, clomipramine, paroxetine, amitriptyline, fluvoxamine, phenelzine, venlafaxine
- Anxiolytics: alprazolam, chlordiazepoxide

For individuals who have SLOS and have responded well to an antipsychotic for the treatment of aggression and/or self-injury but have too much weight gain, there is no contraindication to adding metformin and the usual dosing is metformin 500 mg by mouth twice a day.

Individuals with ADHD symptoms have responded positively to stimulants [28] and to the alpha-adrenergic agonist medications, clonidine and guanfacine (Tierney unpublished observation). Therefore, stimulants, clonidine, and guanfacine can be considered first-line treatments if the individual has ADHD symptoms in the absence of significant self-injurious or other severe maladaptive behavior.

The FDA indication for extended-release guanfacine (Intuniv) for the treatment of ADHD in typically developing individuals is up to a dose of 0.12 mg/kg/day, with the dose being escalated by 1 mg/week. Individuals with SLOS often use the same daily doses of medication as children who do not have special needs, although as in typically developing children, low blood pressure, heart rate, or other side effects may prevent dose escalation. Immediate-release forms of guanfacine are typically dosed once or twice a day in children, with higher amounts of the medication given at a time to target ADHD behavior (morning dosing would help to address this) or sleep impairment (evening dosing would help to address this). If the individual can swallow a capsule whole, the extended-release form of guanfacine (Intuniv) can be administered 1 or 2 times a day. Clonidine and extended-release clonidine (Kapvay) can also be used to treat ADHD symptoms.

Sleep impairment can sometimes be lessened with the use of clonidine, guanfacine, or a combination of the two medications. The use of trazodone for the treatment of sleep impairment should be avoided as it has been shown to increase 7DHC levels [81].

14.7 Common Medical Comorbidities

Medical comorbidities to be considered are recurrent ear infections and pneumonia, partial or full retinal detachment, dental problems secondary to small jaw, swallowing dysfunction, slow gut motility [25], and sometimes Hirschsprung disease [82]. Hearing impairment was detected in 66% of individuals with SLOS, with hearing loss often being related to conduction deficits (such as ear infection or middle ear fluid accumulation), while profound sensorineural hearing loss is rarer [83].

Individuals with SLOS usually have difficulties with weight gain and failure to thrive occurs frequently. Newborns and infants often require tube feeding, which in some cases is permanent. Gastroesophageal reflux with gagging and vomiting is also common.

Hypotonia occurs in infancy but improves with age and may lead to hypertonia, contractures, and orthopedic complications in nonambulatory children that may require the use of splints and braces for feet, standing boards, walkers, wheelchairs, and scooters for individuals who are more severely biochemically impaired [25]. Adrenocortical insufficiency can occur and individuals who were more severely affected biochemically may require fresh frozen plasma and/or stress steroid therapy prior to surgery [84].

Key Points to Remember

- Test for SLOS in all individuals with ASD who have one behavioral or physical aspect.
- Choose medications that do not impair 7DHC production, if possible.
- Cholesterol supplementation is helpful for some individuals.
- Treatment with antioxidants may be helpful.
- Bile acid supplementation may be helpful.
- Clinicians specializing in treating individuals with SLOS can be reached via the Smith-Lemli-Opitz Foundation webpage.

References

1. Irons M, Elias ER, Salen G, Tint GS, Batta AK. Defective cholesterol biosynthesis in Smith-Lemli-Opitz syndrome. Lancet. 1993;341(8857):1414.

2. Fitzky BU, Witsch-Baumgartner M, Erdel M, et al. Mutations in the delta7-sterol reductase gene in patients with the Smith-Lemli-Opitz syndrome. Proc Natl Acad Sci USA. 1998;95(14):8181–6.
3. Wassif CA, Maslen C, Kachilele-Linjewile S, et al. Mutations in the human sterol delta7-reductase gene at 11q12-13 cause Smith-Lemli-Opitz syndrome. Am J Hum Genet. 1998;63(1):55–62.
4. Waterham HR, Wijburg FA, Hennekam RC, et al. Smith-Lemli-Opitz syndrome is caused by mutations in the 7-dehydrocholesterol reductase gene. Am J Hum Genet. 1998;63(2):329–38.
5. Mazein A, Watterson S, Hsieh WY, Griffiths WJ, Ghazal P. A comprehensive machine-readable view of the mammalian cholesterol biosynthesis pathway. Biochem Pharmacol. 2013;86(1):56–66.
6. Griffiths WJ, Abdel-Khalik J, Crick PJ, et al. Sterols and oxysterols in plasma from Smith-Lemli-Opitz syndrome patients. J Steroid Biochem Mol Biol. 2017;169:77–87.
7. Batta AK, Tint GS, Shefer S, Abuelo D, Salen G. Identification of 8-dehydrocholesterol (cholesta-5,8-dien-3 beta-ol) in patients with Smith-Lemli-Opitz syndrome. J Lipid Res. 1995;36(4):705–13.
8. Tint GS, Irons M, Elias ER, et al. Defective cholesterol biosynthesis associated with the Smith-Lemli-Opitz syndrome. N Engl J Med. 1994;330(2):107–13.
9. Opitz JM, Penchaszadeh VB, Holt MC, Spano LM, Smith VL. Smith-Lemli-Opitz (RSH) syndrome bibliography: 1964-1993. Am J Med Genet. 1994;50(4):339–43.
10. Nowaczyk MJ, McCaughey D, Whelan DT, Porter FD. Incidence of Smith-Lemli-Opitz syndrome in Ontario, Canada. Am J Med Genet. 2001;102(1):18–20.
11. Nowaczyk MJ, Zeesman S, Waye JS, Douketis JD. Incidence of Smith-Lemli-Opitz syndrome in Canada: results of three-year population surveillance. J Pediatr. 2004;145(4):530–5.
12. Ryan AK, Bartlett K, Clayton P, et al. Smith-Lemli-Opitz syndrome: a variable clinical and biochemical phenotype. J Med Genet. 1998;35(7):558–65.
13. Lazarin GA, Haque IS, Evans EA, Goldberg JD. Smith-Lemli-Opitz syndrome carrier frequency and estimates of in utero mortality rates. Prenat Diagn. 2017;37(4):350–5.
14. Nowaczyk MJ, Irons MB. Smith-Lemli-Opitz syndrome: phenotype, natural history, and epidemiology. Am J Med Genet C Semin Med Genet. 2012;160C(4):250–62.
15. Porter FD. Smith-Lemli-Opitz syndrome: pathogenesis, diagnosis and management. Eur J Hum Genet. 2008;16(5):535–41.
16. Thurm A, Tierney E, Farmer C, et al. Development, behavior, and biomarker characterization of Smith-Lemli-Opitz syndrome: an update. J Neurodev Disord. 2016;8:12.
17. Tierney E, Nwokoro NA, Porter FD, Freund LS, Ghuman JK, Kelley RI. Behavior phenotype in the RSH/Smith-Lemli-Opitz syndrome. Am J Med Genet. 2001;98(2):191–200.
18. Sikora DM, Pettit-Kekel K, Penfield J, Merkens LS, Steiner RD. The near universal presence of autism spectrum disorders in children with Smith-Lemli-Opitz syndrome. Am J Med Genet A. 2006;140(14):1511–8.
19. Kelley RI. Diagnosis of Smith-Lemli-Opitz syndrome by gas chromatography/mass spectrometry of 7-dehydrocholesterol in plasma, amniotic fluid and cultured skin fibroblasts. Clin Chim Acta. 1995;236(1):45–58.
20. Mueller C, Patel S, Irons M, et al. Normal cognition and behavior in a Smith-Lemli-Opitz syndrome patient who presented with Hirschsprung disease. Am J Med Genet A. 2003;123A(1):100–6.
21. Opitz JM, Zellweger H, Shannon WR, Ptacek LJ. The RSH syndrome. In: Bergsma D, editor. The first conference on the clinical delineation of birth defects part II: malformation syndromes. New York: The National Foundation-March of Dimes; 1969. p. 43–52.
22. Lowry RB, Yong SL. Borderline normal intelligence in the Smith-Lemli-Opitz (RSH) syndrome. Am J Med Genet. 1980;5(2):137–43.
23. Nwokoro NA, Mulvihill JJ. Cholesterol and bile acid replacement therapy in children and adults with Smith-Lemli-Opitz (SLO/RSH) syndrome. Am J Med Genet. 1997;68(3):315–21.

24. Kelley RI. Smith-Lemli-Opitz syndrome. In: Vinken PJ, Bruyn GW, editors. Handbook of clinical neurology. Neurodystrophies and neurolipidoses, vol. 66. Amsterdam: Elsevier; 1996. p. 581–97.
25. Nowaczk MJ, Tierney E. Smith-Lemli-Opitz syndrome. In: Griffiths DM, King R, editors. Demystifying genetic syndromes. Kingston, NY: National Association for the Dually Diagnosed Publishing; 2004. p. 207–23.
26. Elias ER, Irons M. Abnormal cholesterol metabolism in Smith-Lemli-Opitz syndrome. Curr Opin Pediatr. 1995;7(6):710–4.
27. Opitz JM. RSH (so-called Smith-Lemli-Opitz) syndrome. Curr Opin Pediatr. 1999;11(4):353–62.
28. Nowaczyk MJ, Whelan DT, Hill RE. Smith-Lemli-Opitz syndrome: phenotypic extreme with minimal clinical findings. Am J Med Genet. 1998;78(5):419–23.
29. Bukelis I, Porter FD, Zimmerman AW, Tierney E. Smith-Lemli-Opitz syndrome and autism spectrum disorder. Am J Psychiatry. 2007;164(11):1655–61.
30. Schreiber JM, Lanham DC, Trescher WH, et al. Variations in EEG discharges predict ADHD severity within individual Smith-Lemli-Opitz patients. Neurology. 2014;83(2):151–9.
31. Johnson VP. Smith-Lemli-Opitz syndrome: review and report of two affected siblings. Z Kinderheilkd. 1975;119(4):221–34.
32. Porter FD, Herman GE. Malformation syndromes caused by disorders of cholesterol synthesis. J Lipid Res. 2011;52(1):6–34.
33. Tierney E, Nwokoro NA, Kelley RI. Behavioral phenotype of RSH/Smith-Lemli-Opitz syndrome. Ment Retard Dev Disabil Res Rev. 2000;6(2):131–4.
34. Kelley RI, Hennekam RC. The Smith-Lemli-Opitz syndrome. J Med Genet. 2000;37(5):321–35.
35. Zarowski M, Vendrame M, Irons M, Kothare SV. Prevalence of sleep problems in Smith-Lemli-Opitz syndrome. Am J Med Genet A. 2011;155A(7):1558–62.
36. Freeman KA, Olufs E, Tudor M, Roullet JB, Steiner RD. A pilot study of the association of markers of cholesterol synthesis with disturbed sleep in Smith-Lemli-Opitz syndrome. J Dev Behav Pediatr. 2016;37(5):424–30.
37. Smith-Lemli-Opitz Syndrome Foundation, Fargo, ND. Available from: https://www.smithlemliopitz.org/
38. Xiong Q, Ruan B, Whitby FG, et al. A colorimetric assay for 7-dehydrocholesterol with potential application to screening for Smith-Lemli-Opitz syndrome. Chem Phys Lipids. 2002;115(1–2):1–15.
39. Shackleton CH, Roitman E, Kratz LE, Kelley RI. Midgestational maternal urine steroid markers of fetal Smith-Lemli-Opitz (SLO) syndrome (7-dehydrocholesterol 7-reductase deficiency). Steroids. 1999;64(7):446–52.
40. Nowaczyk MJ, Waye JS. The Smith-Lemli-Opitz syndrome: a novel metabolic way of understanding developmental biology, embryogenesis, and dysmorphology. Clin Genet. 2001;59(6):375–86.
41. Honda A, Tint GS, Salen G, et al. Sterol concentrations in cultured Smith-Lemli-Opitz syndrome skin fibroblasts: diagnosis of a biochemically atypical case of the syndrome. Am J Med Genet. 1997;68(3):282–7.
42. Honda M, Tint GS, Honda A, et al. Measurement of 3 beta-hydroxysteroid delta 7-reductase activity in cultured skin fibroblasts utilizing ergosterol as a substrate: a new method for the diagnosis of the Smith-Lemli-Opitz syndrome. J Lipid Res. 1996;37(11):2433–8.
43. Wachtel LE, Hagopian LP. Psychopharmacology and applied behavioral analysis: tandem treatment of severe problem behaviors in intellectual disability and a case series. Isr J Psychiatry Relat Sci. 2006;43(4):265–74.
44. Guinchat V, Cravero C, Lefevre-Utile J, Cohen D. Multidisciplinary treatment plan for challenging behaviors in neurodevelopmental disorders. Handb Clin Neurol. 2020;174:301–21.
45. Svoboda MD, Christie JM, Eroglu Y, Freeman KA, Steiner RD. Treatment of Smith-Lemli-Opitz syndrome and other sterol disorders. Am J Med Genet C Semin Med Genet. 2012;160C(4):285–94.

46. Chan YM, Merkens LS, Connor WE, et al. Effects of dietary cholesterol and simvastatin on cholesterol synthesis in Smith-Lemli-Opitz syndrome. Pediatr Res. 2009;65(6):681–5.
47. Elias ER, Irons MB, Hurley AD, Tint GS, Salen G. Clinical effects of cholesterol supplementation in six patients with the Smith-Lemli-Opitz syndrome (SLOS). Am J Med Genet. 1997;68(3):305–10.
48. Linck LM, Lin DS, Flavell D, Connor WE, Steiner RD. Cholesterol supplementation with egg yolk increases plasma cholesterol and decreases plasma 7-dehydrocholesterol in Smith-Lemli-Opitz syndrome. Am J Med Genet. 2000;93(5):360–5.
49. Pappu AS, Steiner RD, Connor SL, et al. Feedback inhibition of the cholesterol biosynthetic pathway in patients with Smith-Lemli-Opitz syndrome as demonstrated by urinary mevalonate excretion. J Lipid Res. 2002;43(10):1661–9.
50. Sikora DM, Ruggiero M, Petit-Kekel K, Merkens LS, Connor WE, Steiner RD. Cholesterol supplementation does not improve developmental progress in Smith-Lemli-Opitz syndrome. J Pediatr. 2004;144(6):783–91.
51. Pauli RM, Williams MS, Josephson KD, Tint GS. Smith-Lemli-Opitz syndrome: thirty-year follow-up of "S" of "RSH" syndrome. Am J Med Genet. 1997;68(3):260–2.
52. Irons MB, Nores J, Stewart TL, et al. Antenatal therapy of Smith-Lemli-Opitz syndrome. Fetal Diagn Ther. 1999;14(3):133–7.
53. Jira PE, Wevers RA, de Jong J, et al. Simvastatin: a new therapeutic approach for Smith-Lemli-Opitz syndrome. J Lipid Res. 2000;41(8):1339–46.
54. Aman MG, Singh NN, Stewart AW, Field CJ. The aberrant behavior checklist: a behavior rating scale for the assessment of treatment effects. Am J Ment Defic. 1985;89(5):485–91.
55. Wassif CA, Kratz L, Sparks SE, et al. A placebo-controlled trial of simvastatin therapy in Smith-Lemli-Opitz syndrome. Genet Med. 2017;19(3):297–305.
56. Korade Z, Xu L, Shelton R, Porter NA. Biological activities of 7-dehydrocholesterol-derived oxysterols: implications for Smith-Lemli-Opitz syndrome. J Lipid Res. 2010;51(11):3259–69.
57. Xu L, Korade Z, Rosado JDA, Liu W, Lamberson CR, Porter NA. An oxysterol biomarker for 7-dehydrocholesterol oxidation in cell/mouse models for Smith-Lemli-Opitz syndrome. J Lipid Res. 2011;52(6):1222–33.
58. Vaughan DK, Peachey NS, Richards MJ, Buchan B, Fliesler SJ. Light-induced exacerbation of retinal degeneration in a rat model of Smith-Lemli-Opitz syndrome. Exp Eye Res. 2006;82(3):496–504.
59. Korade Z, Xu L, Harrison FE, et al. Antioxidant supplementation ameliorates molecular deficits in Smith-Lemli-Opitz syndrome. Biol Psychiatry. 2014;75(3):215–22.
60. Koczok K, Horváth L, Korade Z, et al. Biochemical and clinical effects of vitamin E supplementation in Hungarian Smith-Lemli-Opitz syndrome patients. Biomol Ther. 2021;11(8):1228.
61. University of Colorado Denver. Cholesterol and antioxidant treatment in patients with Smith-Lemli-Opitz syndrome (SLOS). 2008. Available from: https://ClinicalTrials.gov/show/NCT01773278
62. Insull W Jr. Clinical utility of bile acid sequestrants in the treatment of dyslipidemia: a scientific review. South Med J. 2006;99(3):257–73.
63. Lefebvre P, Cariou B, Lien F, Kuipers F, Staels B. Role of bile acids and bile acid receptors in metabolic regulation. Physiol Rev. 2009;89(1):147–91.
64. Natowicz MR, Evans JE. Abnormal bile acids in the Smith-Lemli-Opitz syndrome. Am J Med Genet. 1994;50(4):364–7.
65. Honda A, Salen G, Shefer S, et al. Bile acid synthesis in the Smith-Lemli-Opitz syndrome: effects of dehydrocholesterols on cholesterol 7alpha-hydroxylase and 27-hydroxylase activities in rat liver. J Lipid Res. 1999;40(8):1520–8.
66. Steiner RD, Linck LM, Flavell DP, Lin DS, Connor WE. Sterol balance in the Smith-Lemli-Opitz syndrome: reduction in whole body cholesterol synthesis and normal bile acid production. J Lipid Res. 2000;41(9):1437–47.
67. University of Nebraska, University of Colorado Denver, Children's Hospital Medical Center, Cincinnati, University of Pittsburgh. Smith-Lemli-Opitz syndrome and cholic acid. 2021. Available from: https://ClinicalTrials.gov/show/NCT03720990

68. Rodrigues CM, Spellman SR, Sola S, et al. Neuroprotection by a bile acid in an acute stroke model in the rat. J Cereb Blood Flow Metab. 2002;22(4):463–71.
69. Pasta S, Akhile O, Tabron D, Ting F, Shackleton C, Watson G. Delivery of the 7-dehydrocholesterol reductase gene to the central nervous system using adeno-associated virus vector in a mouse model of Smith-Lemli-Opitz syndrome. Mol Genet Metab Rep. 2015;4:92–8.
70. Boland MR, Tatonetti NP. Investigation of 7-dehydrocholesterol reductase pathway to elucidate off-target prenatal effects of pharmaceuticals: a systematic review. Pharmacogenomics J. 2016;16(5):411–29.
71. Kim HY, Korade Z, Tallman KA, et al. Inhibitors of 7-dehydrocholesterol reductase: screening of a collection of pharmacologically active compounds in neuro2a cells. Chem Res Toxicol. 2016;29(5):892–900.
72. Korade Z, Tallman KA, Kim HH, et al. Dose-response effects of 7-dehydrocholesterol reductase inhibitors on sterol profiles and vesicular stomatitis virus replication. ACS Pharmacol Transl Sci. 2022;5(11):1086–96.
73. Korade Z, Liu W, Warren EB, Armstrong K, Porter NA, Konradi C. Effect of psychotropic drug treatment on sterol metabolism. Schizophr Res. 2017;187:74–81.
74. Hall P, Michels V, Gavrilov D, et al. Aripiprazole and trazodone cause elevations of 7-dehydrocholesterol in the absence of Smith-Lemli-Opitz syndrome. Mol Genet Metab. 2013;110(1–2):176–8.
75. Lauth M, Rohnalter V, Bergstrom A, Kooshesh M, Svenningsson P, Toftgard R. Antipsychotic drugs regulate hedgehog signaling by modulation of 7-dehydrocholesterol reductase levels. Mol Pharmacol. 2010;78(3):486–96.
76. Genaro-Mattos TC, Anderson A, Allen LB, et al. Maternal cariprazine exposure inhibits embryonic and postnatal brain cholesterol biosynthesis. Mol Psychiatry. 2020;25(11):2685–94.
77. Canfran-Duque A, Casado ME, Pastor O, et al. Atypical antipsychotics alter cholesterol and fatty acid metabolism in vitro. J Lipid Res. 2013;54(2):310–24.
78. Charman CR, Ryan A, Tyrrell RM, et al. Photosensitivity associated with the Smith-Lemli-Opitz syndrome. Br J Dermatol. 1998;138(5):885–8.
79. Drucker AM, Rosen CF. Drug-induced photosensitivity: culprit drugs, management and prevention. Drug Saf. 2011;34(10):821–37.
80. Babes A, Ciotu CI, Hoffmann T, et al. Photosensitization of TRPA1 and TRPV1 by 7-dehydrocholesterol: implications for the Smith-Lemli-Opitz syndrome. Pain. 2017;158(12):2475–86.
81. Korade Z, Allen LB, Anderson A, et al. Trazodone effects on developing brain. Transl Psychiatry. 2021;11(1):85.
82. Lipson A, Hayes A. Smith-Lemli-Opitz syndrome and Hirschsprung disease. J Pediatr. 1984;105(1):177.
83. Zalewski CK, Sydlowski SA, King KA, et al. Auditory phenotype of Smith-Lemli-Opitz syndrome. Am J Med Genet A. 2021;185(4):1131–41.
84. Bianconi SE, Conley SK, Keil MF, et al. Adrenal function in Smith-Lemli-Opitz syndrome. Am J Med Genet A. 2011;155A(11):2732–8.

Further Reading

Balog M, Anderson A, Genaro-Mattos TC, Korade Z, Mirnics K. Individual and simultaneous treatment with antipsychotic aripiprazole and antidepressant trazodone inhibit sterol biosynthesis in the adult brain. J Lipid Res. 2022;63(8):100249.

Freeman KA, Eagle R, Merkens LS, et al. Challenging behavior in Smith-Lemli-Opitz syndrome: initial test of biobehavioral influences. Cogn Behav Neurol. 2013;26(1):23–9.

Genaro-Mattos TC, Anderson A, Allen LB, Korade Z, Mirnics K. Altered cholesterol biosynthesis affects drug metabolism. ACS Omega. 2021;6(8):5490–8.

Guinchat V, Cravero C, Lefevre-Utile J, Cohen D. Multidisciplinary treatment plan for challenging behaviors in neurodevelopmental disorders. Handb Clin Neurol. 2020;174:301–21.

Korade Z, Heffer M, Mirnics K. Medication effects on developmental sterol biosynthesis. Mol Psychiatry. 2022;27(1):490–501.

McGuire K, Fung LK, Hagopian L, et al. Irritability and problem behavior in autism spectrum disorder: a practice pathway for pediatric primary care. Pediatrics. 2016;137(S2):e20152851L.

Newcomb ET, Hagopian LP. Treatment of severe problem behaviour in children with autism spectrum disorder and intellectual disabilities. Int Rev Psychiatry. 2018;30(1):96–109.

Thurm A, Tierney E, Farmer C, et al. Development, behavior, and biomarker characterization of Smith-Lemli-Opitz syndrome: an update. J Neurodev Disord. 2016;8:12.

Tierney E, Conley SK, Goodwin H, Porter FD. Analysis of short-term behavioral effects of dietary cholesterol supplementation in Smith-Lemli-Opitz syndrome. Am J Med Genet A. 2010;152A(1):91–5.

Tierney E, Nwokoro NA, Porter FD, Freund LS, Ghuman JK, Kelley RI. Behavior phenotype in the RSH/Smith-Lemli-Opitz syndrome. Am J Med Genet. 2001;98(2):191–200.

Smith–Magenis Syndrome

15

Diane Treadwell-Deering, Kevin Kaplan, and Lorraine Potocki

15.1 Overview: Epidemiology, Genetic Mechanism, Common Clinical Features

The clinical features now ascribed to the eponymous Smith–Magenis syndrome (SMS) were first associated with an interstitial deletion of the short arm of chromosome 17 in 1982 [1–3]. The molecular mechanism of the SMS chromosomal deletion—non-allelic homologous recombination between flanking repeat gene clusters—was first elucidated over a decade later [4] and proved to be applicable to other common microdeletion and microduplication syndromes [5]. The prevalence of SMS was estimated to be 1 in 25,000 births based on ascertainment data published prior to the implementation of array comparative genomic hybridization (aCGH) [6]; however, more recent estimates suggest a prevalence of 1 in 15,000 [7], owing at least in part to the increased detection of the SMS microdeletion by chromosome microarray analysis (CMA). Another factor is the increased identification of persons with SMS who do not harbor a chromosomal deletion, but who have a pathogenic variant in the dosage-sensitive *RAI1* gene—haploinsufficiency of which is now regarded as the primary driver of the SMS phenotype [8–10]. It is currently estimated that ~5–10% of persons with SMS have pathogenic variants in *RAI1*, detected not by CMA but only by multi-gene panel, genomic sequencing, or gene-targeted deletion/ duplication analysis [11]. In the vast majority of patients, the

D. Treadwell-Deering · K. Kaplan · L. Potocki (✉)
Department of Developmental Pediatrics, Baylor College of Medicine and Texas Children's Hospital, Houston, TX, USA

Department of Sleep Medicine, Baylor College of Medicine and Texas Children's Hospital, Houston, TX, USA

Department of Molecular and Human Genetics, Baylor College of Medicine and Texas Children's Hospital, Houston, TX, USA
e-mail: lpotocki@bcm.edu

R. P. Thom, C. J. McDougle (eds.), *Neuropsychiatric Care for Genetic Syndromes and Other Neurodevelopmental Disorders*,
https://doi.org/10.1007/978-3-031-76269-7_15

microdeletion or *RAI1* variant occurs de novo, though transmission from a mosaic parent has been reported [12].

Clinical features of SMS span multiple organ systems and are variable amongst patients (Table 15.1). Common features that lead to diagnostic testing include infantile hypotonia, global developmental delay, cardiovascular malformations (e.g., septal defects, tetralogy of Fallot), renal and genitourinary anomalies, and dysmorphic craniofacial features (Fig. 15.1). Infants with SMS may have failure to thrive due to hypotonia and oropharyngeal dysphagia, and are typically described as good sleepers. Developmental delay is recognized during infancy with delays in gross motor skills and speech acquisition. Medical concerns such as recurrent otitis media, hearing impairment (conductive, sensorineural, or mixed), and sleep disturbances (frequent nocturnal awakening, excessive daytime sleepiness) emerge in the toddler years. Myopia and short stature may not be recognized until early childhood, though some patients present by 2–3 years of age. Hypercholesterolemia is identified in ~50% of children with SMS [13]. Obesity, which is observed in the majority of patients, typically manifests by late childhood and is often associated with other health issues such as hypercholesterolemia and type 2 diabetes, as well as cardiovascular disease. Scoliosis is present in ~60% of patients and sometimes requires surgical intervention, yet may not be a concern until late childhood or early adolescence. Seizures, while observed in fewer than 20% of patients may not present until adulthood; however, generalized epileptiform patterns were evident in 73% of patients who were systematically evaluated [14, 15]. If the diagnosis of SMS is not suspected based on the physical features and congenital anomalies, it will likely be recognized by the striking neurobehavioral phenotype that includes an array of challenging and disruptive behaviors.

While many of the clinical features observed in SMS were described in case reports and small case series, the first multidisciplinary clinical study of SMS was reported in 1996 [16] and detailed the craniofacial features (Fig. 15.1) and cardinal signs of SMS that are currently recognized (Table 15.1). Subsequent clinical and molecular characterization of patients with SMS determined that despite a common-sized deletion in ~75% of patients, phenotypic variability amongst patients is the rule rather than the exception [17]. Individuals who harbor variants in *RAI1* exhibit the common craniofacial and skeletal appearance, sleep disturbances, and neurobehavioral abnormalities, yet are less likely to have the structural organ system anomalies that are common to those with the 17p11.2 microdeletion [18].

Table 15.1 Clinical features of Smith–Magenis syndrome

Neurologic
• Infantile hypotonia
• Features of peripheral neuropathy
– Hyporeflexia
– Insensitivity to pain
– Decreased muscle mass
• Seizures
Sleep
• Circadian rhythm disorders
• Excessive daytime sleepiness
• Insomnia
• Obstructive sleep apnea
Neurobehavioral
• Developmental delay
• Intellectual disability
• Autism spectrum disorder
• Attention-deficit/hyperactivity disorder
• Self-injurious behavior
• Aggression
• Attention seeking
Ophthalmologic
• Myopia, high myopia (retinal detachment)
• Strabismus
• Microcornea
Otolaryngologic
• Hearing impairment
• Palatal cleft/Velopharygeal insufficiency
• Recurrent/chronic otitis media
• Hoarse, deep voice
• Oral-pharyngeal dysphagia
Organ system anomalies
• Cardiovascular anomalies (tetralogy of Fallot, VSD, ASD)
• Structural renal and GU anomalies
Endocrine
• Hypothyroidism
• Obesity
Gastrointestinal
• Reflux
• Chronic constipation
Other
• Hyperlipidemia
• Immunoglobulin A deficiency
Skeletal
• Short stature
• Brachycephaly
• Midface retrusion
• Prognathism (adulthood)
• Brachydactyly
• Scoliosis

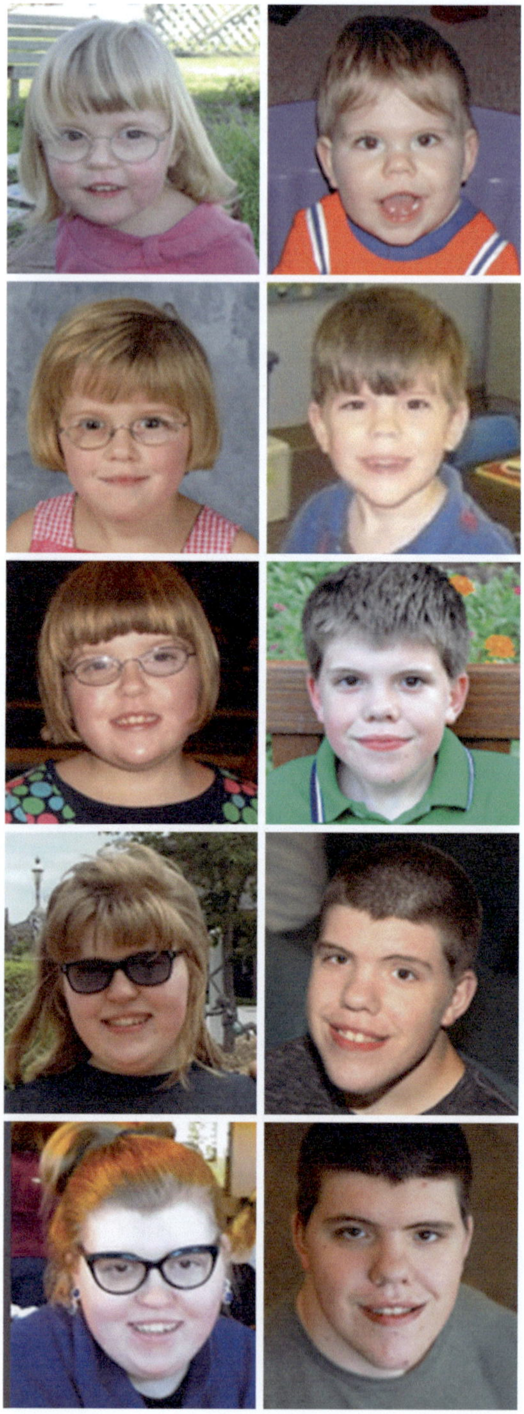

Fig. 15.1 Craniofacial features in SMS. Female (F) and Male (M) individuals at various ages, in years (F: 3.5, 5, 9, 15, 21; M: 2.5, 5, 11, 13, 19). Common features include brachycephaly, synophyrs, full cheeks (most notable in infants and young children), tented upper lip/down-turned mouth, prognathia (in teens and adults)

15.2 Behavior Associated with SMS

Parents of offspring with SMS frequently cite the behavior symptoms associated with the disorder as the most challenging aspect of their child's care [19, 20]. Smith–Magenis syndrome is characterized by several maladaptive behaviors, including stereotypic behavior, self-injurious behavior, aggression toward others, property destruction, non-compliance, temper outbursts, sensory avoidance and seeking, and abnormal eating behaviors.

Although many of these challenging behaviors are seen in other neurodevelopmental disorders, there are some characteristics specific to SMS. Overall, the onset of behavioral symptoms occurs at 18–24 months, which is substantially earlier than in many other neurodevelopmental disorders [14, 19, 21]. The severity of maladaptive behaviors is also greater in SMS patients compared to a reference sample of individuals with heterogeneous intellectual disabilities [19, 20]. This may be due to the high reports of depression and anxiety in parents of SMS individuals. When compared to parents of children with Down syndrome, SMS parents had greater pessimism and more reported family problems [22]. The level of pessimism was correlated with the level of the child's behavioral concerns.

Individuals with SMS frequently demonstrate developmental asynchrony, that is, their emotional maturity is delayed beyond what would be predicted by their level of intellectual functioning. This gap widens as the individual ages and is more prominent in individuals with higher cognitive skills [23]. Social impairment was found in 90% of SMS patients, as measured by the Social Responsiveness Scale (SRS) [21], with more than half of the subjects scoring in the severe range of impairment. Clinicians and educators can easily underestimate the stresses experienced by family members. Adults with SMS often do not perform adaptive life skills such as personal hygiene and activities of daily living independently.

Patients with SMS are described as attention-seeking, which is reported as a problematic behavior by 80% of parent informants [24]. Patients are described as having an unrelenting need for individualized adult attention, with little to no regard for their peers. If there is limited availability for attention, aggressive behavior often ensues. The nature of this dynamic is different from other neurodevelopmental disorders, such as Angelman syndrome with prosocial, friendly attention-seeking or William syndrome with prolonged face-looking directed to adults and peers. Aggressive behaviors include verbal aggression/meanness, hitting, biting, head-butting, and property destruction. Parents of female SMS patients report more behavior problems than parents of male patients [22].

Stereotypic behaviors have been reported in 95% of SMS patients [23], including both self-injurious and less noxious behaviors. Most notably, polyembolokoilamania (inserting foreign bodies into body orifices) occurs in 32% of patients [6, 23], while onychotillomania (yanking out finger- and toenails) occurs in 54% of patients [6, 14, 23]. These behaviors are considered unique to SMS. Other behaviors highly associated with SMS include skin-picking (65%), "self-hugs" (51%), and "lick and flip" (46%) [14, 23, 25]. Self-hugs are specific, spasmodic upper body squeezes; "lick and flip" refers to repetitively licking one's fingers and turning pages [14, 25].

Other stereotypies frequently reported include mouthing objects, teeth grinding, body rocking, spinning or twirling objects, and rubbing surfaces. Other repetitive self-injurious behaviors include self-hitting, self-biting, and self-pinching. Self-injurious behaviors have an earlier age of onset than observed in other neurodevelopmental disorders and are comparable to those reported in Lesch Nyhan syndrome [19].

Sensory issues similar to those observed in ASD are frequently reported. Patients demonstrate both sensory-seeking and sensory-avoidant behaviors, relating to textures, sounds, pressure, and smell. Many demonstrate apparent decreased sensitivity to pain. Rather than complaining of pain, medical issues such as constipation, ear infections, and dental caries or abscesses are often heralded by acute increases in behavior problems.

Disordered eating is directly mediated by *RAI1* haploinsufficiency [23]. After early failure to thrive, elementary school-aged children overeat and forage for food. Ninety percent of children with SMS are overweight or obese by age 10 years [19]. Early and strict management of food intake is crucial to preventing or managing weight issues.

The degree of sleep disturbance is one of the strongest predictors of maladaptive behaviors [14, 19], although impulsivity and anxiety related to change also play significant roles [19]. Garayzabal and colleagues [26] showed positive correlations between multiple categories of sleep problems on the Sleep Disturbance Scale for Children and externalizing behaviors on the Child Behavior Checklist (CBCL) in children with SMS. The severity of sleep disturbance was correlated with the severity of behavior problems. De Leersnyder [27] indicated that behavioral problems diminished when sleep disorders were successfully treated.

15.3 Disordered Sleep in Smith–Magenis Syndrome

The majority of patients with SMS or their caregivers report sleep disturbances [26]. It has been reported that 65–100% of children with SMS experience one or more sleep disorders [7]. Patients typically have difficulty with frequent nocturnal arousals, early morning awakenings, and excessive daytime sleepiness [28]. Alteration of the *RAI1* gene causes dysregulation of several genes responsible for the maintenance of the circadian rhythm including *CLOCK*, *PER1*, *PER2*, and *BMALI1* [29, 30]. One of the best-described consequences of circadian rhythm dysregulation is a chronological inversion of the melatonin pathway in patients with SMS [31] including those with pathogenic variants in *RAI1* [9]. The alteration of the melatonin pathway can only partially explain the sleep disturbances experienced by these patients. However, understanding sleep drive is important to treating the sleep disruptions experienced by this patient population.

Infants with SMS often are reported to sleep well at night by their caregivers. The children will often need to be woken for feeds initially after birth. However, infants with SMS are noted to have a reduction in total sleep time when compared to typically developing peers. Sleep problems often start to arise in early childhood. Typically, children with SMS will wake more often during the night and remain awake for at least 30 min. Early morning awakenings also begin to occur in young children with SMS [32]. Children with SMS generally snore, have difficulty with nocturnal enuresis, and start to exhibit symptoms of daytime sleepiness. In older children and adolescents, difficulty initiating sleep becomes an additional concern. Adolescents often have shortened nighttime sleep duration with an increase in daytime sleep occurring in short, but frequent nap periods. These naps are often described as "sleep attacks" and are difficult to prevent in SMS patients. Often caregivers report that the nocturnal awakenings become less of a burden in the adolescent and teenage years. This pattern of difficulty initiating sleep, early morning awakenings, and sleep attacks often persists through adulthood in SMS patients [33].

Patients with SMS very frequently have obesity as part of their clinical presentation [14]. Obesity is a common risk factor for obstructive sleep apnea (OSA) in both adult and pediatric patients. The pathophysiology of obesity leading to OSA is due to fat deposition in the pharyngeal soft tissue as well as in the thoracic and abdominal walls, all of which contribute to airway collapse [34, 35]. Obstructive sleep apnea can contribute to symptoms of daytime sleepiness, restless sleep, and frequent nocturnal awakenings. As many of the sleep disturbances noted in SMS and OSA can overlap, identifying the correct etiology is important for management.

15.4 Psychiatric Comorbidities: Signs and Symptoms

15.4.1 Attention-Deficit/Hyperactivity Disorder

Before current genetic technology allowed for more rapid diagnosis of SMS, these children were often diagnosed with ASD or attention-deficit/hyperactivity disorder (ADHD) [23]. Symptoms of executive functioning deficits, inattention, distractibility, hyperactivity, and impulsivity often warrant a comorbid diagnosis of ADHD. More than 75% of individuals with SMS demonstrate symptoms of inattention and sometimes also hyperactivity [14].

15.4.2 Developmental Delay

Developmental delay occurs in virtually all patients with SMS. Ambulation occurs at 20–25 months on average. Two-thirds of patients speak their first words by 3 years of age. Daytime toilet training occurs in 78% of children by age 13 years, while nocturnal toilet training is accomplished by 35% of patients at this age. The degree of intellectual disability (ID) ranges from borderline to profound, with the vast majority functioning at the moderate range of intellectual impairment [23]. Cognitively, short-term memory, sequential processing, and math skills are particularly weak. Furthermore, academic performance is negatively impacted by symptoms of hyperactivity, impulsivity and inattention, as well as maladaptive behaviors.

15.4.3 Autism Spectrum Disorder

Fifty to 75% of SMS individuals have features of or meet full diagnostic criteria for ASD [14]. Autism spectrum disorder symptoms appear to be more prominent in female patients [23, 36, 37]. Laje and colleagues [37] found that 90% of their subjects were in the ASD range on the SRS, a 65-item parent questionnaire. Slightly over half were above the autism cut-off on the Social Communication Questionnaire (SCQ). Other authors [38, 39] also found a high association of ASD with SMS based on the Childhood Autism Rating Scales (CARS®).

15.4.4 Anxiety and Mood Disorders

Though less well-described, adolescents and adults with SMS are frequently described as anxious and/or report anxiety, which may meet the criteria for generalized or social anxiety disorders. Parents often report behaviors such as motor mannerisms, pacing, and nail-biting as signs of anxiety in this patient population. However, this comorbidity can be difficult to delineate in the context of comorbid ID and/or ASD. Families may report rapid mood shifts in SMS individuals, for example anger when the patient loses the full attention of adults, but there is little data on the true prevalence of co-occurring mood disorders.

15.5 Assessment: Genetic Testing, Neurobehavioral Analyses, and Objective Measures of Sleep Disturbances

The first-line genetic test for any child or adult with neurodevelopmental and/or clinical features reminiscent of SMS is a CMA, which will detect 100% of the deletions involving the *RAI1* gene. This clinically available laboratory test will not, however, detect single nucleotide variants or many intragenic deletions of *RAI1*; thus, if the diagnosis of SMS is suspected and the CMA is normal or non-diagnostic, further testing is indicated. Single gene testing for pathogenic variants in *RAI1* is available, though a multi-gene panel or exome sequencing offers the advantage of analysis of other genes, variants of which may be associated with features that are observed in SMS. Table 15.2 lists the clinical studies that are recommended at the time of diagnosis and subsequently for medical management. Additionally, clinical assessments for features of Birt-Hogg-Dube syndrome (BHD) are indicated for individuals who harbor a 17p11.2 deletion that encompasses the *FLCN* gene [40]. Features of BHD have been described in several individuals with SMS; however, the risk of cancer in SMS is not increased as compared to the general population [14]. Recommendations related to BHD are to commence in late adolescence or early adulthood or if concerns arise and include dermatologic examination for papules with biopsy of suspicious lesions, chest X-ray and chest computed tomography (CT) in persons with pneumothorax or concerning pulmonary symptoms, and

Table 15.2 Clinical studies

	Initial study/evaluation	Subsequent study/ evaluation
Diagnostic imaging		
CNS imaging	As indicated for seizures, or focal neurologic concern	As indicated
Echocardiogram/ECG	At diagnosis	As indicated
Renal ultrasound	At diagnosis	As indicated
Voiding cysto-urethrogram	As indicated for GU anomalies/UTI	As indicated
Scoliosis survey	As indicated for scoliosis	As indicated
Laboratory studies		
Thyroid function studies	At diagnosis	Annually
Quantitative immunoglobulins	At diagnosis	As indicated
Fasting lipid profile	At diagnosis or at age 4 years	Annually or as indicated
Clinical assessments		
Neurocognitive assessment	At diagnosis	Every 3 years
Autism assessment	As indicated	As indicated
Neurobehavioral rating scales	At diagnosis	Annually
Sleep study	At diagnosis	As indicated
Ophthalmologic	At diagnosis	At least annually
Audiologic	At diagnosis	Pending results and speech
Otolaryngologic	At diagnosis	As indicated
Swallow function study	As indicated	As indicated

abdominal MRI to assess for renal tumors beginning at age 21 years. At this time, there is no consensus on clinical surveillance in BHD syndrome [40].

The assessment of sleep disturbances should begin with a thorough clinical history. The sleep pattern and routine should be elicited as this can further delineate diagnostic decision-making. If daytime sleepiness or sleep fragmentation during the night is reported, then a polysomnogram is recommended. The sleep study will ensure that sleep-disordered breathing is not contributing to the patient's sleep disruptions. Outpatient actigraphy documents sleep occurrence and duration. This information may be useful for monitoring the benefit of medications and behavioral sleep interventions.

The assessment of behavioral difficulties is typically clinical; however, the use of parent- and teacher-rating scales, such as the Behavior Assessment System for Children, Third Edition (BASC™-3) may be useful in establishing the baseline severity and frequency of behaviors and in monitoring changes in behaviors during intervention trials. The Aberrant Behavior Checklist-second Edition (ABC-2) is specifically designed to assess problem behaviors of children and adults with developmental disabilities in a variety of settings. Condition-specific instruments, such as the Childhood Autism Rating Scale, Second Edition (CARS™-2ST) or the Autism Spectrum Rating Scales (ASRS®) and assessment tools, such as the Autism Diagnostic Observation

Schedule ™, Second Edition (ADOS®-2) may be used as part of an assessment for ASD. Rating scales for ADHD and/or anxiety may not be valid in patients with neurodevelopmental disabilities such as SMS and should be used with caution.

Intellectual disability is diagnosed based on individually administered, validated measures of intellectual and adaptive functioning. School systems provide this testing through special education programs designed to meet the parameters of the Individuals with Disabilities Education Act (IDEA), as federal law in the United States guarantees free and appropriate education to children with developmental disabilities. However, the quality of these services is highly variable, and families frequently need support to advocate for appropriate assessments and educational programming. All children with SMS qualify for special education services either based on the genetic diagnosis or as soon as developmental delay is apparent.

15.6 Psychosocial Treatments

15.6.1 Management of Maladaptive Behaviors

Ideally, a comprehensive behavior support plan for home and school should be established and implemented by early elementary school. This requires the input of family, school staff, the community therapy team, the medical team (e.g., developmental pediatrician, clinical psychologist, sleep specialist, etc.), and behavioral therapists. Areas covered may vary based on the individual's presentation but may include attention-seeking behavior, oppositionality, emotional lability, self-harm and aggression toward others, sleep, feeding, and activities of daily living. Consistency across settings is very valuable to the child and family. Considering the child's need for individualized attention, possible accommodations for sleep needs, the benefits of consistent routines, and clear expectations for the child's behavior must be incorporated into every aspect of the plan. Identification and avoidance of triggers are more effective than consequence-based behavior modification approaches, especially regarding self-injury and aggression [21]. Common triggers for challenging behaviors in SMS include losing the full attention of adults, being told "no," and being prevented from engaging in preferred interests. Triggers can be highly individualistic and should be determined through careful observation. Importantly, adapting the environment to avoid triggers and protect the child are a mainstay of intervention [22], as this approach is generally more helpful than consequence-based behavioral modification. Special needs safety beds, specialized restraints in cars, locks, and alarms in the home and other locations may need to be installed. Caretakers, therapists, and teachers need to learn to dampen and extinguish emotional responses to maladaptive behaviors. It is easy to underestimate the level of support the family needs. Respite care is especially welcomed by parents and siblings. Examples include "Parents Night Out" programs and "Creative Writing" activities sponsored by healthcare providers, trainees, and students, as well as family involvement in educational activities for medical and/or genetic counseling students (Potocki, personal communication).

15.6.2 Management of Developmental Delay and Eating Behaviors

Federal law in the United States (IDEA and the Americans with Disabilities Act [ADA]) protects and delineates the rights of SMS individuals in obtaining public special education and supports adults with developmental disabilities.

Psychosocial interventions with regard to abnormal eating center on minimizing weight gain with early and consistent dietary regulation and environmental control of access to food. This may require the entire family to alter their dietary habits, as hiding and/or locking food may not be successful. Patients with SMS may sneak food in the middle of the night or even enter others' homes to eat. High-calorie foods, snack items, and visits to fast food restaurants need to be tightly controlled. Food should not be used as a reward or motivator in any setting. The family may need to collaborate with school staff and behavior therapists to consistently control access to food. Finally, although problematic eating behaviors are a common challenge in SMS, they are not the root cause of all of the behavioral issues.

15.6.3 Management of Sleep Disturbances

Sleep is driven by a variety of behavioral influences. Importantly, behavioral modifications have been shown to be as effective in treating insomnia symptoms as pharmacotherapy in the general population [41]. When focusing on optimizing sleep, experts often start with modifying sleep habits. These recommendations often include maintaining a regular bed and wake time, utilizing the bedroom only for sleep, ensuring a quiet and dark space, ensuring a comfortable sleeping temperature, avoiding bright lights prior to bed, not eating a large meal before bed, exercising regularly, avoiding caffeine in the late afternoon or evenings, and limiting alcohol and excessive fluid intake before bed [42]. Once the sleep routine and behaviors have been optimized, screening for other sleep comorbidities common in patients with SMS is important.

15.7 Biological Treatments for Behavioral Symptoms

There is limited to no research on biological treatments of the behavioral symptoms accompanying SMS. There are no published clinical trials of psychotropic medications with children or adults with SMS [21]. The practitioner caring for these patients must rely on guidelines or best practices for broader indications, such as ASD, ID, or other neurodevelopmental disorders. A small handful of case reports on psychopharmacology in SMS have been published. A case report [43] demonstrated significantly improved aggression and impulsivity in a 12-year-old boy treated with risperidone at a maximum dose of 3 mg daily, after failed trials of paroxetine, carbamazepine, and methylphenidate. Another case report [44] described significant improvement in inattention, impulsivity, and disruptive behavior in a 10-year-old girl treated with a combination of risperidone and extended-release methylphenidate after failed trials of other stimulants, an alpha-$_2$ agonist, another second-generation antipsychotic, and melatonin. Finally, a letter to the editor [45] reported a case of a 4-year-old girl with severe sleep and behavior issues with multiple failed trials of psychotropic medications with and without parent–child interaction therapy (PCIT), highlighting the lack of evidence-based successful treatments for individuals with SMS.

A 2010 retrospective report of psychotropic medication use in 73 individuals was obtained utilizing the natural history of SMS National Institutes of Health (NIH) study [37]. Sixteen participants had never taken any psychotropic medications. Eleven were on sleep agents only. Forty-six participants had used one or more psychotropic medications. Psychotropic medication use started early; sleep medications were used at a mean age of 4.1 years; stimulants and alpha-$_2$ agonists were introduced at a mean age of 7.35 years; and mood stabilizers and anti-psychotics were begun at a mean age of 9.6 years. Polypharmacy was frequent. Most importantly, none of the medication categories showed meaningful improvement in behavior, according to the parents' report.

Müller and colleagues [46] have reported their intention to conduct a series of N-of-1 trials to collect information about the effectiveness of methylphenidate in youngsters with SMS. This approach is appropriate in subjects with rare conditions and for agents with rapid onset and offset of action (e.g., stimulant medications), but may not be so easily applied to other medications.

The lack of evidence to support the use of medication in the management of behaviors associated with SMS does not preclude careful, case-by-case consideration of medication trials to target symptoms with the goals of improving function, relieving distress, and improving the quality of life for the youngster and their family. The judicious use of medications to target symptoms of hyperactivity, impulsivity and inattention, anxiety or aggressive and self-injurious behaviors is warranted. However, the adverse effects on sleep and/or appetite may preclude the use of potentially beneficial agents.

15.8 Biological Treatments for Sleep Disorders

Circadian rhythms are a biological drive that regulates physical, mental, and behavioral processes. Human circadian rhythms need input from our environment, most importantly light, to function properly. Light levels impact our neural anatomy to regulate our internal clock. The photoperception of decreasing light levels allows for the proper release of endogenous melatonin influencing our sleep drive. In patients with a disrupted melatonin pathway, such as in patients with non-24 circadian rhythm disorder or SMS, the subject's circadian rhythm becomes dysfunctional.

Treatment strategies for the sleep disturbances in SMS have sought to correct the melatonin inversion. This can involve melatonin agonists such as over-the-counter melatonin supplements or prescription-based melatonin agonists. Commonly reported side effects of melatonin include nightmares and headaches. More rare side effects include nausea, dizziness, or mood changes. Tasimelteon is currently the only medication approved by the Food and Drug Administration (FDA) for the treatment of sleep disturbances in SMS. Twenty-five patients with SMS were treated with tasimelteon or placebo and tasimelteon was associated with improved sleep quality, total sleep time, and behavioral outcomes [47]. Supplementation with melatonin or melatonin agonists in the evening helps mimic the rise in melatonin levels typically seen in patients with a typically functioning melatonin pathway. Additionally, beta-blockers have been shown to interfere with endogenous melatonin secretion. Utilizing a morning dose of a beta-blocker can suppress the daytime rise in melatonin experienced by individuals with SMS. When treating patients with SMS with the beta-blocker, acebutolol, motor hyperactivity, daytime sleeping and sleep attacks, and behavioral problems all decreased. Sleep patterns were also seen to improve with use of this medication [32]. Although use of these medications helps improve sleep in patients with SMS, caregivers often report ongoing sleep concerns. This is likely due to the complexity and variety of sleep processes.

A variety of other sleep promoting agents have been used off-label for the treatment of insomnia in patients with SMS. Medications that have been used include diphenhydramine, clonidine, trazodone, quetiapine, and gabapentin [33]. Stimulants have also been utilized to reduce the daytime sleepiness experienced by patients with SMS. Medications used in such a manner should be done with caution and by a provider experienced in managing insomnia.

15.9 Common Medical Comorbidities

Of the medical conditions that are common in SMS, sleep disturbances and obesity most greatly impact psychopharmacological interventions. Other comorbidities such as cardiovascular and/or structural genitourinary abnormalities, hypothyroidism, and seizures also warrant consideration when choosing pharmacologic agents. However, none of these is an absolute contraindication. The balance of possible and real benefits versus potential and actual adverse effects is an ongoing challenge. Moreover, normalizing sleep is the first priority, as some behavioral symptoms will subside with improved sleep.

Key Points to Remember

- Smith–Magenis syndrome is more difficult and stressful for families than reported by mixed/general neurodevelopmental disorder parent groups; stress is correlated with the level of child behavior concerns.
- Treating sleep problems should be the priority in order to manage child maladaptive behavior and improve the family's quality of life.
- Tasimelteon, currently the only FDA-approved sleep aid, is a melatonin agonist that has shown benefits in sleep quality and behavioral outcomes.
- Early dietary and behavioral strategies are essential to minimize/manage obesity. This is especially important as the medications that are frequently used to

manage maladaptive behavior may increase appetite and are commonly associated with excessive weight gain.
- No medications for maladaptive behaviors are uniformly effective; there are no published clinical trials of psychotropic medications aside from tasimelteon in individuals with SMS.

References

1. Smith ACM, Mc Gavran L, Waldstein G. Deletion of the 17 short arm in two patients with facial clefts and congenital heart disease. Am J Hum Genet. 1982;34:A410.
2. Smith AC, McGavran L, Robinson J, et al. Interstitial deletion of (17)(p11.2p11.2) in nine patients. Am J Med Genet. 1986;24(3):393–414.
3. Stratton RF, Dobyns WB, Greenberg F, et al. Interstitial deletion of (17)(p11.2p11.2): report of six additional patients with a new chromosome deletion syndrome. Am J Med Genet. 1986;24(3):421–32.
4. Chen KS, Manian P, Koeuth T, et al. Homologous recombination of a flanking repeat gene cluster is a mechanism for a common contiguous gene deletion syndrome. Nat Genet. 1997;17(2):154–63.
5. Harel T, Lupski JR. Genomic disorders 20 years on-mechanisms for clinical manifestations. Clin Genet. 2018;93(3):439–49.
6. Greenberg F, Guzzetta V, Montes de Oca-Luna R, et al. Molecular analysis of the Smith-Magenis syndrome: A possible contiguous-gene syndrome associated with del(17)(p11.2). Am J Hum Genet. 1991;49(6):1207–18.
7. Smith AC, Magenis RE, Elsea SH. Overview of Smith-Magenis syndrome. J Assoc Genet Technol. 2005;31(4):163–7.
8. Slager RE, Newton TL, Vlangos CN, Finucane B, Elsea SH. Mutations in RAI1 associated with Smith-Magenis syndrome. Nat Genet. 2003;33(4):466–8.
9. Boone PM, Reiter RJ, Glaze DG, Tan DX, Lupski JR, Potocki L. Abnormal circadian rhythm of melatonin in Smith-Magenis syndrome patients with RAI1 point mutations. Am J Med Genet A. 2011;155A(8):2024–7.
10. Elsea SH, Williams SR. Smith-Magenis syndrome: haploinsufficiency of RAI1 results in altered gene regulation in neurological and metabolic pathways. Expert Rev Mol Med. 2011;13:e14.
11. Falco M, Amabile S, Acquaviva F. RAI1 gene mutations: mechanisms of Smith-Magenis syndrome. Appl Clin Genet. 2017;10:85–94.
12. Campbell IM, Yuan B, Robberecht C, et al. Parental somatic mosaicism is underrecognized and influences recurrence risk of genomic disorders. Am J Hum Genet. 2014;95(2):173–82.
13. Smith AC, Gropman AL, Bailey-Wilson JE, et al. Hypercholesterolemia in children with Smith-Magenis syndrome: del (17) (p11.2p11.2). Genet Med. 2002;4(3):118–25.
14. Smith ACM, Boyd KE, Brennan C, et al. Smith-Magenis syndrome. In: Adam MP, Mirzaa GM, Pagon RA, et al., editors. GeneReviews((R)). Seattle (WA): University of Washington, Seattle; 1993.
15. Goldman AM, Potocki L, Walz K, et al. Epilepsy and chromosomal rearrangements in Smith-Magenis syndrome [del(17)(p11.2p11.2)]. J Child Neurol. 2006;21(2):93–8.
16. Greenberg F, Lewis RA, Potocki L, et al. Multi-disciplinary clinical study of Smith-Magenis syndrome (deletion 17p11.2). Am J Med Genet. 1996;62(3):247–54.
17. Potocki L, Shaw CJ, Stankiewicz P, Lupski JR. Variability in clinical phenotype despite common chromosomal deletion in Smith-Magenis syndrome [del(17)(p11.2p11.2)]. Genet Med. 2003;5(6):430–4.
18. Bi W, Saifi GM, Shaw CJ, et al. Mutations of RAI1, a PHD-containing protein, in nondeletion patients with Smith-Magenis syndrome. Hum Genet. 2004;115(6):515–24.

19. Shayota BJ, Elsea SH. Behavior and sleep disturbance in Smith-Magenis syndrome. Curr Opin Psychiatry. 2019;32(2):73–8.
20. Alaimo JT, Barton LV, Mullegama SV, Wills RD, Foster RH, Elsea SH. Individuals with Smith-Magenis syndrome display profound neurodevelopmental behavioral deficiencies and exhibit food-related behaviors equivalent to Prader-Willi syndrome. Res Dev Disabil. 2015;47:27–38.
21. Smith ACM, Boyd KE, Brennan C, et al. Medical management guidelines for an individual diagnosed with SMS. PRISMS; 2018.
22. Nag HE, Hoxmark LB, Naerland T. Parental experiences with behavioural problems in Smith-Magenis syndrome: the need for syndrome-specific competence. J Intellect Disabil. 2019;23(3):359–72.
23. Rinaldi B, Villa R, Sironi A, Garavelli L, Finelli P, Bedeschi MF. Smith-Magenis syndrome: clinical review, biological background and related disorders. Genes (Basel). 2022;13(2):335.
24. Wilde L, Silva D, Oliver C. The nature of social preference and interactions in Smith-Magenis syndrome. Res Dev Disabil. 2013;34(12):4355–65.
25. Finucane BM, Konar D, Haas-Givler B, Kurtz MB, Scott CI Jr. The spasmodic upper-body squeeze: a characteristic behavior in Smith-Magenis syndrome. Dev Med Child Neurol. 1994;36(1):78–83.
26. Garayzabal E, Hidalgo I, Miranda de Souza ALD, da Silva NC, Giacheti CM, Pinato L. Sleep disturbances and behavior in Smith-Magenis syndrome. Res Dev Disabil. 2022;128:104286.
27. De Leersnyder H, Bresson JL, de Blois MC, et al. Beta 1-adrenergic antagonists and melatonin reset the clock and restore sleep in a circadian disorder, Smith-Magenis syndrome. J Med Genet. 2003;40(1):74–8.
28. Trickett J, Heald M, Oliver C, Richards C. A cross-syndrome cohort comparison of sleep disturbance in children with Smith-Magenis syndrome, Angelman syndrome, autism spectrum disorder and tuberous sclerosis complex. J Neurodev Disord. 2018;10(1):9.
29. Williams SR, Zies D, Mullegama SV, Grotewiel MS, Elsea SH. Smith-Magenis syndrome results in disruption of CLOCK gene transcription and reveals an integral role for RAI1 in the maintenance of circadian rhythmicity. Am J Hum Genet. 2012;90(6):941–9.
30. Mullegama SV, Alaimo JT, Fountain MD, et al. RAI1 overexpression promotes altered circadian gene expression and dyssomnia in Potocki-Lupski syndrome. J Pediatr Genet. 2017;6(3):155–64.
31. Potocki L, Glaze D, Tan DX, et al. Circadian rhythm abnormalities of melatonin in Smith-Magenis syndrome. J Med Genet. 2000;37(6):428–33.
32. De Leersnyder H, de Blois MC, Vekemans M, et al. Beta(1)-adrenergic antagonists improve sleep and behavioural disturbances in a circadian disorder, Smith-Magenis syndrome. J Med Genet. 2001;38(9):586–90.
33. Kaplan KA, Elsea SH, Potocki L. Management of sleep disturbances associated with Smith-Magenis syndrome. CNS Drugs. 2020;34(7):723–30.
34. Arens R, Sin S, Nandalike K, et al. Upper airway structure and body fat composition in obese children with obstructive sleep apnea syndrome. Am J Respir Crit Care Med. 2011;183(6):782–7.
35. Van de Graaff WB. Thoracic traction on the trachea: mechanisms and magnitude. J Appl Physiol (1985). 1991;70(3):1328–36.
36. Laje G, Morse R, Richter W, Ball J, Pao M, Smith AC. Autism spectrum features in Smith-Magenis syndrome. Am J Med Genet C Semin Med Genet. 2010;154C(4):456–62.
37. Laje G, Bernert R, Morse R, Pao M, Smith AC. Pharmacological treatment of disruptive behavior in Smith-Magenis syndrome. Am J Med Genet C Semin Med Genet. 2010;154C(4):463–8.
38. Martin SC, Wolters PL, Smith AC. Adaptive and maladaptive behavior in children with Smith-Magenis syndrome. J Autism Dev Disord. 2006;36(4):541–52.
39. Wolters PL, Gropman AL, Martin SC, et al. Neurodevelopment of children under 3 years of age with Smith-Magenis syndrome. Pediatr Neurol. 2009;41(4):250–8.
40. Sattler EC, Steinlein OK. Birt-Hogg-Dube syndrome. In: Adam MP, Mirzaa GM, Pagon RA, et al., editors. GeneReviews((R)). Seattle (WA): University of Washington, Seattle; 1993.

41. Edinger JD, Arnedt JT, Bertisch SM, et al. Behavioral and psychological treatments for chronic insomnia disorder in adults: an American Academy of Sleep Medicine systematic review, meta-analysis, and GRADE assessment. J Clin Sleep Med. 2021;17(2):263–98.
42. Medicine AAoS. Healthy sleep habits. 2020. Available from: https://sleepeducation.org/healthy-sleep/healthy-sleep-habits/
43. Niederhofer H. Efficacy of risperidone treatment in Smith-Magenis syndrome (del 17 pll. 2). Psychiatr Danub. 2007;19(3):189–92.
44. Narlesky MR, McDonald D, Bradford B, Sukpraprut-Braaten S, Strayhan R. Management of attention deficits and behavioral dyscontrol with an evening-dosed methylphenidate formulation in Smith-Magenis syndrome. Cureus. 2022;14(1):e21255.
45. Khan SS, Pradhan T. Case of Smith-Magenis syndrome. J Clin Psychopharmacol. 2019;39(5):525–7.
46. Muller AR, Zinkstok JR, Rommelse NNJ, et al. Methylphenidate for attention-deficit/hyperactivity disorder in patients with Smith-Magenis syndrome: protocol for a series of N-of-1 trials. Orphanet J Rare Dis. 2021;16(1):380.
47. Polymeropoulos CM, Brooks J, Czeisler EL, et al. Tasimelteon safely and effectively improves sleep in Smith-Magenis syndrome: a double-blind randomized trial followed by an open-label extension. Genet Med. 2021;23(12):2426–32.

Further Reading

American Academy of Sleep Medicine: https://aasm.org
PRISMS; Parents and Researchers Interested in Smith-Magenis Syndrome: https://www.prisms.org/
SMS Research Foundation: https://smsresearchfoundation.org/
Sabus A, Feinstein J, Romani P, Goldson E, Blackmer A. Management of self-injurious behaviors in children with neurodevelopmental disorders: a pharmacotherapy overview. Pharmacotherapy. 2019;39(6):645–64.
Smith E, Stogios N, Au E, et al. The metabolic adverse effects of antipsychotic use in individuals with intellectual and/or developmental disability: a systematic review and meta-analysis. Acta Psychiatr Scand. 2022;146:201–14.

Klinefelter Syndrome

16

David S. Hong

16.1 Overview

47,XXY, or Klinefelter syndrome (KS), is a common genetic variation. Best estimates of prevalence are derived from prenatal and newborn studies [1–4], which indicate that ~1/650 males are affected. The underlying genetic etiology associated with the syndrome arises from a nondisjunction event in germ cells during meiosis. Either an X-X or X-Y pair remains together during gamete formation, which pairs with a haploid gamete (sperm or egg) to result in a triploid 47,XXY zygote [5]. The majority of individuals with 47,XXY tend to have a monosomic phenotype (80–90%), though ~5–10% of males may have a mosaic karyotype (e.g., 47,XXY/46,XY) [6]. Serial examinations of live births indicate a high prevalence in the general population, which contrasts with surprisingly low ascertainment of individuals with a confirmed clinical diagnosis. The penetrance of this genetic variation is variable and has been challenging to estimate given the low diagnostic yield for this condition, but suggests that many individuals with the karyotype may experience a relatively low symptom burden. However, when symptoms are present, the literature indicates that they tend to cluster in relatively consistent phenotypic and neurocognitive domains.

Regarding the physical phenotype, individuals with 47,XXY may demonstrate hypotonia (62%) and motor developmental delays in infancy and childhood, as well as delays in speech and language development (>40%) [6]. In adulthood, males with KS are typically found to have taller stature (>30%), gynecomastia (28–75%), decreased muscle mass (~40%), and aberrant body hair distribution (30–80%) [6]. Importantly, 47,XXY is the most common diagnosis associated with primary hypogonadism, which in KS occurs as a result of the involution of testicular seminal

D. S. Hong (✉)
Department of Psychiatry and Behavioral Sciences, Stanford University, Stanford, CA, USA
e-mail: dshong@stanford.edu

R. P. Thom, C. J. McDougle (eds.), *Neuropsychiatric Care for Genetic Syndromes and Other Neurodevelopmental Disorders*,
https://doi.org/10.1007/978-3-031-76269-7_16

vesicles during puberty. As such, males with KS may have smaller testes (>95%), azoospermia (>95%), and infertility (>99%) [6]. Autoimmune conditions, such as systemic lupus erythematosus (SLE) and rheumatoid arthritis, as well as metabolic syndrome (elevated glucose, lipids, and blood pressure) are also thought to occur more frequently in males with KS relative to unaffected males.

A characteristic neurocognitive phenotype has also been consistently identified in KS; among the most common findings is a full-scale IQ in the average to low-average range. A closer examination of subdomains indicates a split between verbal and nonverbal IQ, where verbal IQ is a relative weakness, compared to nonverbal IQ which is generally intact [5, 7]. It should also be noted that some other studies have not identified a split between verbal and nonverbal IQ [8, 9], indicating both a need for further research, as well as the potential variance in phenotype in this condition. However, when deficits in verbal domains are present, affected functions typically include verbal fluency, syntactic processing, semantic memory, and articulation, among others. Interestingly, expressive language is disproportionately affected relative to receptive language [10]. In addition to verbal domains, the neurocognitive profile is also frequently associated with deficits in executive function, including lower scores in the domains of inhibition, sustained attention, and working memory. Social cognitive vulnerabilities have also been consistently identified, including face recognition, emotion identification, and theory of mind tasks [11, 12]. Notably, these neurocognitive findings are further supported by a number of neuroimaging studies that demonstrate both structural differences in brain regions [13] associated with these cognitive functions, as well as differences in connectivity within related neural networks [14]. Biological mechanisms underlying the observed phenotype likely arise both from genetic etiologies (i.e., sex chromosome "dosage effects" from surplus gene products on the additional X chromosome [15, 16]), as well as hormonal effects (i.e., downstream end-organ impact from testosterone deficiency that typically arises during the pubertal period). Together, both genetic and hormonal effects indicate an overarching framework by which genetic and epigenetic processes stemming from the additional X chromosome ultimately manifest in a behavioral phenotype characteristic of KS.

16.2 Psychiatric Comorbidities

Based on the underlying neurocognitive profile that emerges early and tends to persist across developmental stages, it is unsurprising to find that a number of psychiatric diagnoses are also frequently diagnosed in people with KS. Among the most commonly identified is the presence of a language-based specific learning disorder (SLD). This includes findings from early longitudinal studies of boys with KS showing that 70–80% demonstrated vulnerabilities in language domains [7, 17], and 60–80% of individuals in various studies met clinical criteria for a language-based SLD [18–20], many of whom required psychoeducational support services in school settings. Also, executive function deficits associated with KS translate to a much higher prevalence of attention-deficit/hyperactivity disorder (ADHD), with an estimated 5.6-fold increased likelihood of an ADHD diagnosis [21]. The prevalence of ADHD is ~35–65% [20, 22], which vastly exceeds population estimates for ADHD in euploid individuals. Interestingly, symptoms associated with ADHD in KS skew toward the inattentive presentation, with a lower proportion presenting with combined symptoms [20]. Further, social skills deficits correlate with a higher incidence of autism spectrum disorder (ASD) diagnoses—with an average of ~18% meeting full criteria for ASD, while closer to ~25% of individuals may have symptoms consistent with the broader autism phenotype [23].

There additionally appears to be a higher risk for schizophrenia spectrum disorders in KS. Despite a relatively low overall prevalence of schizophrenia spectrum disorder, the odds ratio for a diagnosis of schizophrenia in KS was four times higher than expected for the general population in one sample of adults [21]. Similarly, studies of children indicate a higher incidence of reporting psychotic symptoms or "thought problems" on dimensional scales [20, 24]. Rates of bipolar disorder are also reportedly higher than expected, with an odds ratio of 3.8 relative to matched population controls [21]. Broadly, the prevalence of mood and anxiety disorders in KS is mixed, with estimates of depressive disorders averaging ~25% and anxiety disorders ~20% in pediatric samples [23], though it is less clear how much this diverges from expected rates in the general population. However, given the high overall incidence of mood and anxiety disorders, these symptoms should be accounted for in the clinical management of patients with KS.

Overall, there is a significant symptom burden across a range of psychiatric diagnoses in KS. Several of these diagnoses putatively demonstrate a mechanistic link to the underlying genetic etiology of the condition (extra X chromosome effects and testosterone deficiency), while others may represent more generalized associations with living with a chronic medical condition. Also, it should be kept in mind that while comorbid psychiatric conditions are more frequent, a sizable proportion of individuals with KS do not meet the criteria for psychiatric diagnoses, again underscoring the significant inter-individual variation within this phenotype which should also be taken into consideration in clinical management.

16.3 Assessment

Klinefelter syndrome is typically identified by standard karyotype analysis, a relatively straightforward diagnostic procedure in clinical laboratories. When suspicion of the condition is present, based on phenotypic traits on clinical assessment, providers may order a karyotype. A karyotype reports the number of cells with additional chromosomes, indicating the presence of XXY cells relative to the total number of cells counted. Additionally, fluorescence in situ hybridization (FISH) may be performed which allows for the detection of chromosome deletions or duplications that cannot be detected with standard karyotyping. Notably, the genetic etiology for KS arises from de novo nondisjunction events. Thus, postnatal testing commonly arises from clinical suspicion, such as hypogonadism, small testes and behavioral traits in boys, or infertility in adult men. Genetic testing should occur in coordination with appropriate counseling services and multidisciplinary clinical referrals.

In contrast, recent advances in cell-free noninvasive prenatal testing (NIPT) have increasingly allowed for the detection of chromosomal aneuploidy prior to the emergence of clinical symptoms, and hence free of selection bias. Positive predictive value is high with 74% of fetuses with XXY karyotypes being detected, prompting the American College of Medical Genetics (ACMG) to recommend NIPT screening for XXY (and other sex chromosome aneuploidy) as a routine, though optional, part of prenatal care [25]. As such, early detection will putatively result in the detection of a higher proportion of individuals with a 47,XXY karyotype who may not demonstrate symptoms typically associated with KS. Parents receiving a prenatal diagnosis of an 47,XXY karyotype will typically have genetic counseling services available. Parent advocacy organizations, such as the Association for X and Y Chromosome Variations (AXYS) (www.genetic.org), additionally provide educational resources and support for expecting parents.

Whether the diagnosis is made pre- or postnatally, further assessment entails ongoing anticipatory guidance and routine screening for symptom domains commonly associated with the KS phenotype as outlined above. This includes the early assessment of developmental milestones, with a focus on motor, social, and cognitive trajectories. When signs are present, there is a low threshold to pursue a comprehensive assessment to determine if a psychiatric diagnosis should be made and thereby initiate the process for early intervention and evidence-based treatment. In the absence of psychometric tools specific to KS, standard assessment procedures for relevant symptom domains are appropriate, including ASD, ADHD, mood and anxiety screening questionnaires, as well as comprehensive neuropsychological testing when available.

16.4 Psychosocial Treatments

Unfortunately, randomized controlled trials specifically examining the efficacy of psychosocial treatments in individuals with KS are lacking. As a result, when psychiatric conditions are identified in individuals with KS, treatment selection is reliant on the broader clinical literature. Therefore, among the most common diagnoses associated with KS, standard clinical approaches to psychotherapy should be followed. As an example, individuals with KS with a comorbid diagnosis of ASD may benefit from applied behavioral analysis (ABA) or social skills-based group interventions. Similarly, individuals with mood or anxiety disorders may benefit from cognitive-behavioral therapy or other similar evidence-based psychosocial approaches. While the evidence for the efficacy of these interventions specific to KS is lacking, there is also no evidence to suggest that standard therapy approaches would not be effective in this cohort. However, the full spectrum of potential comorbid conditions associated with KS should be taken into account—for instance, ASD and anxiety symptoms should be considered jointly as treatment targets when both are present, and the adaptation of psychotherapy approaches may be indicated to accommodate comorbid symptoms. Clinical research examining the impact or utility of adapting clinical protocols to be more specifically tailored to individuals with 47,XXY is an important area of future study.

Further, while not part of traditional psychotherapy per se, there is a significant need for interdisciplinary coordination when SLDs, motor, and/or speech deficits are present. This includes collaboration with schools to coordinate psychoeducational intervention and accommodations, as well as referrals to speech, occupational and physical therapy when issues arise during routine developmental surveillance.

16.5 Biological Treatments

Similar to psychosocial therapies, rigorous examination of psychopharmacology specific to KS is scarce. Relatedly, there is limited understanding of whether the additional X chromosome influences the mechanism of action and/or efficacy of traditional psychotropic medications. Biological treatment selection therefore generally follows the same principles as for equivalent diagnoses in the broader population.

Given ADHD is among the most common psychiatric conditions associated with KS, medications are often indicated, including the use of stimulants. There is some evidence for structural cardiac abnormalities in KS relative to 46XY males [26], as well as evidence for the increased risk for thromboembolic disease, hypertrophic cardiomyopathy, and atrial fibrillation [27], though mechanisms for these cardiac conditions remain unclear. Interestingly, it also appears that the QTc interval may actually be shortened in KS [28]. As such, if increased cardiac risk is present, a referral should be made for a cardiac consultation and/or electrocardiogram consistent with existing ADHD treatment guidelines. However, case reports indicate that when used, stimulants are effective in this population of youth, indicating that the appropriate use of stimulants may be of benefit. There is limited to no data on other commonly used psychotropic medications, including selective serotonin reuptake inhibitors (SSRIs), alpha agonists, and mood stabilizers in KS. However, when atypical antipsychotics are indicated, additional consideration is needed given substantially higher rates of metabolic impairments in this population, including increased risk for obesity, dyslipidemia, insulin resistance, and thromboembolic disorders [6, 29].

As hypogonadism is a central characteristic for many individuals with KS, testosterone replacement is a routine component of broader treatment. While hormone replacement therapy is not directly part of psychiatric treatment, studies indicate that exogenous testosterone may have neurocognitive effects. This includes findings that exogenous androgen administration in the first few years of life may impact language, motor, and behavioral performance [30, 31], while administration in middle childhood was associated with positive effects on visuomotor and psychosocial function [32]. However, a study of early adolescents demonstrated no association between testosterone levels and neurocognitive outcomes [33], and a history of testosterone replacement was not found to significantly improve quality of life across the lifespan in KS [33–35]. Further prospective research is needed to determine whether these neuroendocrine interventions are developmentally specific, as well as to better understand the longitudinal effects of exogenous androgens on psychosocial and neurocognitive outcomes.

16.6 Common Medical Comorbidities

There are a number of medical comorbidities that are frequently encountered in KS. Foremost is primary hypogonadism which likely drives other downstream phenotypes. This endocrinological disturbance typically emerges during the pubertal period and not uncommonly results in exogenous hormone replacement therapy. Relatedly, most men with a monosomic 47,XXY will experience fertility issues due to azoospermia. Issues with bone metabolism and musculoskeletal issues are likely also a consequence of hypogonadism, and include associations with lower bone mineral density, increased rates of osteoporosis and fractures, reduced muscle strength, and poor motor coordination [36]. As outlined above, frequent comorbidities also include cardiometabolic concerns, including increased risk of obesity, diabetes, dyslipidemia, thromboembolic disease, and atrial fibrillation [26, 27]. Furthermore, men with KS are at increased risk for gynecomastia and breast cancer, and have a higher-than-expected incidence of autoimmune conditions including SLE, hypothyroidism, multiple sclerosis, and rheumatological conditions, relative to the general male population [37, 38].

Key Points to Remember

- Having the 47,XXY genetic variation is not deterministic: there is variable penetrance of symptoms associated with this condition. Some individuals are unaffected and others have a characteristic profile.
- Provide anticipatory guidance throughout development.
- This includes diagnostic assessment including genetic testing, as well as routine screening throughout development, i.e., neurocognitive testing at various junctures during educational pathway, and clinical evaluation for symptoms of ADHD, social cognitive difficulties, mood and anxiety symptoms, and evidence for psychosis in adolescence and young adulthood.
- Routine monitoring for features associated with KS allows for early and prompt intervention when symptoms manifest.
- Standard psychosocial and pharmacological treatment algorithms should be used when Diagnostic and Statistical Manual of Mental Disorders (DSM)-based psychiatric diagnoses are present.

References

1. Berglund A, Viuff MH, Skakkebæk A, Chang S, Stochholm K, Gravholt CH. Changes in the cohort composition of Turner syndrome and severe non-diagnosis of Klinefelter, 47,XXX and 47,XYY syndrome: a nationwide cohort study. Orphanet J Rare Dis. 2019;14(1):16.
2. Berglund A, Stochholm K, Gravholt CH. The epidemiology of sex chromosome abnormalities. Am J Med Genet C Semin Med Genet. 2020;184(2):202–15.
3. Bojesen A, Juul S, Gravholt CH. Prenatal and postnatal prevalence of Klinefelter syndrome: a national registry study. J Clin Endocrinol Metab. 2003;88(2):622–6.
4. Coffee B, Keith K, Albizua I, et al. Incidence of Fragile X syndrome by newborn screening for methylated FMR1 dNA. Am J Hum Genet. 2009;85(4):503–14.
5. Hong DS, Reiss AL. Cognitive and neurological aspects of sex chromosome aneuploidies. Lancet Neurol. 2014;13(3):306–18.
6. Gravholt CH, Chang S, Wallentin M, Fedder J, Moore P, Skakkebæk A. Klinefelter syndrome: integrating genetics, neuropsychology, and endocrinology. Endocr Rev. 2018;39(4):389–423.
7. Boada R, Janusz J, Hutaff-Lee C, Tartaglia N. The cognitive phenotype in Klinefelter syndrome: a review of the literature including genetic and hormonal factors. Dev Disabil Res Rev. 2009;15(4):284–94.
8. Nielsen J, Pelsen B. Follow-up 20 years later of 34 Klinefelter males with karyotype 47,XXY and 16 hypogonadal males with karyotype 46,XY. Hum Genet. 1987;77(2):188–92.
9. Ross JL, Roeltgen DP, Stefanatos G, et al. Cognitive and motor development during childhood in boys with Klinefelter syndrome. Am J Med Genet A. 2008;146A(6):708–19.
10. St John M, Ponchard C, van Reyk O, et al. Speech and language in children with Klinefelter syndrome. J Commun Disord. 2019;78:84–96.
11. van Rijn S, de Sonneville L, Swaab H. The nature of social cognitive deficits in children and adults with Klinefelter syndrome (47,XXY). Genes Brain Behav. 2018;17(6):e12465.
12. Melogno S, Pinto MA, Badolato F, et al. High-level language competencies and theory of mind in a group of children with Klinefelter syndrome. Am J Med Genet A. 2019;179(2):183–9.
13. Foland-Ross LC, Gil M, Shrestha SB, Chromik LC, Hong D, Reiss AL. Cortical gray matter structure in boys with Klinefelter syndrome. Psychiatry Res Neuroimaging. 2021;313:111299.
14. Whitman ET, Liu S, Torres E, et al. Resting-state functional connectivity and psychopathology in Klinefelter syndrome (47, XXY). Cereb Cortex. 2021;31(9):4180–90.
15. Zhang X, Hong D, Ma S, et al. Integrated functional genomic analyses of Klinefelter and Turner syndromes reveal global network effects of altered X chromosome dosage. Proc Natl Acad Sci USA. 2020;117(9):4864–73.
16. Raznahan A, Parikshak NN, Chandran V, et al. Sex-chromosome dosage effects on gene expression in humans. Proc Natl Acad Sci USA. 2018;115(28):7398–403.
17. Geschwind DH, Boone KB, Miller BL, Swerdloff RS. Neurobehavioral phenotype of Klinefelter syndrome. Ment Retard Dev Disabil Res Rev. 2000;6(2):107–16.
18. Geschwind DH, Gregg J, Boone K, et al. Klinefelter's syndrome as a model of anomalous cerebral laterality: testing gene dosage in the X chromosome pseudoautosomal region using a DNA microarray. Dev Genet. 1998;23(3):215–29.
19. Bender BG, Puck MH, Salbenblatt JA, Robinson A. Dyslexia in 47,XXXY boys identified at birth. Behav Genet. 1986;16(3):343–54.
20. Bruining H, Swaab H, Kas M, van Engeland H. Psychiatric characteristics in a self-selected sample of boys with Klinefelter syndrome. Pediatrics. 2009;123(5):e865–70.
21. Cederlöf M, Ohlsson Gotby A, Larsson H, et al. Klinefelter syndrome and risk of psychosis, autism and ADHD. J Psychiatr Res. 2014;48(1):128–30.
22. Tartaglia NR, Ayari N, Hutaff-Lee C, Boada R. Attention-deficit hyperactivity disorder symptoms in children and adolescents with sex chromosome aneuploidy: XXY, XXX, XYY, and XXYY. J Dev Behav Pediatr. 2012;33(4):309–18.
23. van Rijn S. A review of neurocognitive functioning and risk for psychopathology in sex chromosome trisomy (47,XXY, 47,XXX, 47, XYY). Curr Opin Psychiatry. 2019;32(2):79–84.

24. van Rijn S, Swaab H. Executive dysfunction and the relation with behavioral problems in children with 47,XXY and 47,XXX. Genes Brain Behav. 2015;14(2):200–8.
25. Dungan JS, Klugman S, Darilek S, et al. Noninvasive prenatal screening (NIPS) for fetal chromosome abnormalities in a general-risk population: an evidence-based clinical guideline of the American College of Medical Genetics and Genomics (ACMG). Genet Med. 2023;25(2):100336. Available from: https://www.gimjournal.org/article/S1098-3600(22)01004-8/fulltext
26. Accardo G, Amoresano Paglionico V, Di Fraia R, et al. Management of cardiovascular complications in Klinefelter syndrome patients. Expert Rev Endocrinol Metab. 2019;14(2):145–52.
27. Wren G, Davies W. Sex-linked genetic mechanisms and atrial fibrillation risk. Eur J Med Genet. 2022;65(4):104459.
28. Skakkebæk A, Kjær-Sørensen K, Matchkov VV, et al. Dosage of the pseudoautosomal gene SLC25A6 is implicated in QTc interval duration. Sci Rep. 2023;13:12089.
29. Kanakis GA, Nieschlag E. Klinefelter syndrome: more than hypogonadism. Metabolism. 2018;86:135–44.
30. Samango-Sprouse C, Stapleton EJ, Lawson P, et al. Positive effects of early androgen therapy on the behavioral phenotype of boys with 47,XXY. Am J Med Genet C Semin Med Genet. 2015;169(2):150–7.
31. Samango-Sprouse CA, Sadeghin T, Mitchell FL, et al. Positive effects of short course androgen therapy on the neurodevelopmental outcome in boys with 47,XXY syndrome at 36 and 72 months of age. Am J Med Genet A. 2013;161(3):501–8.
32. Ross JL, Kushner H, Kowal K, et al. Androgen treatment effects on motor function, cognition, and behavior in boys with Klinefelter syndrome. J Pediatr. 2017;185:193–199.e4.
33. Jordan TL, Foland-Ross LC, Wun VL, Ross JL, Reiss AL. Cognition, academic achievement, adaptive behavior, and quality of life in child and adolescent boys with Klinefelter syndrome. J Dev Behav Pediatr. 2023;44(7):e476–85.
34. Close S, Fennoy I, Smaldone A, Reame N. Phenotype and adverse quality of life in boys with Klinefelter syndrome. J Pediatr. 2015;167(3):650–7.
35. Skakkebæk A, Moore PJ, Chang S, Fedder J, Gravholt CH. Quality of life in men with Klinefelter syndrome: the impact of genotype, health, socioeconomics, and sexual function. Genet Med. 2018;20(2):214–22.
36. Grande G, Graziani A, Mambro AD, Selice R, Ferlin A. Osteoporosis and bone metabolism in patients with Klinefelter syndrome. Endocr Connect. 2023;12(8):e230058. Available from: https://ec.bioscientifica.com/view/journals/ec/12/8/EC-23-0058.xml
37. Seminog OO, Seminog AB, Yeates D, Goldacre MJ. Associations between Klinefelter's syndrome and autoimmune diseases: English national record linkage studies. Autoimmunity. 2015;48(2):125–8.
38. Bojesen A, Juul S, Birkebæk NH, Gravholt CH. Morbidity in Klinefelter syndrome: a Danish register study based on hospital discharge diagnoses. J Clin Endocrinol Metab. 2006;91(4):1254–60.

Further Reading

Cederlöf M, Ohlsson Gotby A, Larsson H, et al. Klinefelter syndrome and risk of psychosis, autism and ADHD. J Psychiatr Res. 2014;48(1):128–30.

Gravholt CH, Chang S, Wallentin M, Fedder J, Moore P, Skakkebæk A. Klinefelter syndrome: integrating genetics, neuropsychology, and endocrinology. Endocr Rev. 2018;39(4):389–423.

Hong DS, Reiss AL. Cognitive and neurological aspects of sex chromosome aneuploidies. Lancet Neurol. 2014;13(3):306–18.

van Rijn S. A review of neurocognitive functioning and risk for psychopathology in sex chromosome trisomy (47,XXY, 47,XXX, 47, XYY). Curr Opin Psychiatry. 2019;32(2):79–84.

Lesch–Nyhan Syndrome

17

Lydia J. Fischer and David W. Dunn

17.1 Overview

Lesch–Nyhan syndrome was first described by Michael Lesch and William Nyhan in 1964 in a case report of two brothers noted to have problems with hyperuricemia, choreoathetosis, and intellectual disability [1]. In 1967, Seegmiller et al. found that the syndrome is caused by a near-complete deficiency of hypoxanthine-guanine phosphoribosyltransferase (HGPRT), an enzyme involved in purine metabolism, and which when deficient, results in excess uric acid [2]. Specifically, HGPRT converts guanine and hypoxanthine into guanosine monophosphate and inosine monophosphate. The lack of HGPRT therefore causes increased levels of guanine and hypoxanthine, which is then converted into uric acid. Also in 1967, partial HGPRT deficiency was described in a population of adult males with gouty arthritis and was initially termed Kelly Seegmiller syndrome [3]. HGPRT deficiency occurs along a spectrum, where enzyme activity of <1–2% of normal and is associated with more severe symptoms and is classically called Lesch–Nyhan syndrome [4]. Currently, there have been more than 300 described genetic mutations that result in some level of deficiency of the HGPRT enzyme, now referred to as Lesch–Nyhan variants [5]. Common clinical features include hyperuricemia, motor and cognitive impairment, and in severe cases, the classic, recurrent, and oftentimes severe self-injurious behaviors. There is significant variability in phenotype, as cases of mild Lesch–Nyhan variants may only present with hyperuricemia [6].

L. J. Fischer
Department of Psychiatry, Indiana University School of Medicine, Indianapolis, IN, USA
e-mail: lydfisch@iu.edu

D. W. Dunn (✉)
Department of Psychiatry, Indiana University School of Medicine, Indianapolis, IN, USA

Department of Neurology, Indiana University School of Medicine, Indianapolis, IN, USA
e-mail: ddunn@iu.edu

R. P. Thom, C. J. McDougle (eds.), *Neuropsychiatric Care for Genetic Syndromes and Other Neurodevelopmental Disorders*,
https://doi.org/10.1007/978-3-031-76269-7_17

17.2 Epidemiology

The HGPRT enzyme is encoded on the *HPRT1* gene located on the X chromosome, and so is inherited in an X-linked recessive manner [7]. For this reason, Lesch–Nyhan syndrome and Lesch–Nyhan syndrome variants are almost exclusively expressed in males, while women generally carry the gene as asymptomatic carriers. There have been case reports of women with Lesch–Nyhan syndrome, though these reports are extremely rare [8–15]. Currently, there are more than 300 described genetic mutations that result in some level of HGPRT enzyme deficiency with varying levels of symptom manifestation [5]. This can create some difficulty in describing the prevalence of Lesch–Nyhan syndrome and Lesch–Nyhan syndrome variants. In an early study done in 1972, it was thought that the prevalence of Lesch–Nyhan syndrome was 1 per 380,000 [16]. Studies since then indicate that the syndrome may actually be more rare. A population-based study in the UK from 1988 to 2008, for example, showed an incidence rate of 0.18 per 100,000 live births, giving a prevalence rate of one in two million people [17]. Patients with partial HGPRT enzyme function are more difficult to diagnose, as some patients may only present with symptoms of hyperuricemia. For this reason, Lesch–Nyhan syndrome variants are most likely underrecognized.

17.3 Underlying Genetic and Neurobiological Mechanisms

Lesch–Nyhan syndrome is a metabolic disorder that results in a deficiency of hypoxanthine-guanine phosphoribosyltransferase (HGPRT). HGPRT is an enzyme in the purine salvage pathway that is encoded by the *HPRT1* gene. It is inherited via an X-linked inheritance pattern and has been localized to the long arm of the X chromosome. A study looking at the genetic variability in *HGPRT1* gene mutations including 75 new cases and 196 previously reported cases found significant variability in both the location and type of mutation, though these factors do not seem to reliably predict clinical phenotype [5, 18]. While there are already hundreds of identified mutations, new mutations resulting in impaired HGPRT enzyme function continue to be found and described in the literature [19]. The severity of the clinical phenotype does generally seem to be related to the level of impairment of the HGPRT enzyme, with the most severe clinical features seen in patients with little to no activity [20]. Severe phenotypes exhibit hyperuricemia, motor and cognitive impairment, as well as the classic recurrent and severe self-injurious behaviors, while a mild phenotype may present only with hyperuricemia [6]. Hyperuricemia is present in all patients with Lesch–Nyhan syndrome or Lesch–Nyhan variant and causes the classic sequelae of elevated uric acid levels including arthritis, tophi, nephrolithiasis, and if left untreated, renal disease or failure. The mechanism of elevated uric acid in these patients is well understood. HGPRT is the enzyme that catalyzes the salvage of inosine monophosphate and guanosine monophosphate. A deficit of this enzyme results in an increase in guanine and hypoxanthine which are then converted into uric acid [21]. Additionally, failure of hypoxanthine and guanine recycling causes increased synthesis of purines by the de novo pathway which further results in the overproduction of uric acid in HGPRT deficiency at a rate thought to be 5–10 times that of a healthy individual [20].

The exact mechanism of the neurologic and neuropsychiatric symptoms of Lesch–Nyhan syndrome remains somewhat unclear, though several theories have been advanced. While the high levels of serum uric acid in patients with Lesch–Nyhan syndrome were initially thought to directly relate to impairments in neurodevelopment and self-injurious behavior, it was found that even patients with prenatal diagnosis and treatment with allopurinol at birth, who therefore entirely avoided hyperuricemia, continued to experience the neurologic symptoms of the disease [22]. While the HGPRT enzyme is needed in both guanine and hypoxanthine recycling, it is not clear if hypoxanthine or guanine recycling is more important in relation to phenotypic severity. A study looking at hypoxanthine and guanine recycling activity in skin fibroblasts indicated that loss of guanine recycling may be more closely linked to the neurologic (dystonia and cognitive impairment) and behavioral phenotype than hypoxanthine recycling [23].

While some early studies assessed how low levels of adenine or serotonin could contribute to the neurologic symptoms of Lesch–Nyhan syndrome, the most promising research has concentrated on dopamine and the basal ganglia [22]. The exact mechanism is not well understood, but is thought to be due to the effect of HGPRT deficiency on the developing brain [24, 25]. A neuroimaging study showed reductions in intracranial volume, with the most significant difference in the basal ganglia [26]. An autopsy study showed functional loss of 65–90% of nigrostriatal and mesolimbic dopamine terminals, but with normal dopamine levels in the substantia nigra. The main dopamine metabolite, homovanillic acid, was found in the caudate nucleus, putamen, and nucleus accumbens. Together, these changes may suggest diminished branching of dendrites rather than cell loss in the substantia nigra [27].

Another study by Bell et al. using stem cells and genetic engineering technologies indicated that HGPRT deficiency results in impaired energy metabolism and reduced developmental potential in midbrain dopaminergic cells [28]. Neurological manifestations may also be related to HGPRT deficiency causing increased amounts of hypoxanthine in the extracellular medium which may then cause transcriptional errors in genes needed for striatal progenitor cell development [6]. More research is needed to understand the mechanisms of the neurologic and behavioral symptoms of Lesch–Nyhan syndrome and Lesch–Nyhan variants.

17.4 Common Clinical Features

Lesch–Nyhan syndrome is considered the severe end of a spectrum of clinical presentations and is usually thought to represent enzyme activity of <1.5%. The characteristic defining symptoms are hyperuricemia, neurodevelopmental abnormalities including severe motor and cognitive impairment, involuntary movements (dystonia, choreoathetosis, ballism), and in the most severe cases, self-injurious behaviors.

At birth, patients are often asymptomatic with an initially normal prenatal growth and development curve though may have symptomatic hyperuricemia. In severe cases, neurocognitive and motor symptoms can present as early as 3–6 months of age and may include hypotonia or developmental delay. In a study of 44 patients, ages 2–38 years old with Lesch–Nyhan syndrome, all but two patients first presented with delayed motor skills. While dystonia was the most common motor symptom and was present in all patients, choreoathetosis was present in 50% and ballism was observed in 30% [24]. In a study of Korean patients with Lesch–Nyhan syndrome, the median age at diagnosis was 2.3 years (range 4 months to 22.6 years) with the initial presenting features including developmental delay, orange-colored urine, and self-injurious behaviors [29]. Extrapyramidal symptoms may begin to appear at 6–24 months of age, with the most common extrapyramidal symptom being dystonia, followed by choreoathetosis and ballism. In classic Lesch–Nyhan syndrome, the severity of motor impairment almost always interferes with the acquisition of gross motor milestones like crawling and walking, and patients largely become wheelchair dependent and need significant help with their activities of daily living. Speech delay is also common and presents along a spectrum with multiple contributing factors. Speech is often difficult to understand and thought to be due to striatal dysarthria with excessive activation of pharyngeal, lingual, and perioral muscles leading to slow and irregular enunciation [24]. Chewing and swallowing can also be impaired, and for this reason, patients may need a gastrostomy tube for nutrition [24].

Once fully developed, motor impairment is thought to remain relatively stable with the most pronounced deficits resulting from severe action dystonia superimposed on baseline hypotonia. While some literature describes spasticity in Lesch–Nyhan syndrome, it is likely more accurately described as dystonia. Spasticity is an abnormality of muscle tone with a velocity-dependent increase in resistance to externally imposed movement and is evidence of corticospinal dysfunction. In contrast, dystonia is involuntary, sustained, patterned, and sometimes repetitive contractions of opposing muscles often leading to twisting movements or abnormal posturing, and results from impairment of the extrapyramidal system. Differentiating spasticity and dystonia can be challenging for clinicians who don't specialize in movement disorders and has resulted in discrepancies in the literature regarding motor dysfunction in Lesch–Nyhan syndrome. For example, scissoring of the legs is commonly seen in cerebral palsy and is caused by spasticity, but can also be seen in severe dystonia. Likewise, the extensor plantar reflex or Babinski sign is a sign of corticospinal dysfunction but is easily confused with the "striatal toe" which is a form of dystonia [24].

Patients with Lesch–Nyhan syndrome and Lesch–Nyhan variants characteristically have hyperuricemia that can result in gout, tophi, nephrolithiasis, and eventually even renal impairment or failure. If diagnosis is delayed, and allopurinol is not readily started in infancy, patients can present with end-stage renal failure [30–32]. Hyperuricemia and subsequent sequelae are exceedingly rare in childhood, and the presence of these symptoms should prompt a thorough metabolic workup.

It has been suggested that the phenotypic spectrum of patients with impaired HGPRT enzyme function can be roughly divided into three groups. Patients with severe neurological deficiencies and self-injurious behaviors typically have nearly undetectable HGPRT activity and are referred to classically as having Lesch–Nyhan syndrome. A second set of patients have a spectrum of neuromuscular symptoms, but no self-injury, and usually have residual HGPRT activity. A third group has no neurobehavioral disturbance and symptoms are only secondary to hyperuricemia, and usually have HGPRT activity of at least 10% of normal [33].

Patients with Lesch–Nyhan variant phenotypes exhibit deficits in the same domains as those with Lesch–Nyhan syndrome, but to varying digress. All Lesch–Nyhan syndrome and Lesch–Nyhan variant patients have some degree of hyperuricemia. Jinna et al. describe a cohort of Lesch–Nyhan variant patients and found that in 46 patients, 91% had some degree of motor abnormality and 67% had some level of cognitive impairment. The most frequent presenting problem for these cases was neurological (59%), though motor impairment in this study group was as mild as clumsiness of fine dexterous movements of the fingers and hands, or an awkward or stiff appearing gait. The same article summarizes previously reported cases of 109 patients with Lesch–Nyhan syndrome variants with an average age of diagnosis of 12.4 years. Sixty-nine percent of these patients presented with a problem related to hyperuricemia. Mild cognitive impairment was common, but severe cognitive impairment was uncommon [34]. This suggests that patients with more mild cases of Lesch–Nyhan variant who were diagnosed with hyperuricemia may also have mild symptoms of motor or cognitive impairment that go undetected until a diagnosis of the Lesch–Nyhan variant is considered.

Patients with Lesch–Nyhan syndrome almost invariably have macrocytic red blood cells. In a study which assessed 257 complete blood counts from 65 patients over a 23-year period, 81–92% of patients had macrocytic erythrocytes. Excluding cases with iron deficiency (since this pseudonormalizes erythrocyte volume), macrocytosis occurred in 97% of subjects [35].

17.5 Signs and Symptoms of Common Psychiatric Comorbidities

The classic and frequent cause of psychiatric involvement of Lesch–Nyhan syndrome is self-injurious behavior which includes severe self-mutilation. Self-injury is present in Lesch–Nyhan syndrome, but is not present in Lesch–Nyhan variants where some enzyme activity is maintained.

The most common types of self-injury include finger, lip, and tongue biting [36]. Other types of self-injury are also common including head, arm, and leg banging as well as inserting fingers or extremities into dangerous or painful places. Patients typically report a sense of frustration or sorrow after an event of self-injury but feel incapable of preventing the behavior. Like many self-injurious behaviors, they often seem to be worse during times of stress. Aggression has been found to be as common as self-injury in some studies [37]. Schretlen et al. described behavioral aspects of Lesch–Nyhan syndrome and its variants using well-validated rating scales and found patterns of severe self-injury, problematic aggression, anxious-depressive symptoms, distractibility/inattention, and disturbing interpersonal behaviors [38]. Bozano et al. published a careful description of behaviors seen in three children with Lesch–Nyhan syndrome including antecedent conditions, consequent reactions, and emotions of the child as well as caregiver management strategies. They confirmed that patients do experience pain associated with self-harm behaviors, and the most common emotional reactions of the patient were regret and shock, as well as increased anxiety rather than satisfaction after a self-injurious behavior [39]. Self-injury in three relatively young boys (age 17, 25, and 30 months) with Lesch–Nyhan syndrome is described in another study, suggesting that it differs from that seen in young children with autism or other developmental disabilities, both in its abrupt onset and severity [40]. The compulsion for self-injury in patients with Lesch–Nyhan syndrome can be so strong and severe that even after total dental extraction, new behaviors such as rubbing one foot against the other, scratching toenails with hands, and sticking legs and feet against hard objects may appear [41].

Patients with Lesch–Nyhan syndrome exhibit mild-to-moderate cognitive impairment, another frequent symptom leading to psychiatric involvement. Deficits in cognition are thought to be due to a static insult rather than a progressive or degenerative disease [24]. In one study of 42 patients with Lesch–Nyhan syndrome, cognitive impairment was not readily described by caregivers observing activities of daily living, though only 15% of these patients were at grade level for math and reading [42]. In patients with Lesch–Nyhan variants, cognitive deficits may be subtle or not present at all, and may not be reported unless the patient is specifically referred for neuropsychiatric testing.

In addition to self-injury, patients with Lesch–Nyhan syndrome are thought to be more anxious, and may have increased emotional lability, which can be particularly pronounced at the time of a medical encounter [24].

17.6 Assessment, Including Genetic Testing and Other Recommended Diagnostic Assessments

The differential diagnosis of the presenting symptoms of Lesch–Nyhan syndrome varies by age. During the first months of life, prior to the appearance of self-injury, children with Lesch–Nyhan syndrome have been incorrectly diagnosed with cerebral palsy. The absence of prenatal or postnatal neurological insult should point away from a cerebral palsy diagnosis. When dystonia appears, early-onset isolated or inherited dystonia should be considered. Segawa syndrome, or Dopa-responsive dystonia, is included in the differential diagnosis for early-onset dystonia. The presence of hyperuricemia helps rule out these disorders. Once self-injury starts, the differential diagnosis includes autism spectrum disorder with intellectual disability and several genetic disorders. The incidence of self-injury is highest in Smith-Magenis syndrome, Cri du Chat syndrome, and Prader-Willi syndrome. The presence of dystonia and hyperuricemia helps rule out these disorders [43]. Self-injurious behavior also occurs in hereditary sensory and autonomic neuropathies characterized by loss of pain sensitivity. In contrast, children with Lesch–Nyhan syndrome have intact sensation.

While a patient with hyperuricemia and developmental delay should prompt a workup for Lesch–Nyhan syndrome, these are both non-specific findings. Definitive diagnosis is made by either enzymatic testing to estimate the HGPRT enzyme activity level or with molecular genetic testing sequencing the *HPRT1* gene. The main problem with gene testing is that mutations are heterogeneous so can be time-consuming and expensive to complete, and new unique mutations continue to be described, so even with comprehensive genetic testing, it is possible to miss a diagnosis. Enzymatic testing is most accurately done with live cells, typically cultured skin fibroblasts, to mimic natural enzyme environments. Enzyme function can be underestimated if using the technically simpler and less expensive process using cell lysates that less closely resemble the natural environment but does not require the more tedious cell culture process [34].

There has been some research into identifying biomarkers that would facilitate earlier diagnosis and treatment for patients with Lesch–Nyhan syndrome and Lesch–Nyhan syndrome variants. Ceballos-Picot et al. published a study in 2015 demonstrating a highly significant correlation between six metabolites (AICAR mono- and tri-phosphate, nicotinamide, nicotinic acid, ATP, and Succinyl-AMP) and HGPRT deficiency that may represent future avenues for early and reliable diagnosis [33].

Prenatal testing is available by chorionic villus sampling or amniocentesis and can be done in male patients with a family history of Lesch–Nyhan syndrome. It is also possible to determine the carrier status of a potential mother to facilitate family planning in affected families [44].

17.7 Psychosocial Treatments

The psychosocial treatments for Lesch–Nyhan syndrome are often focused on interventions to prevent self-injury. Many patients utilize protective devices that may include helmets, arm and leg pads, or mouth guards that prevent damage from biting. Similarly, restraints can be used to prevent the patient from harming themself or others. Patients with Lesch–Nyhan syndrome have been known to feel the compulsion for self-harm and request interventions such as restraints [37]. Specialized equipment including intraoral resin mouthguards to prevent injury from teeth has been shown to have some efficacy [45, 46], though often even with these devices, dental extraction is still pursued because of the severity of the injuries. In a group of five patients with Lesch–Nyhan syndrome who initially used mouth guards to avoid removal of the teeth, success was variable and four of these patients eventually needed dental extraction [47].

Olson et al. summarize behavioral interventions that have been used to target the particularly difficult-to-treat self-injurious behaviors associated with Lesch–Nyhan syndrome. The authors outline case reports and case series targeting various forms of self-injury (biting, head banging, finger biting, skin picking/ripping) and subsequently use a variety of behavioral techniques including extinction, systematic desensitization, punishment, play therapy, positive reinforcement, differential reinforcement of other behaviors, differential reinforcement of incompatible behavior, and relaxation with variable success in reducing the frequency and severity of the target behaviors. In their conclusion, the authors of this report note that the most common behavioral intervention is restraint, and while effective, is also the most restrictive. Although less restrictive behavioral interventions can be difficult to employ for a variety of reasons (maintaining behavioral intervention across treatment settings, severity of tissue damage caused by self-injury requiring immediate intervention, etc.), they can be effective and with individualization and adjustment, can provide benefit to patients with Lesch–Nyhan syndrome [48].

17.8 Biological Treatments

Allopurinol is a mainstay of treatment and blocks the conversion of hypoxanthine and xanthine to uric acid. Decreasing the uric acid burden prevents nephrolithiasis, gout, and kidney disease caused by uncontrolled uric acid levels. Though treatment with allopurinol does not prevent neurologic dysfunction, it should be started immediately upon diagnosis to protect kidney function. In adults, colchicine and nonsteroidal anti-inflammatory drugs (NSAIDs) are used to prevent gout flares. Though levels of uric acid may be higher than in other diseases resulting in gout, allopurinol dosing does not differ significantly and can begin at 5–10 mg/kg, with final total doses ranging from 50 to 600 mg per day. This is thought to result in a mean 50% reduction of serum urate and a 74% reduction in urinary uric acid:creatinine ratio [49]. Though nephrolithiasis in Lesch–Nyhan syndrome is often due to uric acid, stones can also be comprised of xanthine or other oxypurines. In more common cases of gout, treatment with allopurinol increases HGPRT-mediated recycling of hypoxanthine and subsequent feedback inhibition of de novo purine synthesis. In HGPRT-deficient patients, hypoxanthine cannot be recycled, and purine synthesis is upregulated. This may result in increased concentrations of xanthine to a point of lithiasis (crystallization of a substance into a solid mass or "stone"). Without examining the stones for their composition, a clinician may increase allopurinol assuming the stone is due to hyperuricemia when the more effective approach would be to decrease the dose [49, 50]. Febuxostat is a newer non-purine inhibitor that is used in the treatment of gout and works by inhibiting both the oxidized and reduced forms of xanthine oxidase. While allopurinol is more commonly prescribed, there has been much research in the safety and efficacy of febuxostat, and it therefore, would be a reasonable alternative to allopurinol for the treatment of hyperuricemia [51–54].

Unfortunately, even with allopurinol treatment starting at birth, the neurologic effects of Lesch–Nyhan syndrome still occur. While there are hypotheses that the neurological dysfunction is related to dopaminergic neuron concentration in the basal ganglia, supplemental dopamine has had inconsistent effects ranging from slightly positive to a significantly negative effect on self-mutilation and aggressive behavior and is not considered to be a reliable treatment [22].

Movement disorders resulting in dystonia may be managed with medications such as baclofen or benzodiazepines in addition to assistive devices such as wheelchairs, walkers, or canes. Intrathecal baclofen therapy for generalized dystonia has been trialed with some success in case reports [55, 56].

A common treatment for oral self-injury is the extraction of teeth, which limits the amount of damage during self-injury events [36, 41, 57, 58]. Some patients with a severe pattern of oral self-injurious behavior may cause damage to the teeth that results in extraction or may self-extract teeth as a form of self-injury. Botulinum toxin is also showing promise as a more conservative approach to self-mutilation when injected into the masticatory muscles. Additional case reports support this finding [59, 60].

Deep brain stimulation (DBS) has been studied in Lesch–Nyhan syndrome with some efficacy. Though the studies have been relatively small and limited in scope, there is evidence that deep brain stimulation may improve both the motor and behavioral symptoms of Lesch–Nyhan syndrome [61, 62]. A recent systematic review looked at the results of eight publications describing a total of 12 patients and showed that DBS improved dystonia in all patients to varying degrees. Likewise, all patients also reported partial or complete control of self-injurious behavior, indicating that DBS may be an effective treatment, though there were high rates of adverse events such as infections involving DBS leads or hardware-related issues such as broken wires [63]. In one case report, improvements in dystonia and self-injurious behaviors were maintained at a 5-year follow-up [64]. Deep brain stimulation may be considered in some patients with Lesch–Nyhan syndrome but must be weighed against the risk of adverse events. Further studies on this treatment modality may help inform these recommendations.

There is very little evidence to guide psychotropic prescribing in patients with Lesch–Nyhan syndrome. Pharmacotherapy in children with neurodevelopmental disorders has successfully targeted irritability and hyperactivity but has shown limited efficacy in reducing self-injurious behaviors. Second-generation antipsychotics and N-acetylcysteine have low levels of evidence in patients with developmental disabilities. The evidence for clonidine, amantadine, naltrexone, and mood stabilizers is very low and inconsistent [43]. Serotonin reuptake inhibitors can be used for comorbid anxiety but will probably have little effect on self-injurious behavior.

The common medical comorbidities of Lesch–Nyhan syndrome need to be considered when prescribing pharmacotherapy to this patient population. Careful consideration of renal function is important to consider when prescribing medications that are renally metabolized or excreted. It would be important to work closely with a patient's nephrologist prior to prescribing medications that affect or are affected by the kidneys.

Another important consideration is the overlap between the side effect profile of psychotropic medications commonly prescribed for aggression in intellectual disability and the underlying motor symptoms caused by Lesch–Nyhan syndrome. First- and second-generation antipsychotics can cause extrapyramidal motor symptoms including dystonic reactions that may be difficult to differentiate from symptoms of the primary disorder. Given this, having a clear understanding of baseline motor function, impairment, and symptoms would be important prior to prescribing medications known to cause extrapyramidal side effects.

Key Points to Remember

- Lesch–Nyhan syndrome is a rare, X-linked metabolic disorder related to deficits in HGPRT enzyme which is involved in the purine salvage pathway and results in symptoms of hyperuricemia, intellectual disability, motor impairment, and in severe cases, self-mutilation.
- There is a phenotypic spectrum of patients with impaired HGPRT enzyme function which can range from severe neurological deficiencies and self-injurious behaviors along with hyperuricemia to mild hyperuricemia alone on the mild end of the spectrum.
- Self-injurious behaviors in patients with Lesch–Nyhan syndrome can be extremely severe and difficult to treat.
- Kidney function should be appropriately monitored when treating self-injurious behaviors or comorbid psychiatric conditions with psychotropic medications given the known association with hyperuricemia and subsequent kidney disease.
- A clear understanding of baseline motor function and impairment will help a clinician when prescribing medications that can cause dystonia since extrapyramidal symptoms can also be a part of the underlying primary disorder and are unrelated to medication side effects.

References

1. Lesch MNW. A familial disorder of uric acid metabolism and central nervous system function. Am J Med. 1964;36:561–70.
2. Seegmiller JE, Rosenbloom FM, Kelley WN. Enzyme defect associated with a sex-linked human neurological disorder and excessive purine synthesis. Science. 1967;155(3770):1682–4.
3. Kelley WN, Rosenbloom FM, Henderson JF, Seegmiller JE. A specific enzyme defect in gout associated with overproduction of uric acid. Proc Natl Acad Sci USA. 1967;57(6):1735–9.
4. Fu R, Sutcliffe D, Zhao H, et al. Clinical severity in Lesch-Nyhan disease: the role of residual enzyme and compensatory pathways. Mol Genet Metab. 2015;114(1):55–61.
5. Sampat R, Fu R, Larovere LE, et al. Mechanisms for phenotypic variation in Lesch-Nyhan disease and its variants. Hum Genet. 2011;129(1):71–8.
6. Torres RJ, Puig JG. Hypoxanthine deregulates genes involved in early neuronal development. Implications in Lesch-Nyhan disease pathogenesis. J Inherit Metab Dis. 2015;38(6):1109–18.
7. Hoefnagel D. Lesch-Nyhan syndrome. Pathology and pathologic physiology. Summary. Fed Proc. 1968;27(4):1042–6.
8. Ogasawara N, Stout JT, Goto H, Sonta S, Matsumoto A, Caskey CT. Molecular analysis of a female Lesch-Nyhan patient. J Clin Invest. 1989;84(3):1024–7.
9. Rinat C, Zoref-Shani E, Ben-Neriah Z, et al. Molecular, biochemical, and genetic characterization of a female patient with Lesch-Nyhan disease. Mol Genet Metab. 2006;87(3):249–52.

10. De Gregorio L, Jinnah HA, Harris JC, et al. Lesch-Nyhan disease in a female with a clinically normal monozygotic twin. Mol Genet Metab. 2005;85(1):70–7.
11. De Gregorio L, Nyhan WL, Serafin E, Chamoles NA. An unexpected affected female patient in a classical Lesch-Nyhan family. Mol Genet Metab. 2000;69(3):263–8.
12. Aral B, de Saint BG, Al-Garawi S, Kamoun P, Ceballos-Picot I. Novel nonsense mutation in the hypoxanthine guanine phosphoribosyltransferase gene and nonrandom X-inactivation causing Lesch-Nyhan syndrome in a female patient. Hum Mutat. 1996;7(1):52–8.
13. Yukawa T, Akazawa H, Miyake Y, Takahashi Y, Nagao H, Takeda E. A female patient with Lesch-Nyhan syndrome. Dev Med Child Neurol. 1992;34(6):543–6.
14. van Bogaert P, Ceballos I, Desguerre I, Telvi L, Kamoun P, Ponsot G. Lesch-Nyhan syndrome in a girl. J Inherit Metab Dis. 1992;15(5):790–1.
15. AlBakheet A, AlQudairy H, Alkhalifah J, Almoaily S, Kaya N, Rahbeeni Z. Detailed genetic and clinical analysis of a novel de novo variant in HPRT1: case report of a female patient from Saudi Arabia with Lesch-Nyhan syndrome. Front Genet. 2022;13:1044936.
16. Crawhall JC, Henderson JF, Kelley WN. Diagnosis and treatment of the Lesch-Nyhan syndrome. Pediatr Res. 1972;6(5):504–13.
17. McCarthy GT, Green EM, Ogunbona O, et al. A population study of Lesch-Nyhan disease in the UK. Dev Med Child Neurol. 2011;53(1):34–9.
18. Jinnah HA, De Gregorio L, Harris JC, Nyhan WL, O'Neill JP. The spectrum of inherited mutations causing HPRT deficiency: 75 new cases and a review of 196 previously reported cases. Mutat Res. 2000;463(3):309–26.
19. Li L, Qiao X, Liu F, et al. Description of the molecular and phenotypic spectrum of Lesch-Nyhan disease in eight Chinese patients. Front Genet. 2022;13:868942.
20. Fu R, Chen CJ, Jinnah HA. Genotypic and phenotypic spectrum in attenuated variants of Lesch-Nyhan disease. Mol Genet Metab. 2014;112(4):280–5.
21. Torres RJ, Puig JG. Hypoxanthine-guanine phosophoribosyltransferase (HPRT) deficiency: Lesch-Nyhan syndrome. Orphanet J Rare Dis. 2007;2:48.
22. Bell S, Kolobova I, Crapper L, Ernst C. Lesch-Nyhan syndrome: models, theories, and therapies. Mol Syndromol. 2016;7(6):302–11.
23. Schretlen DJ, Callon W, Ward RE, et al. Do clinical features of Lesch-Nyhan disease correlate more closely with hypoxanthine or guanine recycling? J Inherit Metab Dis. 2016;39(1):85–91.
24. Jinnah HA, Visser JE, Harris JC, et al. Delineation of the motor disorder of Lesch-Nyhan disease. Brain. 2006;129(Pt 5):1201–17.
25. Visser JE, Bar PR, Jinnah HA. Lesch-Nyhan disease and the basal ganglia. Brain Res Brain Res Rev. 2000;32(2–3):449–75.
26. Schretlen DJ, Varvaris M, Ho TE, et al. Regional brain volume abnormalities in Lesch-Nyhan disease and its variants: a cross-sectional study. Lancet Neurol. 2013;12(12):1151–8.
27. Harris JC. Lesch-Nyhan syndrome and its variants: examining the behavioral and neurocognitive phenotype. Curr Opin Psychiatry. 2018;31(2):96–102.
28. Bell S, McCarty V, Peng H, et al. Lesch-Nyhan disease causes impaired energy metabolism and reduced developmental potential in midbrain dopaminergic cells. Stem Cell Reports. 2021;16(7):1749–62.
29. Cho JH, Choi JH, Heo SH, et al. Phenotypic and molecular spectrum of Korean patients with Lesch-Nyhan syndrome and attenuated clinical variants. Metab Brain Dis. 2019;34(5):1335–40.
30. Yang L, Guo H. Case report: early-onset renal failure as presenting sign of Lesch-Nyhan disease in infancy. Front Pediatr. 2022;10:1080486.
31. Kollios K, Savvidou P, Karipiadou A, et al. Lesch-Nyhan syndrome due to a splice-site mutation in a 14-month-old boy presenting as acute renal failure. Clin Nephrol. 2021;96(2):120–3.
32. Ambarsari CG, Cahyadi D, Sari L, et al. Late diagnosis of Lesch-Nyhan disease complicated with end-stage renal disease and tophi burst: a case report. Ren Fail. 2020;42(1):113–21.
33. Ceballos-Picot I, Le Dantec A, Brassier A, et al. New biomarkers for early diagnosis of Lesch-Nyhan disease revealed by metabolic analysis on a large cohort of patients. Orphanet J Rare Dis. 2015;10:7.

34. Jinnah HA, Ceballos-Picot I, Torres RJ, et al. Attenuated variants of Lesch-Nyhan disease. Brain. 2010;133(Pt 3):671–89.
35. Cakmakli HF, Torres RJ, Menendez A, et al. Macrocytic anemia in Lesch-Nyhan disease and its variants. Genet Med. 2019;21(2):353–60.
36. Isola G, Piccardo I, De Mari A, Alberti G, Migliorati M. Oral self-mutilation in Lesch-Nyhan patients: a cross-sectional study. J Clin Med. 2022;11(20):5981.
37. Anderson LT, Ernst M. Self-injury in Lesch-Nyhan disease. J Autism Dev Disord. 1994;24(1):67–81.
38. Schretlen DJ, Ward J, Meyer SM, et al. Behavioral aspects of Lesch-Nyhan disease and its variants. Dev Med Child Neurol. 2005;47(10):673–7.
39. Bozano A, Schiaffino A, Spessa A, et al. Description of the Lesch-Nyhan neurobehavioral disorder and its management through participant observation of three young individuals. JIMD Rep. 2020;52(1):63–71.
40. Hall S, Oliver C, Murphy G. Self-injurious behaviour in young children with Lesch-Nyhan syndrome. Dev Med Child Neurol. 2001;43(11):745–9.
41. Gisbert de la Cuadra L, Torres RJ, Beltran LM, Sanchez A, Puig JG. Development of new forms of self-injurious behavior following total dental extraction in Lesch-Nyhan disease. Nucleosides Nucleotides Nucleic Acids. 2016;35(10–12):524–8.
42. Anderson LT, Ernst M, Davis SV. Cognitive abilities of patients with Lesch-Nyhan disease. J Autism Dev Disord. 1992;22(2):189–203.
43. Sabus A, Feinstein J, Romani P, Goldson E, Blackmer A. Management of self-injurious behaviors in children with neurodevelopmental disorders: a pharmacotherapy overview. Pharmacotherapy. 2019;39(6):645–64.
44. O'Neill JP. Mutation carrier testing in Lesch-Nyhan syndrome families: HPRT mutant frequency and mutation analysis with peripheral blood T lymphocytes. Genet Test. 2004;8(1):51–64.
45. Ragazzini G, Delucchi A, Calcagno E, Servetto R, Denotti G. A modified intraoral resin mouthguard to prevent self-mutilations in lesch-nyhan patients. Int J Dent. 2014;2014:396830.
46. Arhakis A, Topouzelis N, Kotsiomiti E, Kotsanos N. Effective treatment of self-injurious oral trauma in Lesch-Nyhan syndrome: a case report. Dent Traumatol. 2010;26(6):496–500.
47. Goodman EM, Torres RJ, Puig JG, Jinnah HA. Consequences of delayed dental extraction in Lesch-Nyhan disease. Mov Disord Clin Pract. 2014;1(3):225–9.
48. Olson L, Houlihan D. A review of behavioral treatments used for Lesch-Nyhan syndrome. Behav Modif. 2000;24(2):202–22.
49. Torres RJ, Puig JG, Jinnah HA. Update on the phenotypic spectrum of Lesch-Nyhan disease and its attenuated variants. Curr Rheumatol Rep. 2012;14(2):189–94.
50. Sikora P, Pijanowska M, Majewski M, Bienias B, Borzecka H, Zajczkowska M. Acute renal failure due to bilateral xanthine urolithiasis in a boy with Lesch-Nyhan syndrome. Pediatr Nephrol. 2006;21(7):1045–7.
51. Kang SH, Kim BY, Son EJ, Kim GO, Do JY. Comparison between the effects of allopurinol and febuxostat on the survival of patients on maintenance hemodialysis. Am J Nephrol. 2023;54(3–4):117–25.
52. Park S, Lee JP, Kim DK, Kim YS, Lim CS. Superior effect of allopurinol compared to febuxostat on the retardation of chronic kidney disease progression. PLoS One. 2022;17(2):e0264627.
53. Liao Z, Xu L, Wan B, et al. Comparison of febuxostat and allopurinol in the treatment of patients with chronic kidney disease stage 3~5 with hyperuricemia. Emerg Med Int. 2022;2022:1177946.
54. Suzuki S, Yoshihisa A, Yokokawa T, et al. Comparison between febuxostat and allopurinol uric acid-lowering therapy in patients with chronic heart failure and hyperuricemia: a multicenter randomized controlled trial. J Int Med Res. 2021;49(12):3000605211062770.
55. Satow T, Ogawa M, Komuro T. Intrathecal baclofen therapy for Lesch-Nyhan disease: illustrative case. J Neurosurg Case Lessons. 2021;1(1):CASE202.
56. Pozzi M, Piccinini L, Gallo M, Motta F, Radice S, Clementi E. Treatment of motor and behavioural symptoms in three Lesch-Nyhan patients with intrathecal baclofen. Orphanet J Rare Dis. 2014;9:208.

57. Rashid N, Yusuf H. Oral self-mutilation by a 17-month-old child with Lesch-Nyhan syndrome. Int J Paediatr Dent. 1997;7(2):115–7.
58. Campolo Gonzalez A, Vargas Diaz A, Fontbote Riesco D, Hernandez CM. Oral self-mutilation in Lesch-Nyhan syndrome. Case report. Rev Chil Pediatr. 2018;89(1):86–91.
59. Ferrao J, Rodrigues Barros C, Figueiredo L, Fernandes A. Oral self-mutilation in Lesch-Nyhan syndrome: a case report. Cureus. 2022;14(8):e27874.
60. Gilbert C, Sauer M, Cheng J. Reduction of self-mutilating behavior and improved oromotor function in a patient with Lesch-Nyhan syndrome following botulinum toxin injection: a case report. J Pediatr Rehabil Med. 2021;14(1):133–6.
61. Visser JE, Cotton AC, Schretlen DJ, et al. Deep brain stimulation in Lesch-Nyhan disease: outcomes from the patient's perspective. Dev Med Child Neurol. 2021;63(8):963–8.
62. Tambirajoo K, Furlanetti L, Hasegawa H, et al. Deep brain stimulation of the internal pallidum in Lesch-Nyhan syndrome: clinical outcomes and connectivity analysis. Neuromodulation. 2021;24(2):380–91.
63. Deng H, Xiong BT, Wu Y, Wang W. Deep brain stimulation in Lesch-Nyhan syndrome: a systematic review. Neurosurg Rev. 2023;46(1):40.
64. Piedimonte F, Andreani JC, Piedimonte L, Micheli F, Graff P, Bacaro V. Remarkable clinical improvement with bilateral globus pallidus internus deep brain stimulation in a case of Lesch-Nyhan disease: five-year follow-up. Neuromodulation. 2015;18(2):118–22; discussion 22.

Further Reading

Bell S, Kolobova I, Crapper L, Ernst C. Lesch-Nyhan syndrome: models, theories, and therapies. Mol Syndromol. 2016;7(6):302–11.

Fu R, Chen CJ, Jinnah HA. Genotypic and phenotypic spectrum in attenuated variants of Lesch-Nyhan disease. Mol Genet Metab. 2014;112(4):280–5.

Harris JC. Lesch-Nyhan syndrome and its variants: examining the behavioral and neurocognitive phenotype. Curr Opin Psychiatry. 2018;31(2):96–102.

Jinnah HA, Ceballos-Picot I, Torres RJ, et al. Attenuated variants of Lesch-Nyhan disease. Brain. 2010;133(Pt 3):671–89.

Jinnah HA, Visser JE, Harris JC, et al. Delineation of the motor disorder of Lesch-Nyhan disease. Brain. 2006;129(Pt 5):1201–17.

Cornelia de Lange Syndrome

18

Marco A. Grados, Sid Srivastava, Pratik Agarwal, and Antonie D. Kline

18.1 Overview

18.1.1 History

Cornelia de Lange syndrome (CdLS) is a rare genetic disorder, affecting up to 1/10,000 live births, resulting from a deficit in genetic substrates including *NIPBL, HDAC8, SMC1A, SMC3*, and other cohesin-related genes. The main downstream effect of CDLS transcriptional deficits (transcriptomopathy) includes "cohesinopathies" as a cardinal finding in CdLS [1], with cohesinopathies having a large spectrum of clinical manifestations [2]. As a consequence of transcriptional dysfunction, multiple organ systems, including brain, bone, gastrointestinal, immune, and endocrine systems are affected [3]. Manifestations include malformation of the upper limbs; gastroesophageal dysfunction; cardiac, ophthalmologic, and genitourinary anomalies; and hirsutism [4]. The condition is named for the Dutch pediatrician, Cornelia de Lange, who described a phenotype of facial features including long eyelashes, confluent eyebrows (synophrys), long philtrum, thin lips, and crescent-shaped mouths in 1933 [5]. However, the syndrome had been recognized earlier by the German physician-in-training, W. Brachmann, who reported on a neonate

M. A. Grados (✉)
Johns Hopkins University School of Medicine, Baltimore, MD, USA
e-mail: mgrados1@jhmi.edu

S. Srivastava
Harvard Medical School, Boston, MA, USA

P. Agarwal
Lokmanya Tilak Municipal Medical College, Mumbai, India

A. D. Kline
Greater Baltimore Medical Center, Baltimore, MD, USA

R. P. Thom, C. J. McDougle (eds.), *Neuropsychiatric Care for Genetic Syndromes and Other Neurodevelopmental Disorders*,
https://doi.org/10.1007/978-3-031-76269-7_18

deceased at 19 days of age from pneumonia as a child with "symmetrical monodactyly…dwarfism, cervical ribs, and hirsutism [Zwerghaftigkeit, Halsrippen, Behaarung]," with an emphasis on the limb malformations [6]. In an editorial in 1985, Opitz thus advocated for the denomination of Brachmann-de Lange syndrome to recognize the facial and limb manifestations, after reporting having seen approximately 100 cases [7]. The behavioral phenotype was noted by William Nyhan to be prototypic for conditions with developmental delay which had significant repetitive behaviors, including the malignant self-injurious behaviors (SIB) with self-biting, skin picking, head banging [8], and other behaviors including "circling, twirling and whirling" [9]. Nyhan observed that children with CdLS appeared to be "[have] self-programmed … stereotyped patterns of unusual behavior [which] could represent the presence of structural defects in the central nervous system, just as there are structural defects in the hair, the bones, and the dermatoglyphics" [9]. The complex behavioral phenotype of CdLS, however, is difficult to capture in discrete categories. As stated by Gualtieri in his text on developmental disorders, his experience with a large number of children with CdLS led him to describe the phenotype as "immature, hypersensitive and dysrhythmic," emphasizing their ability to relate, but also to overreact to small stimuli and engage in episodic bodily and emotional dysregulation. Therapeutically, this framework leads to a call for "developmentally appropriate programming, structure, stability, and family support" as the primary tools for the management of behavioral challenges in individuals with CdLS [10].

18.1.2 Pathophysiology

The involvement of *NIBPL* as the main affected gene in CdLS [11] led to the notion of a range of cohesinopathies, as similar phenotypes to classic CdLS which were then linked to pathogenic variants in the other cohesin-related genes including *SMC1A*, *SMC3*, *RAD21*, and *HDAC8* [12]. The known variants of these cohesin-related genes account for approximately 80% of clinical CdLS cases, and more recently "deep intronic" changes in *NIPBL* leading to aberrant transcripts have been found to account for an additional proportion [13]. However, it was soon recognized that other elements were also involved in the genesis of the CdLS phenotype [14]. In terms of animal developmental research, the analog of *NIPBL*, *nipped-b*, has been studied extensively in Drosophila models by Dale Dorsett at Washington University. *Nipped-b* heterozygous mutant Drosophila show reduced growth, learning, and memory, and altered circadian rhythms. Importantly, the growth deficits are not caused by changes in systemic growth controls, but rather, by reductions in cell number and size due to reduced expression of *myc* and other growth control genes [15]. In the fruit fly model, *nipped-b* mutation deficits may respond to the role of *nipped-b* in promoting enhancer–promoter communication in gene developmental systems [16], which by extension suggests that this mutated gene can widely impact developmental systems in humans. In a mouse model of heterozygous *Nibpl* deficiency, gene expression profiling leads to modest but significant transcriptional dysregulation of many genes, including genes that would support a role for *Nipbl* in long-range chromosomal regulatory interactions [17]. In concordance with the key role of *NIPBL* in the CdLS phenotype, studies have shown that many *NIPBL* variants, in contrast with variants in other cohesin-related genes, are associated with lower self-help and verbal skills, leading to lower mood states and increased insistence on sameness with older age [18]. Similar but lesser deficits are observed in individuals with *SMC1A* gene disruption in somatic, cognitive, and behavioral domains [19]. Thus, the effect of *NIPBL* gene deficits leads to transcriptional dysregulation and changes in multiple organ systems, with major targets being limb formation and brain development.

Brain involvement in CdLS as a result of developmental dysregulation is, to date, not well characterized. An anatomical report of a deceased neonate with CdLS showed significant brain abnormalities including hypoplasia of the anterior thalamic nuclei, neurohypophysis, lateral geniculate body, cerebral peduncle, ventral pons, and cerebellar internal granular layer, as well as heterotopic cell nests in the cerebellar white matter and immature or simple convolution pattern of the cerebral gyri [20]. An autopsy of a 35-year-old adult with CdLS demonstrated abnormal convolution patterns of the cerebral gyri, frontal lobe hypoplasia, and focal lack of myelination in layers V and VI of the left temporal cortex [21], while a series of 15 MRI scans completed for clinical reasons in a cohort of individuals with CdLS showed cerebral atrophy, white matter changes, cerebellar hypoplasia, and enlarged ventricles with foci of gliosis [22]. There is an interesting observation related to the developmental system confluence of brain and limb structures. For example, the manifestation of simple convolution patterns is reminiscent of lissencephaly due to underdeveloped cerebral gyri due to mutations in *GLI3* [23]. Tanaka reports that the fin-to-limb transition in autopods (hand or foot) is influenced by *GLI3* and *SHH*, two genes that are highly influential in gyri formation (hence lissencephaly in *GLI3* mutations) and structural brain formation (*SHH* guiding brain and limb patterning), which are similar to those changes in CdLS autopsy results. It should be noted that *GLI3*, a zinc finger transcription factor, belongs to a genetic network that determines limb formation [24], another important clinical feature in CdLS [25, 26]. An additional gene network implicated in CdLS and affecting brain development is the Wnt pathway, identified as abnormal in cell studies of CdLS as well as in animal models [27]. The investigation into limb and brain development [28, 29] being affected by similar genetic networks implicating *SHH*, *GLI*, *WNT*, and *BMP* genes can set the groundwork for investigations into the developmental connections between limb and brain development, with CdLS as a model disease.

18.2 Signs and Symptoms of Psychiatric Comorbidities

The behavioral phenotype of CdLS can be parsed into the following categories: autism spectrum disorder (ASD), general developmental/intellectual delay, anxiety, repetitive behaviors, speech difficulties, and sleep problems.

18.2.1 Autism Spectrum Disorder

The diagnosis of ASD hinges on the core deficit of impaired social reciprocity. This major symptom complex in idiopathic ASD follows from widespread developmental brain insults or more specific social brain network abnormalities [30]. Known genetic syndromes, such as Fragile X syndrome (FXS), tuberous sclerosis complex, and CdLS have been posited as models for ASD research; however, it is germane to point out that these genetic syndromes display mostly atypical autism features. These differences in clinical presentation appear to follow morphological and functional brain differences. In FXS, for example, examination of brain structure in idiopathic ASD and individuals with FXS show notable differences in caudate and amygdala volumes between the two groups [31]. A study of clinical ASD features in CdLS confirms that an atypical pattern of symptoms characterizes this genetic condition. Forty-one children with CdLS (23 females and 18 males) aged 5–18 years were studied using the Childhood Autism Rating Scale (CARS). The CARS classified 17% as having no autism, 41% with moderate autism, and another 41% with severe autism. From a symptom perspective, absent or poor expressive language was most prominent, along with rigid, stereotypical movements, and behaviors. Social deficits were less prominent, although remained a clinical concern [32]. In another study, 49 caregivers of individuals with mild-to-severe phenotypic CdLS completed the Social Communication Questionnaire and the Autism Diagnostic Interview-Revised; 49% of the cohort had significant autistic features. In both studies, as expected, a higher number of autistic features correlated with lower adaptive and intellectual functioning [33]. An earlier study also using the CARS, identified 32% of 54 individuals with CdLS as having ASD, compared with 7% of a comparison group with intellectual disability [34], suggesting that autistic features are common in CdLS, often in conjunction with lower adaptive functioning [35]. The comparison of different genetic syndromes in relation to autistic features has also been instructive. In a study of FXS, Cri du chat syndrome, and CdLS, cohorts examined at baseline (Time 1) and 30-months later (Time 2), it was found that individuals with FXS and CdLS initially had a higher number of autism features (Time 1), but at 30-month follow-up (Time 2), individuals with CdLS had the most autism-related clinical features [36].

18.2.2 Intellectual Disability

Individuals with CdLS are broadly affected with a range of intellectual deficits. As a group, the average IQ reflects moderate intellectual disability (range of 55–70) [37]. Earlier reports suggested that intellectual disability was universal in CdLS [38]; however, more recent reports consistently show a subtype of CdLS that is less affected with mild or no intellectual disability. From a molecular perspective, it has been consistently shown that larger *NIPBL* gene insults, such as truncations affecting multiple exons, result in a more severe phenotype, in both somatic and cognitive domains. For example, in an individual with a deletion of only exon 11 from *NIPBL*, resulting in an in-frame deletion, there was only mild intellectual impairment [39]. Similarly, greater intellectual disability often co-occurs with greater maladaptive behaviors [34], exerting an important influence on the behavioral phenotype of CdLS. In this manner, lower levels of adaptive functioning, which strongly correlate with IQ, are strongly associated with more autistic traits [32], hyperactivity, SIB and aggressive behaviors [40], as well as general behavior problems [41]. In an important association study of type of variant with phenotype severity, missense variants were associated with least affected, while other types of variants (e.g., frameshift) were associated with more severely affected somatically and cognitively [42]. In another interesting study, correlating physical features of CdLS with prognostic utility, limb and palate malformations appeared to carry the higher valence for poor prognosis, with cleft palate affecting approximately 20% of individuals with CdLS [43]. In summary, intellectual disability is a common feature in CdLS with specific somatic differences and a greater portion of gene involvement being associated with general cognitive deficits.

18.2.3 Anxiety

The behavioral phenotype of CdLS is characterized by a very high frequency of anxiety disorders [44]. While free-floating anxiety is commonly observed, the data strongly point to social anxiety, in particular, as a salient clinical feature in CdLS. This form of anxiety takes the guise of social avoidance, reduced verbal interactions, or even selective mutism. The free-floating anxiety may respond more to mounting anxiety when routines or ritualistic behaviors are incomplete. In one study, there were notable differences showing reduced eye contact and lower use of speaking turns in the context of social demands for 12 youth with CdLS compared to the other developmental disorders [45]. In comparison to Down syndrome, similarly, less speech initiation is seen in youth with CdLS, not related to cognitive level, but concurrent with the level of working memory [46]. While in comparison to Rubinstein–Taybi syndrome and FXS, individuals with CdLS show heightened social anxiety and reduced social motivation only during interactions with an unfamiliar adults—but not familiar adults [47]. In addition, more manifestations of generalized anxiety and separation anxiety appear with increased age in individuals with CdLS [48]. Additional research exploring social anxiety and other forms of anxiety in CdLS is needed to characterize this impairing behavioral feature of the disorder in order to implement targeted treatments.

18.2.4 Repetitive and Self-Injurious Behaviors

Restrictive and repetitive behaviors (RRBs) are, aside from anxiety, among the most common phenotypic features in individuals with CdLS. William Nyhan singled out CdLS and Lesch–Nyhan syndrome as two disorders displaying paradigmatic forms of SIB, as evidenced by the compulsive, relentless forms of SIB displayed by both disorders [8, 49]. In clinical reports of CdLS, forms of RRBs appear to be almost universally present, whereas frank SIB is reported in approximately 40% of cases. Importantly, clinicians familiar with CdLS emphasize that bouts of SIB are often associated with somatic complaints, especially gastroesophageal reflux disease (GERD), a common medical condition in CdLS [50]. On the other hand, the amount of repetitive and compulsive, ritualistic behavior is also associated with the degree of SIB observed [33, 51, 52]. These behavioral observations are concordant with an earlier study by Hyman et al., who reported a significant association between SIB and physical self-restraint to not self-injury, as well as compulsions [53]. Another factor associated with an increase in SIB in CdLS is older age [40], a clinical phenomenon largely understudied to date [54]. Environmental factors have also been examined as a contributing factor for increased SIB in CdLS, with one study comparing individuals with CdLS to individuals with intellectual disability and no CdLS, with no difference in the influence of environmental events and SIB [55]. Among the cohesinopathies, *SMC1A*-related disorders due to missense variants have a phenotype that is milder in severity with less frequency of SIB when compared to those with *NIPBL* variants; however, *SMC1A* loss of function gene variants can also result in a Rett-like syndrome with lower cognitive function and high levels of SIB [56]. In summary, RRBs and SIB are important clinical features of the behavioral phenotype of CdLS, causing significant dysfunction and at times bodily harm. While endogenous SIB is a potential SIB type in CdLS (automatic reinforcement), the response of individuals with CdLS to somatic complaints such as GERD [57] ostensibly plays a larger role in the origin of SIB in CdLS compared to other SIB-prone developmental conditions such as Lesch–Nyhan syndrome.

18.2.5 Hyperactivity

Many clinicians have noted that a proportion of youth with CdLS present with a hyperactive behavioral phenotype. Reports of hyperactivity are widely prevalent in CdLS research [58], a behavior that is noted to occur spontaneously, possibly as a need for intense vestibular stimulation. This behavior has also been noted to be increased in the presence of GERD [50]. Especially with advancing age, individuals with CdLS are noted to have increased deficits in attention (digit span), inhibition, and flexibility compared to individuals with Down syndrome [59].

18.2.6 Mood Disorders and Psychosis

Depressive illness and/or bipolar disorder (manic-like episodes) are present in a select group of individuals with CdLS, often manifesting in the adolescent years. No extant literature so far has been published on mood disorders in CdLS. Similarly, there are no published reports of frank psychosis or schizophrenic-like illness in CdLS; however, perceptual disturbances and delusional thinking accompany clinical presentations of mood disorders, heightened anxiety states, and manic-like states.

18.2.7 Speech and Language

Individuals with CdLS have notable expressive language difficulties which, in addition to social anxiety and/or selective mutism, pose significant challenges in expressive communication. Early reports noted the low verbal output or selective mutism compared to receptive language [60]. In a comprehensive study of 116 individuals with CdLS, 2 months–29 years of age, Goodban et al. reported stronger receptive than expressive language skills, as well as poor syntactic ability despite vocabulary skills. Also present were articulation errors, as well as distortion or missing consonants sounds. Correlates of worse language included lower birth weight, more hearing impairment, greater upper limb malformations, more social deficits, and more severe motor delays [61]. A survey of 27 youth with CdLS noted that only four were able to produce functional speech, with older children using nonverbal means to communicate needs [62]. A case report of a 2-year, 7-month old child with CdLS noted that early language therapeutic interventions produced a favorable outcome [63], possibly based on strengthening the vocalization musculature. In CdLS, a glottal "fry" (a nonperiodical phonation of the vocal folds in a frequency below the normal pitch register) can be present, along with hoarseness in older individuals [64]. Importantly, in a study of 15 individuals with CdLS, compared to an equal number of neurotypical individuals and individuals with Down syndrome, individuals with CdLS used a higher number of gestures to communicate compared to both other groups [65], suggesting that training in gestural communication might alleviate expressive language deficits. In summary, expressive deficits are a hallmark of the phenotype of CdLS, and this deficit may benefit from early intervention to enhance expressive skills and/or usage of alternate communication strategies such as gestures.

18.2.8 Sleep

Sleep difficulties are notably prevalent in individuals with CdLS. Over half of individuals with CdLS suffer from sleep disturbances according to survey data [40, 66]. In a study of 46 individuals with CdLS, the Sleep Disturbance Scale for Children was administered to caretakers. Of this sample, up to 15% showed an abnormal total sleep score, with another 56% showing borderline abnormal scores. Sleep disturbance was associated with epilepsy, GERD, intellectual disability, and maladaptive behaviors [67]. Similarly, using a sleep history questionnaire, Rajan et al. queried 31 caretakers of individuals with CdLS across the age span. Sleep onset and maintenance insomnia were noted in over half of the respondents, with children having approximately twice the rate of sleep disturbance as adults [68]. An exploration of the occurrence of sleep disordered breathing, to include obstructive sleep apnea (OSA), was carried out in 22 individuals with CdLS. Using three questionnaires (the Pediatric Sleep Questionnaire (PSQ), Pediatric Daytime Sleepiness Scale (PDSS), and OSA), moderate to severe disordered breathing conditions were found in up to one-third of this cohort, almost ten times higher than in the general population [69]. However, this rate of sleep disorder in CdLS has not been found to be different from other groups with intellectual disability [67].

18.3 Assessment and Early Management

The diagnosis of CdLS spectrum disorder relies on cardinal symptoms and secondary symptoms, with a scoring system developed by the CdLS World Federation [70]. The cardinal symptoms (2 points each) include synophrys/thick eyebrows; short nose/concave nasal ridge/upturned nasal tip; long/smooth philtrum; hand oligodactyly/adactyly; and congenital diaphragmatic hernia. The suggestive features (1 point each) include global developmental delay/intellectual disability; prenatal growth restriction; postnatal growth restriction; microcephaly; small hand/feet; short fifth finger; and hirsutism. A score of 11 points or more with three cardinal symptoms is diagnostic of classic CdLS. Indications for a prenatal work-up include an earlier child with CdLS, a new pregnancy in a family with a known genetic alteration in a CdLS gene or, as occurs most frequently, no family history but features suggestive of CdLS on fetal ultrasonography. Postnatal molecular testing should include at least the seven genes known to cause the CdLS phenotype using next-generation sequencing methods to cover *NIPBL, SMC1A, SMC3, RAD21, BRD4, HDAC8,* and *ANKRD11* to confirm the diagnosis. As many children with CdLS are diagnosed early in life, the pediatric management from an early age should include routine echocardiography (25% affected) and renal sonography (10% affected), with central nervous system testing if seizures are present (20% affected). Weight at birth is usually below the fifth percentile, and monitoring of feeding patterns and weight gain with dietician involvement is an important aspect of early management. Oral feeding is often difficult in children with CdLS, with enteral feeding remaining an option if feed time intervals are >3 hours. Teeth malformations, cleft palate (20%), and gastrointestinal conditions such as GERD are common and should be managed [70].

18.4 Psychosocial Treatments

The behavioral challenges in CdLS can benefit from standard behavioral management strategies for individuals with developmental disability. A functional analysis (FA) of behavior is indicated when maladaptive behaviors are life impairing or altering [71]. From the array of behavioral and psychiatric symptoms acknowledged in the above section, which affect a significant proportion of individuals with CdLS across the lifespan, it is important for families to strategically avail themselves to access behavioral specialists to aid in implementing innovative behavioral treatments [72]. No clinical trials specifically targeting problem behaviors in individuals with CdLS using applied behavior analysis techniques are available to date. However, isolated case reports indicate that behavioral management methods can be of great utility in problem behaviors, especially, those concerning SIB.

18.5 Biological Treatments

The pharmacological treatment of challenging behaviors in individuals with CdLS should follow guiding principles based on safety and efficacy. First, there is substantial empirical evidence that individuals with CdLS are especially sensitive to side effects of psychotropics, beyond what is expected in intellectual disability-related conditions. There is also a range of "paradoxical" reactions observed in individuals with CdLS, with reactions opposite to those expected from the psychotropic dispensed. Hence the use of psychotropics should be undertaken with special caution in individuals with CdLS. These empirical observations led to an early commentary from Gualtieri where individuals with CdLS will benefit mostly from seeking an underlying medical cause of the behavioral challenges (pain) and a psychoeducational programmatic approach [10]. On the other hand, general schemes of psychopharmacologic treatment as indicated for ASD and other developmental disability-related conditions can be applied to individuals with CdLS, including alpha agonists for disruptive behaviors, antidepressants for anxiety/depression, and at times, and antipsychotics for psychosis and SIB.

18.5.1 Anxiety

The use of selective serotonin reuptake inhibitors (SSRIs) is empirically supported in individuals with CdLS, although no case series or controlled trials are available. As with other developmental disabilities, "start low and go slow" is an imperative approach in the dosing of SSRIs in individuals with CdLS. The use of citalopram (Celexa) or fluvoxamine (Luvox) may be preferable to the more activating SSRIs, such as sertraline (Zoloft) or fluoxetine (Prozac), but a highly individualized and personalized approach is required in the use of SSRIs for the management of anxiety and mood states such as depressive disorders.

18.5.2 Repetitive Behaviors

RRBs are challenging to treat pharmacologically in genetic syndromes due to the need for higher doses required for the amelioration of perseverative behaviors. While high dose SSRIs can be used in these instances, care must be taken to avoid the induction of activated or manic states.

18.5.3 Self-Injurious Behaviors

The use of antipsychotics to treat SIB in individuals with CdLS remains an option of last resort, with risperidone being the most utilized drug. Haloperidol (Haldol) is relatively contraindicated due to the reports of poor outcomes in some instances.

Use of other antipsychotics is based on empirical evidence, such as quetiapine for anxiety, sleep and mild psychotic symptoms.

18.6 Common Medical Comorbidities

When prescribing psychotropics in individuals with CdLS, care must be taken for those who have GI difficulties such as GERD (with SSRIs), growth retardation (with stimulants), unstable gait (with alpha agonists), and seizures (with any seizure-threshold lowering agent).

18.7 Conclusion

Cornelia de Lange syndrome is a genetic condition which affects multiple organ systems impacting communication, behavioral and emotional domains of function. In particular, expressive language, repetitive behaviors and social anxiety characterize the phenotype. Mapping the behavioral and psychiatric manifestations for each individual with CdLS becomes critically important in order to offer the most effective individualized treatment approach.

Key Points to Remember

- CdLS is a genetic disorder with multiple neuropsychiatric manifestations such as social anxiety, hyperactivity, self-injurious, and aggressive behaviors, as well as restrictive and repetitive behaviors.
- Individuals with CdLS can have a large range of medical conditions which affect multiple organ systems. Medical care is essential with early detection and treatment being an important aspect of the general management of individuals with CdLS.
- Psychoeducational and programmatic approaches that support developmental trajectories are highly advised for youth with CdLS. Team-based care is essential to cover the multiple needs that may arise due to medical, psychological, and behavioral concerns.

Photographs of Individuals with the Syndrome

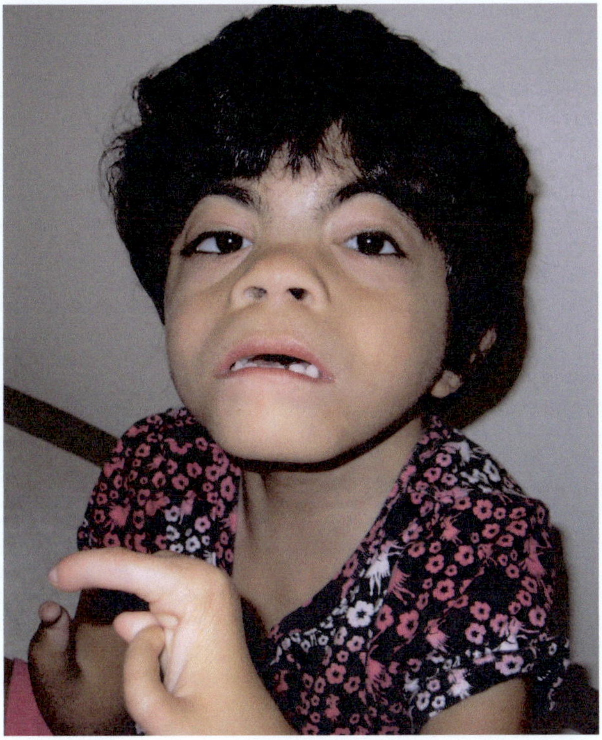

References

1. García-Gutiérrez P, García-Domínguez M. Betting on a transcriptional deficit as the main cause for Cornelia de Lange syndrome. Front Mol Biosci. 2021;8:709232.
2. Piché J, Van Vliet PP, Pucéat M, Andelfinger G. The expanding phenotypes of cohesinopathies: one ring to rule them all! Cell Cycle. 2019;18(21):2828–48.
3. Gause M, Webber HA, Misulovin Z, et al. Functional links between Drosophila Nipped-B and cohesin in somatic and meiotic cells. Chromosoma. 2008 Feb;117(1):51–66.
4. Jackson L, Kline AD, Barr MA, Koch S. de Lange syndrome: a clinical review of 310 individuals. Am J Med Genet. 1993;47(7):940–6.
5. De Lange C. Sur un type nouveau de degeneration (Typus Amstelodamensis). Arch d Med d Enf. 1933;36:713–9.
6. Brachmann W. Ein Fall von symmetrischer Monodaktylie durch Ulnadefekt, mit symmetrischer Flughautbildung in den Ellenbeugen, sowie anderen Abnormitaten (Zwerghaftigkeit, Halsrippen, Behaarung). J b Kinderheilkd. 1916;84:225–35.
7. Opitz JM. The Brachmann-de Lange syndrome. Am J Med Genet. 1985;22:89–102.
8. Shear CS, Nyhan WL, Kirman BH, Stern J. Self-mutilative behavior as a feature of the de Lange syndrome. J Pediatr. 1971;78(3):506–9.
9. Nyhan WL. Behavioral phenotypes in organic genetic disease. Presidential address to the Society for Pediatric Research, May 1, 1971. Pediatr Res. 1972;6(1):1–9.

10. Gualtieri T. Neuropsychiatry and behavioral pharmacology. New York: Springer-Verlag; 1991. p. 173–86.
11. Krantz ID, McCallum J, DeScipio C, et al. Cornelia de Lange syndrome is caused by mutations in NIPBL, the human homolog of Drosophila melanogaster Nipped-B. Nat Genet. 2004;36(6):631–5.
12. Mannini L, Cucco F, Quarantotti V, Krantz ID, Musio A. Mutation spectrum and genotype-phenotype correlation in Cornelia de Lange syndrome. Hum Mutat. 2013;34(12):1589–96.
13. Coursimault J, Cassinari K, Lecoquierre F, et al. Deep intronic NIPBL de novo mutations and differential diagnoses revealed by whole genome and RNA sequencing in Cornelia de Lange syndrome patients. Hum Mutat. 2022;43(12):1882–97.
14. Liu J, Krantz ID. Cornelia de Lange syndrome, cohesin, and beyond. Clin Genet. 2009;76(4):303–14.
15. Wu Y, Gause M, Xu D, et al. Drosophila nipped-b mutants model Cornelia de Lange syndrome in growth and behavior. PLoS Genet. 2015;11(11):e1005655.
16. Rollins RA, Morcillo P, Dorsett D. Nipped-B, a Drosophila homologue of chromosomal adherins, participates in activation by remote enhancers in the cut and Ultrabithorax genes. Genetics. 1999;152(2):577–93.
17. Kawauchi S, Calof AL, Santos R, et al. Multiple organ system defects and transcriptional dysregulation in the Nipbl(+/−) mouse, a model of Cornelia de Lange syndrome. PLoS Genet. 2009;5(9):e1000650.
18. Moss J, Penhallow J, Ansari M, et al. Genotype-phenotype correlations in Cornelia de Lange syndrome: behavioral characteristics and changes with age. Am J Med Genet A. 2017;173(6):1566–74.
19. Huisman S, Mulder PA, Redeker E, et al. Phenotypes and genotypes in individuals with SMC1A variants. Am J Med Genet A. 2017;173(8):2108–25.
20. Yamaguchi K, Ishitobi F. Brain dysgenesis in Cornelia de Lange syndrome. Clin Neuropathol. 1999;18(2):99–105.
21. Vuilleumier N, Kövari E, Michon A, et al. Neuropathological analysis of an adult case of the Cornelia de Lange syndrome. Acta Neuropathol. 2002;104(3):327–32.
22. Roshan Lal TR, Kliewer MA, Lopes T, et al. Cornelia de Lange syndrome: correlation of brain MRI findings with behavioral assessment. Am J Med Genet C Semin Med Genet. 2016;172(2):190–7.
23. Tanaka M. Fins into limbs: autopod acquisition and anterior elements reduction by modifying gene networks involving 5'Hox, Gli3, and Shh. Dev Biol. 2016;413(1):1–7.
24. Abbasi AA, Minhas R, Schmidt A, Koch S, Grzeschik K. Cis-regulatory underpinnings of human GLI3 expression in embryonic craniofacial structures and internal organs. Develop Growth Differ. 2013;55(8):699–709.
25. Hayashi S, Akiyama R, Wong J, Tahara N, Kawakami H, Kawakami Y. Gata6-dependent GLI3 repressor function is essential in anterior limb progenitor cells for proper limb development. PLoS Genet. 2016;12(6):e1006138.
26. Anwar S, Minhas R, Ali S, et al. Identification and functional characterization of novel transcriptional enhancers involved in regulating human GLI3 expression during early development. Develop Growth Differ. 2015;57(8):570–80.
27. Avagliano L, Grazioli P, Mariani M, Bulfamante GP, Selicorni A, Massa V. Integrating molecular and structural findings: Wnt as a possible actor in shaping cognitive impairment in Cornelia de Lange syndrome. Orphanet J Rare Dis. 2017;12(1):174.
28. Parga JA, Rodriguez-Pallares J, Blanco V, Guerra MJ, Labandeira-Garcia JL. Different effects of anti-sonic hedgehog antibodies and the hedgehog pathway inhibitor cyclopamine on generation of dopaminergic neurons from neurospheres of mesencephalic precursors. Dev Dyn. 2008;237(4):909–17.
29. Abeliovich A, Hammond R. Midbrain dopamine neuron differentiation: factors and fates. Dev Biol. 2007;304(2):447–54.
30. Elsabbagh M, Johnson MH. Autism and the social brain: the first-year puzzle. Biol Psychiatry. 2016;80(2):94–9.

31. Hazlett HC, Poe MD, Lightbody AA, et al. Teasing apart the heterogeneity of autism: same behavior, different brains in toddlers with fragile X syndrome and autism. J Neurodev Disord. 2009;1(1):81–90.
32. Srivastava S, Landy-Schmitt C, Clark B, Kline AD, Specht M, Grados MA. Autism traits in children and adolescents with Cornelia de Lange syndrome. Am J Med Genet A. 2014;164A(6):1400–10.
33. Nakanishi M, Deardorff MA, Clark D, Levy SE, Krantz I, Pipan M. Investigation of autistic features among individuals with mild to moderate Cornelia de Lange syndrome. Am J Med Genet A. 2012;158A(8):1841–7.
34. Oliver C, Arron K, Sloneem J, Hall S. Behavioural phenotype of Cornelia de Lange syndrome: case-control study. Br J Psychiatry. 2008;193(6):466–70.
35. Ajmone PF, Rigamonti C, Dall'Ara F, et al. Communication, cognitive development and behavior in children with Cornelia de Lange syndrome (CdLS): preliminary results. Am J Med Genet B Neuropsychiatr Genet. 2014;165B(3):223–9.
36. Cochran L, Moss J, Nelson L, Oliver C. Contrasting age related changes in autism spectrum disorder phenomenology in Cornelia de Lange, Fragile X, and Cri du Chat syndromes: results from a 2.5 year follow-up. Am J Med Genet C Semin Med Genet. 2015;169(2):188–97.
37. Kline AD, Krantz ID, Sommer A, et al. Cornelia de Lange syndrome: clinical review, diagnostic and scoring systems, and anticipatory guidance. Am J Med Genet A. 2007;143A(12):1287–96.
38. Hawley PP, Jackson LG, Kurnit DM. Sixty-four patients with Brachmann-de Lange syndrome: a survey. Am J Med Genet. 1985;20(3):453–9.
39. Pehlivan D, Hullings M, Carvalho CMB, et al. NIPBL rearrangements in Cornelia de Lange syndrome: evidence for replicative mechanism and genotype-phenotype correlation. Genet Med. 2012;14(3):313–22.
40. Berney TP, Ireland M, Burn J. Behavioural phenotype of Cornelia de Lange syndrome. Arch Dis Child. 1999;81(4):333–6.
41. Bhuiyan ZA, Klein M, Hammond P, et al. Genotype-phenotype correlations of 39 patients with Cornelia De Lange syndrome: the Dutch experience. J Med Genet. 2006;43(7):568–75.
42. Gillis LA, McCallum J, Kaur M, et al. NIPBL mutational analysis in 120 individuals with Cornelia de Lange syndrome and evaluation of genotype-phenotype correlations. Am J Hum Genet. 2004;75(4):610–23.
43. Cereda A, Mariani M, Rebora P, et al. A new prognostic index of severity of intellectual disabilities in Cornelia de Lange syndrome. Am J Med Genet C Semin Med Genet. 2016;172(2):179–89.
44. Giani L, Michelini G, Nobile M, Ajmone PF, Vizziello PG, Scaini S. Behavioral markers of social anxiety in Cornelia de Lange syndrome: a brief systematic review. J Affect Disord. 2022;299:636–43.
45. Richards C, Moss J, O'Farrell L, Kaur G, Oliver C. Social anxiety in Cornelia de Lange syndrome. J Autism Dev Disord. 2009;39(8):1155–62.
46. Nelson L, Crawford H, Reid D, Moss J, Oliver C. An experimental study of executive function and social impairment in Cornelia de Lange syndrome. J Neurodev Disord. 2017;9(1):33.
47. Crawford H, Moss J, Groves L, et al. A behavioural assessment of social anxiety and social motivation in Fragile X, Cornelia de Lange and Rubinstein-Taybi syndromes. J Autism Dev Disord. 2020;50(1):127–44.
48. Crawford H, Waite J, Oliver C. Diverse profiles of anxiety related disorders in Fragile X, Cornelia de Lange and Rubinstein-Taybi syndromes. J Autism Dev Disord. 2017;47(12):3728–40.
49. Schretlen DJ, Ward J, Meyer SM, et al. Behavioral aspects of Lesch-Nyhan disease and its variants. Dev Med Child Neurol. 2005;47(10):673–7.
50. Luzzani S, Macchini F, Valadè A, Milani D, Selicorni A. Gastroesophageal reflux and Cornelia de Lange syndrome: typical and atypical symptoms. Am J Med Genet A. 2003;119A(3):283–7.
51. Oliver C, Sloneem J, Hall S, Arron K. Self-injurious behaviour in Cornelia de Lange syndrome: 1. Prevalence and phenomenology. J Intellect Disabil Res. 2009;53(7):575–89.
52. Parisi L, Di Filippo T, Roccella M. Behavioral phenotype and autism spectrum disorders in Cornelia de Lange syndrome. Ment Illn. 2015;7(2):5988.

53. Hyman P, Oliver C, Hall S. Self-injurious behavior, self-restraint, and compulsive behaviors in Cornelia de Lange syndrome. Am J Ment Retard. 2002;107(2):146–54.
54. Kline AD, Grados M, Sponseller P, et al. Natural history of aging in Cornelia de Lange syndrome. Am J Med Genet C Semin Med Genet. 2007;145C(3):248–60.
55. Sloneem J, Arron K, Hall SS, Oliver C. Self-injurious behaviour in Cornelia de Lange syndrome: association with environmental events. J Intellect Disabil Res. 2009;53(7):590–603.
56. Mulder PA, Huisman S, Landlust AM, et al. Development, behaviour and autism in individuals with SMC1A variants. J Child Psychol Psychiatry. 2019;60(3):305–13.
57. Mariani M, Decimi V, Bettini LR, et al. Adolescents and adults affected by Cornelia de Lange syndrome: a report of 73 Italian patients. Am J Med Genet C Semin Med Genet. 2016;172(2):206–13.
58. Basile E, Villa L, Selicorni A, Molteni M. The behavioural phenotype of Cornelia de Lange syndrome: a study of 56 individuals. J Intellect Disabil Res. 2007;51(Pt 9):671–81.
59. Reid D, Moss J, Nelson L, Groves L, Oliver C. Executive functioning in Cornelia de Lange syndrome: domain asynchrony and age-related performance. J Neurodev Disord. 2017;9(1):29.
60. Joubin J, Pettrone CF, Pettrone FA. Cornelia de Lange's syndrome. A review article (with emphasis on orthopedic significance). Clin Orthop Relat Res. 1982;(171):180–5.
61. Goodban MT. Survey of speech and language skills with prognostic indicators in 116 patients with Cornelia de Lange syndrome. Am J Med Genet. 1993;47(7):1059–63.
62. Sarimski K. Communication, social-emotional development and parenting stress in Cornelia-de-Lange syndrome. J Intellect Disabil Res. 1997;41(Pt 1):70–5.
63. Cameron TH, Kelly DP. Normal language skills and normal intelligence in a child with de Lange syndrome. J Speech Hear Disord. 1988;53(2):219–22.
64. Fraser WI, Campbell BM. A study of six cases of de Lange Amsterdam dwarf syndrome, with special attention to voice, speech and language characteristics. Dev Med Child Neurol. 1978;20(2):189–98.
65. Pearson E, Nielsen E, Kita S, et al. Low speech rate but high gesture rate during conversational interaction in people with Cornelia de Lange syndrome. J Intellect Disabil Res. 2021;65(6):601–7.
66. Hall SS, Arron K, Sloneem J, Oliver C. Health and sleep problems in Cornelia de Lange syndrome: a case control study. J Intellect Disabil Res. 2008;52(Pt 5):458–68.
67. Zambrelli E, Fossati C, Turner K, et al. Sleep disorders in Cornelia de Lange syndrome. Am J Med Genet C Semin Med Genet. 2016;172(2):214–21.
68. Rajan R, Benke JR, Kline AD, et al. Insomnia in Cornelia de Lange syndrome. Int J Pediatr Otorhinolaryngol. 2012;76(7):972–5.
69. Stavinoha RC, Kline AD, Levy HP, Kimball A, Mettel TL, Ishman SL. Characterization of sleep disturbance in Cornelia de Lange syndrome. Int J Pediatr Otorhinolaryngol. 2011;75(2):215–8.
70. Kline AD, Moss JF, Selicorni A, et al. Diagnosis and management of Cornelia de Lange syndrome: first international consensus statement. Nat Rev Genet. 2018;19(10):649–66.
71. Melanson IJ, Fahmie TA. Functional analysis of problem behavior: a 40-year review. J Appl Behav Anal. 2023;56(2):262–81.
72. Hall SS, Monlux KD, Rodriguez AB, Jo B, Pollard JS. Telehealth-enabled behavioral treatment for problem behaviors in boys with fragile X syndrome: a randomized controlled trial. J Neurodev Disord. 2020;12(1):31–4.

Further Reading

Kline AD, Moss JF, Selicorni A, et al. Diagnosis and management of Cornelia de Lange syndrome: first international consensus statement. Nat Rev. Genet. 2018;19(10):649–66.

Gillis LA, McCallum J, Kaur M, et al. NIPBL mutational analysis in 120 individuals with Cornelia de Lange syndrome and evaluation of genotype-phenotype correlations. Am J Hum Genet. 2004;75(4):610–23.

Index

A
Absolute neutrophil count (ANC), 147
Acceptance and commitment therapy (ACT), 97
Actigraphy, 81
Active chromosome, 110
Adaptive functioning, 28, 31
Adaptive skills, 27
Adolescents, 251
Aggression, 74–76, 79–83, 85
Alpha agonists, 265
Alpha-2 agonists, 11, 118
Alzheimer's disease (AD), 63, 67
American Sign Language (ASL), 215
Angelman syndrome (AS), 130
  ABA, 78
  anxiety, 75
  biological treatments, 82–84
  FCT, 79
  functional analysis, 79
  hyperactivity, 74, 75
  medical co-morbidities, 84–86
  non-pharmacological interventions, 80–82
  sleep disorders, 76
  social interest, 79
  treatment plan, 77
  UBE3A gene, 74
  UBE3A sequencing tests, 77
Antidepressants, 119, 148, 237
Antipsychotics, 4, 11, 120, 147, 237
Antiseizure, 166
Anxiety, 6, 42–43, 61, 66, 74–76, 82, 83, 85, 86, 143, 162, 176, 208, 287, 291
Applied behavior analysis (ABA), 78–80, 146, 213
Applied behavioral analysis (ABA)-based interventions, 64
Aripiprazole, 4, 11, 15, 98, 166
Arrythmias, 50
Atomoxetine, 11, 166
Attention-deficit/hyperactivity disorder (ADHD), 5, 43, 47, 60, 82, 112, 131, 142, 148, 159, 175, 232, 251
Auditory hypersensitivity, 232
Augmentative and alternative communication (AAC), 215
Autism spectrum disorder (ASD), 60–61, 65–66, 92, 109, 111–112, 129, 144–145, 159, 162, 175, 206, 231, 252, 286
  ADHD, 5
  anxiety disorders, 6
  assessment, 8–9
  behavioral interventions, 10
  depression, 7
  diagnostic criteria for, 2
  gastrointestinal (GI) issues, 13
  immune dysregulation, 14
  intellectual disability, 3–4
  irritability, 4
  OCD, 7
  pharmacological treatment, 10–13
  prevalence of, 1
  seizures/epilepsy, 13
  self-injurious behaviors, 5
  sleep disorders, 8
  social deficits, 7
Autoimmune thyroiditis, 182
Automatisms, 6
Azoospermia, 266

B
Behavioral interventions, 10
Bile acids, 236
Bipolar disorder, 62, 66, 207, 208

R. P. Thom, C. J. McDougle (eds.), *Neuropsychiatric Care for Genetic Syndromes and Other Neurodevelopmental Disorders*, https://doi.org/10.1007/978-3-031-76269-7

Birt-Hogg-Dube syndrome (BHD), 252
Body-focused repetitive behaviors, 48
Buspirone, 46, 82

C
Cannabidiol, 160, 165
Carbamazepine, 135
Cardiac rhabdomyoma, 159
Cardinal symptoms, 290
Cardiology, 212
Cardiovascular disease, 48–50
Caregivers, 75
Catatonia, 63, 67, 207, 208
Cerebral gyri, 285
Childhood Autism Rating Scale (CARS), 286
Childhood- or adolescent-onset psychosis, 196
Choreoathetosis, 269
Chorionic villus sampling (CVS), 64
Chromosome microarray analysis (CMA), 77, 209, 245
Circadian rhythms, 256
Clozapine, 166
Cognitive abilities, 27
Cognitive behavioral therapy (CBT), 33, 46, 97, 146, 148
Composite sleep disturbance index (CSDI), 13
Comprehensive testing, 31
Comprehensive treatment models (CTMs), 10
Conceptual domain, 27
Congenital heart disease (CHD), 68, 180
Constipation, 75
Cornelia de Lange syndrome (CdLS)
  anxiety, 287, 291
  ASD, 286
  assessment and early management, 290
  biological treatments, 291
  history, 283, 284
  hyperactivity, 288
  intellectual disability, 286, 287
  medical comorbidities, 292
  mood disorders and psychosis, 288
  pathophysiology, 284, 285
  psychosocial treatments, 290
  repetitive and self-injurious behaviors, 287, 288, 291
  sleep, 289, 290
  speech and language, 289
Cortical tubers, 159
Cubitus valgus, 172

D
Deep brain stimulation (DBS), 277
Dehydrocholesterol (DHC), 233
Depression, 7, 47–48, 61, 66, 162
Developmental therapy, 64
DHCR7 mutational analysis, 234
Diabetes, 181
Dialectical behavioral therapy (DBT), 33, 97
Diarrhea, 165
DiGeorge syndrome, 141
Distinctive facial features, 171
Divalproex, 148
Diverse symptoms, 149
DNA copy number variations (CNVs), 28–29
DNA markers, 29
Down syndrome (DS), 28, 149, 287, 289
  ADHD, 60
  anxiety, 61
  ASD, 60
  assessment, 64
  biological treatments, 65–67
  bipolar disorder, 62
  catatonia, 63
  CHD, 68
  depression, 61
  hearing impairment, 69
  non-pharmacological treatments, 64
  OCD, 62
  OSA, 68
  physical examination, 59
  psychiatric disorders, 67
  psychosis, 63
  regression, 62
  thyroid disease, 68
  visual problems, 69
Drosophila models, 284
Dysmenorrhea, 75
Dysregulation, 159

E
Early Intervention (EI) services, 215
Electrocardiogram (EKG), 148, 178
Electroconvulsive therapy (ECT), 67
Electroencephalogram (EEG), 73, 121
Endocrine abnormalities, 51, 149
Epilepsy, 84
Everolimus, 160
Exposure therapy, 45
Extrapyramidal symptoms (EPS), 6

F
FLCN gene, 252
Flexible testing, 4
Fluorescent in situ hybridization (FISH), 173, 263
Fluoxetine, 119

Follicle-stimulating hormone (FSH), 172
Food and Drug Administration (FDA), 82, 192
FORWARD dataset, 113
Fragile X Clinical and Research Consortium (FXCRC), 110
Fragile X syndrome (FXS), 28
 ADHD, 112
 ASD, 112
 assessment/diagnosis of, 114
 biological treatments, 117–120
 developmental and cognitive characteristics, 110
 educational interventions, 115
 language development, 111
 supportive behavioral approaches, 116
 supportive therapies, 114–115
Free-floating anxiety, 287
Functional analysis (FA), 79
Functional communication training (FCT), 79
Functional neurological symptom disorder (FNSD), 44

G
Gas-chromatography-mass spectroscopy (GC-MS), 233
Gastroenterology, 212–213
Gastroesophageal reflux disease (GERD), 50, 75, 121, 133, 212, 288
Gastrointestinal (GI) problems, 133
Gastrointestinal abnormalities, 50
Gastrointestinal disorders, 13–14
Gene therapy, 236
Genetic syndromes, 286
Genetic testing, 209
Gestures, 289
Giant cell astrocytoma, 161
Glucose intolerance, 181
Grave's disease, 182
Growth hormone (GH), 100
Growth hormone (GH) therapy, 172, 179
Guanfacine, 166
Guanfacine extended release, 99
Gynecomastia, 266

H
Hearing impairment, 69
Hormone replacement therapy (HRT), 180
Human chorionic gonadotropin (hCG), 174
Hydroxyzine, 238
Hyperactive and agitated behaviors, 207
Hyperactivity, 74–76, 80, 82, 85, 86, 288
Hyperarousal, 116
Hypercalcemia, 52
Hypercholesterolemia, 246
Hypermotoric behavior, 73, 74
Hyperphagia, 92
Hypertension, 49
Hyperuricemia, 269, 270, 275
Hypocalcemia, 149
Hypogonadism, 265
Hypoparathyroidism, 149
Hypopigmented macule, 161
Hypothyroidism, 61, 68, 100, 213
Hypotonia, 239
Hypoxanthine-guanine phosphoribosyltranferase deficiency, 271
Hypoxanthine-guanine phosphoribosyltranferase (HGPRT), 269, 276

I
Immune dysfunction, 13
Immune system dysregulation, 14–15
Inattention, 74, 82
Individualized education programs (IEPs), 216
Individuals with Disabilities Education Act (IDEA), 254
Insulin-like growth factor 1 (IGF-1), 179
Intellectual deficits, 175
Intellectual disability (ID), 41, 73, 191, 203, 254, 269, 286, 287
 assessment of, 31, 32
 biological treatments, 34–35
 environmental and genetic factors, 28
 genetics of, 28–29
 medical co-morbidities, 35, 36
 psychosocial supports, 32–34
 signs and symptoms, 29–31
Intelligence quotient (IQ), 28
Interictal epileptiform discharges (IEDs), 232
Irritability, agitation, aggression and self-injurious (IAAS) behaviors, 113
Isochromosome Xq, 173

K
Kandutsch-Russel pathway, 229
Karyotyping, 174
Klinefelter syndrome (KS)
 assessment, 263–264
 biological treatments, 265–266
 genetic variation, 261
 medical co-morbidities, 266
 nonverbal IQ, 262
 psychiatric co-morbidities, 262–263
 psychosocial treatments, 264
 social cognitive vulnerabilities, 262

L
Lamotrigine, 238
Lesch-Nyhan syndrome, 250, 287
  biological treatments, 276–278
  clinical features, 271–273
  epidemiology, 270
  genetic and neurobiological mechanisms, 270–271
  genetic testing, 274–275
  HGPRT deficiency, 271
  psychiatric co-morbidities, 273–274
  psychosocial treatments, 275
Low cholesterol, 233
Luteinizing hormone (LH), 172
Lymphangiomyomatosis (LAM), 159, 160

M
Madelung's deformity, 172
Mammalian target of rapamycin (mTOR), 159
Maternal 15q duplication syndrome (Dup15q), 130
  anxiety, 131
  attention-deficit/hyperactivity disorder, 131
  bipolar disorder, 135
  dysmorphic features, 130
  epidemiology, 129
  epilepsy, 132
  genetic testing, 133
  genetic/neurobiological mechanisms, 129–130
  mood disorders, 131
  multidisciplinary assessments, 133
  psychopharmacology, 135
  psychosocial treatment, 134
  psychotic symptoms, 132
  seizure management, 134
MECP2 duplication syndrome, 192, 193
MECP2 mutations, 191, 192
MECP2-related disorders, 194
Medical co-morbidities, 28, 35, 36
Melatonin, 13
Metabolic syndrome, 13, 147
Methylphenidate (MPH), 65
Micrognathia, 172
Mineral and vitamin deficiencies, 13
Mitochondrial disorders, 13
Mood disorders, 30, 131, 135, 143, 144, 176, 195, 288
Mood stabilizers, 148, 265
Motor dysfunction, 214
Mouse models, 99
Myopia, 246

N
N-acetylcysteine (NAC), 99
Nail hypoplasia, 172
National Fragile X Foundation (NFXF), 110
Neuroinflammation, 159
Neuropsychiatric disorders, 143, 208
Neuropsychological evaluation, 31
NIPBL gene, 284–286
Non-invasive prenatal screening (NIPS), 64
Noninvasive prenatal testing (NIPT), 264
Non-steroidal anti-inflammatory drugs (NSAIDs), 276
Nonsyndromic intellectual disability, 28

O
Obesity, 66, 181
Obsessive-compulsive disorder (OCD), 6, 62
Obstructive sleep apnea (OSA), 43, 121, 251, 289
Occupational therapy (OT), 114, 214
Olanzapine, 166
Oligomenorrhoea, 92
Oral sirolimus, 165

P
Parent child interaction therapy (PCIT), 256
Parkinson's disease, 149
Pervasive developmental disorders (PDDs), 2
Pharmacotherapy, 277
Phelan-McDermid syndrome (PMS)
  ABA therapy, 214
  anxiety, 208
  ASD, 206
  assessments, 208–213
  biological treatments, 216–218
  bipolar disorder, 207
  catatonia, 207
  clinical characteristics, 205–206
  educational services, 215
  epidemiology, 203
  epilepsy and seizures, 211
  genetic mutations, 204
  genetic/neurobiological mechanisms, 203–205
  genetic testing, 209, 210
  hyperactive and agitated behaviors, 207
  medical comorbidities, 219
  occupational therapy, 214
  physical therapy, 214
  primary care, 210
  psychiatric comorbidities, 217–218

psychiatry and psychology, 212
schizophrenia spectrum, 208
sleep disturbances, 206, 216
verbal and non-verbal communication skills, 215
Photoperception, 256
Photosensitivity, 238
Physical therapy (PT), 64, 214
Picture Exchange Communication Systems (PECS), 215
Pitt-Hopkins and Peters plus syndrome, 29
Poorly-controlled epilepsy, 132
Positron emission topography (PET), 11
Prader-Willi syndrome (PWS), 129
anxiety disorders, 94
assessment, 95
behavioral dysregulation, 93
biological treatments, 97–99
manifestation of, 91
medical comorbidities, 99
psychiatric co-morbidities, 93–95
psychosis, 95
psychosocial treatments, 96–97
skin picking behavior, 94
social difficulties, 94
Pre-diabetes and diabetes, 51
Proton pump inhibitors (PPI), 134
Psychiatric co-morbidities, 29–31, 217–218
Psychiatric disorders, 67
Psychosis, 30, 63, 208, 288
Psychotic disorders, 136–137
Puberty, 180

Q

Quantitative trait locus (QTL) analysis, 29

R

RAI1 gene, 245
RAS homolog expressed in brain (Rheb), 159
Regression, 62, 67
Renal angiomyolipoma, 160
Renal carcinoma, 160
Repetitive behavior, 81
Restrictive and repetitive behaviors (RRBs), 2, 4, 6, 287, 288, 291
Rett syndrome
anxiety disorder, 194
assessment, 196–197
biological treatments, 198
clinical features, 193
MECP2 duplication syndrome, 193
MECP2-related disorders, 194
mood disorders, 195
psychiatric medications, 199
psychosis, 196
psychosocial treatments, 197
Rheumatoid arthritis, 262
Rhythm disturbances, 50
Risperidone, 4, 11, 15, 98, 120, 166
Routine chromosome analysis, 64
Rubinstein–Taybi syndrome, 287

S

Schizophrenia, 143
Schizophrenia spectrum disorders, 136–137, 208, 263
Selective serotonin reuptake inhibitors (SSRIs), 11, 46, 119, 135, 148, 198, 265, 291
Self-help skills, 78
Self-injurious behaviors (SIB), 75, 82–83, 287, 288, 291
Self-injury, 232
Sensory stimulation abnormalities, 2
Serotonin-norepinephrine reuptake inhibitors (SNRIs), 148
Serotonin reuptake inhibitors, 277
7-dehydrocholesterol reductase (DHCR7), 230
Severe sleep cycle disturbances, 232
Sexual abuse, 34
Sexually transmitted diseases (STDs), 34
SHANK3 gene, 203, 204
Sirolimus, 160
Skin lesions, 159
Skin picking behavior, 94
Sleep and nap diary (SND), 13
Sleep apnea, 100
Sleep diaries, 81
Sleep disorders, 8, 43, 76, 81–84, 86
Sleep disturbances, 47, 206
Sleep hygiene, 216
SMC1A-related disorders, 288
Smith-Lemli-Opitz syndrome (SLOS)
behavioral assessments, 234
biological treatments, 235–236
clinical features of, 231
distinct facial features, 230
incidence of, 229
medical comorbidities, 239
oral malformations, 230
psychopharmacological intervention, 236–239
psychosocial treatments, 234–235

Smith-Magenis syndrome (SMS)
ADHD, 251
anxiety and mood disorders, 252
ASD, 252
assessment of behavioral difficulties, 253
assessment of sleep disturbances, 253
behavioral symptoms, 249, 250, 255, 256
biological treatments, 256–257
clinical features of, 246, 247
clinical studies, 253
craniofacial features, 248
developmental delay, 251
disordered sleep, 250–251
medical co-morbidities, 257–258
psychosocial treatments, 254–255
Social communication questionnaire (SCQ), 252
Social deficits, 7
Social difficulties, 94
Social responsiveness scale (SRS), 249
Social skills training, 45
Solid tumors, 67
Spasticity, 272
Speech-language therapy (ST), 64
Stereotypic behaviors, 249
Stereotypies, 6
Stimulants, 12
Subclinical hypothyroidism, 51
Sudden unexpected death in epilepsy (SUDEP), 132
Systemic lupus erythematosus (SLE), 262

T
Tasimelteon, 257
Tauroursodeoxycholic acid (TUDCA), 236
Thyroid disease, 68
Thyroid dysfunction, 149
Topiramate, 98, 100
Transthoracic echocardiogram (TTE), 181
Trisomy 21, 64
TSC1 gene, 158
TSC-associated neuropsychiatric disorders (TAND), 162
Tuberous sclerosis complex (TSC)
assessments, 163–164
biological treatments, 164
characteristic features of, 159
definite diagnosis of, 157
diagnostic criteria, 158
genetic/neurobiological mechanisms, 158–159
medical co-morbidities, 166–167
psychosocial treatments, 164
signs and symptoms of, 162–163
TAND, 162
Turner syndrome (TS)
autoimmune comorbidities, 182
cardiovascular anomalies, 180
clinical features, 171–172
diagnosis of, 173–175
epidemiological analysis, 172
genetic mosaicism, 173
GH therapy, 179
hepatic comorbidities, 182–183
karyotype analysis, 174
metabolic comorbidities, 181–182
neurocognitive disorders, 175–176
neuropsychiatric testing, 177
otolaryngological comorbidities, 183
psychiatric comorbidities, 177
psychosocial challenges, 176, 177
psychosocial interventions, 177
puberty, 180
renal comorbidities, 182
22q11.2 deletion syndrome
ADHD, 142
anxiety disorders, 143
ASD, 144
biological treatments, 147–148
CBT, 146
clinical features, 142
diagnostic tests, 146
intellectual and learning disabilities, 145
medical co-morbidities, 148–153
medical complications, 150
metabolic monitoring, 147
mood disorders, 143
prenatal screening, 145
psychosocial treatments, 146
schizophrenia, 143

U
UBE3A gene, 74, 77
Ungual fibroma, 160
Urinary tract infections (UTIs), 182

V
Valvar involvement, 50
Vascular stenoses, 48
Verbal and physical aggression, 4
Videosomnography, 81
Vigabatrin, 160, 165
Viloxazine, 82

W

Williams syndrome (WS)
ADHD, 43, 47
anxiety, 42–43, 46–47
cardiovascular disease, 48–50
CBT, 46
depression, 47–48
endocrine abnormalities, 51
epidemiology, 41–42
FNSD, 44
gastrointestinal problems, 50
genetics and diagnostic testing, 44–45
medical features of, 49
psychosocial treatments, 45
sleep disorders, 43
sleep disturbances, 47
weight, 51

X

X-active specific transcript (XIS), 173
X chromosome, 172, 173, 191, 192, 263, 270

Y

Y-chromosome mosaicism (45X/46XY), 173

MIX
Papier aus verantwortungsvollen Quellen
Paper from responsible sources
FSC® C105338

If you have any concerns about our products,
you can contact us on
ProductSafety@springernature.com

In case Publisher is established outside the EU,
the EU authorized representative is:
Springer Nature Customer Service Center GmbH
Europaplatz 3, 69115 Heidelberg, Germany

Printed by Libri Plureos GmbH
in Hamburg, Germany